# 60 HIKES
## WITHIN 60 MILES
### 2ND Edition

## BOSTON

### Including Coastal and Interior Regions and New Hampshire

**Lafe Low and Helen Weatherall**

**MENASHA RIDGE PRESS**
Your Guide to the Outdoors Since 1982

## 60 Hikes Within 60 Miles: Boston

Published by Menasha Ridge Press

Second edition, first printing

Project editors: Holly Cross and Kate Johnson
Cover and interior design: Jonathan Norberg
Interior photos: Lafe Low, except where noted
Cartography and elevation profiles: Scott McGrew and Tim Kissel
Copy editor: Kate Johnson
Proofreader: Emily Beaumont
Indexing: Rich Carlson

*Front cover:* View of Spectacle Island photographed by Ilaria Ranieri
*Back cover:* Top, Spectacle Island (see Hike 3, page 29); bottom left, World's End (see Hike 9, page 60); bottom center, Mount Watatic Reservation (see Hike 54, page 272); bottom right, Hemlock Gorge Reservation (see Hike 51, page 258). All photos by Lafe Low.

### Library of Congress Cataloging-in-Publication Data

Names: Low, Lafe, 1962- author.
Title: 60 hikes within 60 miles. Boston : including Coastal and Interior Regions and New Hampshire / Lafe Low.
Other titles: Sixty hikes within sixty miles
Description: Second Edition. | Birmingham, Alabama : Menasha Ridge Press, [2018] |
    Previous edition published: Birmingham, Alabama : Menasha Ridge Press, 2008. |
    "Distributed by Publishers Group West"—T.p. verso.
Identifiers: LCCN 2018008764| ISBN 9780897324557 (paperback) | ISBN 9780897324564 (ebook)
Subjects: LCSH: Hiking—Massachusetts—Boston Region—Guidebooks. | Walking—Massachusetts—Boston
    Region—Guidebooks. | Trails—Massachusetts—Boston Region—Guidebooks. | Outdoor recreation—
    Massachusetts—Boston Region—Guidebooks. | Hiking—New Hampshire—Guidebooks. |
    Walking—New Hampshire—Guidebooks. | Trails—New Hampshire—Guidebooks. | Outdoor recreation—
    New Hampshire—Guidebooks. | Boston Region (Mass.)—Guidebooks. | New Hampshire—Guidebooks.
Classification: LCC GV199.42.M42 B67 2018 | DDC 796.5109744—dc23
LC record available at https://lccn.loc.gov/2018008764

**MENASHA RIDGE PRESS**
An imprint of AdventureKEEN
2204 First Ave. S., Ste. 102
Birmingham, Alabama 35233

Visit menasharidge.com for a complete listing of our books and for ordering information. Contact us at our website, at facebook.com/menasharidge, or at twitter.com/menasharidge with questions or comments. To find out more about who we are and what we're doing, visit our blog, blog.menasharidge.com.

**DISCLAIMER** This book is meant only as a guide to select trails in the Boston area and does not guarantee hiker safety in any way—you hike at your own risk. Neither Menasha Ridge Press nor Helen Weatherall nor Lafe Low is liable for property loss or damage, personal injury, or death that result in any way from accessing or hiking the trails described in the following pages. Please be aware that hikers have been injured in the Boston area. Be especially cautious when walking on or near boulders, steep inclines, and drop-offs, and do not attempt to explore terrain that may be beyond your abilities. To help ensure a safe and enjoyable hike, please carefully read the introduction to this book, and perhaps get further safety information and guidance from other sources. Familiarize yourself thoroughly with the areas you intend to visit before venturing out. Ask questions, and prepare for the unforeseen. Familiarize yourself with current weather reports, maps of the area you intend to visit, and any relevant park regulations.

## *Dedication*

This book is dedicated, as always, to my best hiking, skiing, and camping buddy—my son, Devin Low.

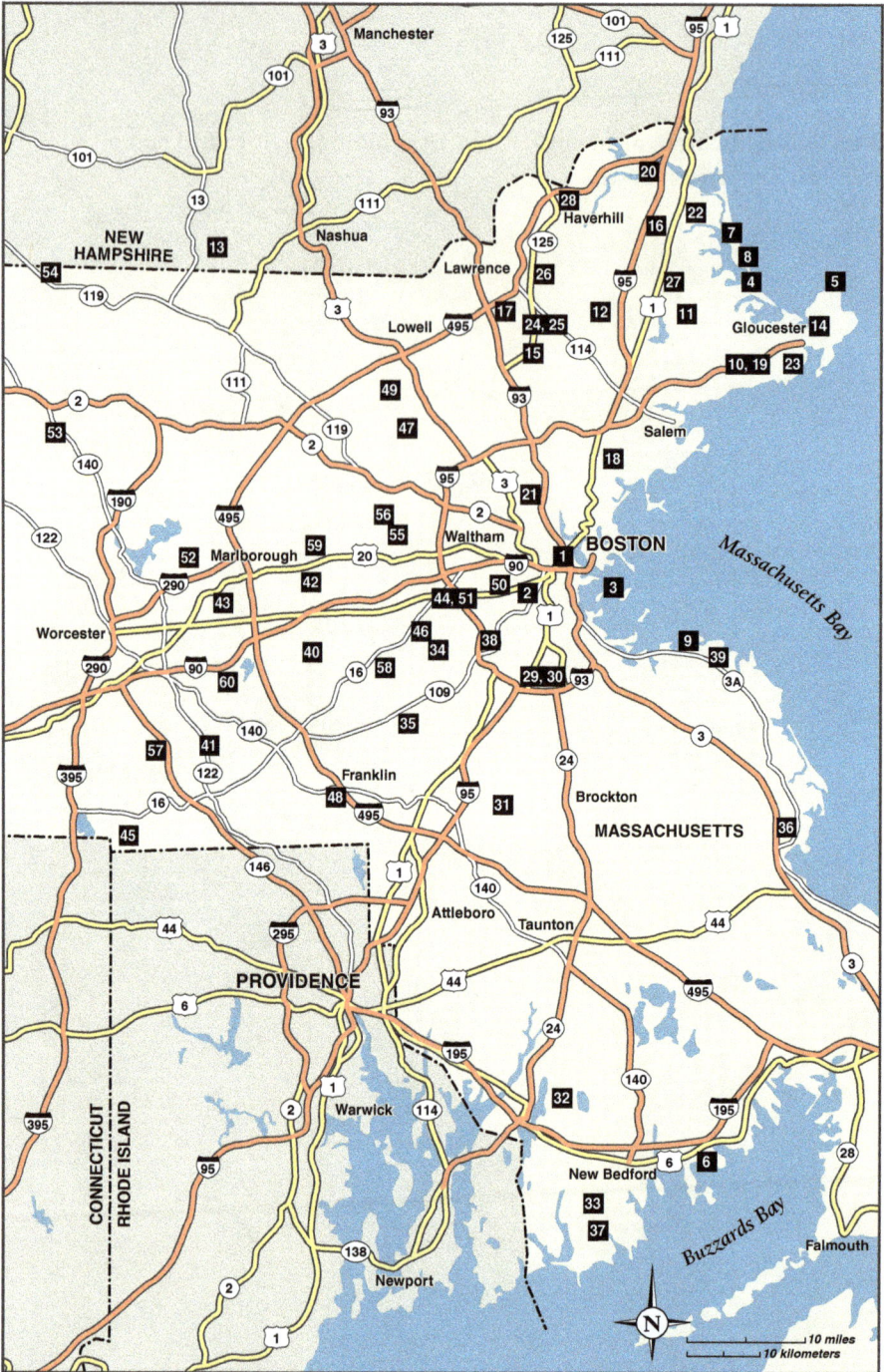

# TABLE OF CONTENTS

# MAP LEGEND

|  |  |  |
|---|---|---|
| ←→ ➡ Directional arrows | Featured trail | Alternate trail |
| Freeway | Highway with bridge | Minor road |
| Boardwalk | Unpaved road | |
| Railroad | Power line | Boundary line |
| Park/forest | Water body | River/creek/ intermittent stream |

| | | |
|---|---|---|
| ♨ Amphitheater | •→ Gate | ▲ Peak/hill |
| ⛱ Beach access | ● General point of interest | ⛩ Picnic area |
| ⌐ Bench | ⓘ Information/kiosk | ⛺ Picnic shelter |
| 🚤 Boat launch | ♜ Lookout tower | ⚘ Playground |
| ⛺ Campground | ✕ Mine/quarry | 📡 Radio tower |
| 🛶 Canoe launch | ⚱ Monument | 🚻 Restroom |
| ⚰ Cemetery | ◄ One-way (road) | 🏔 Scenic view |
| ✏ Dam | ⛩ Outhouse | 🏃 Trailhead |
| ⛲ Drinking water | ⌂ Park office | ⌒ Tunnel (pedestrian) |
| 🎣 Fishing | 🅿 Parking | 🔭 Viewing platform |
| ⋈ Footbridge | | ♿ Wheelchair access |
| ✳ Garden | | |

# ACKNOWLEDGMENTS

From Helen Weatherall: Many of the most wonderful places in Massachusetts likely would not exist as open space if not for Charles Eliot, landscape architect and founder of The Trustees of Reservations. In the interest of fostering support, I would also like to acknowledge the Essex County Greenbelt Association; the Sudbury Valley Trustees; the Andover Village Improvement Society (AVIS); the Dartmouth Natural Resource Trust; the Trust for Public Land; the Charles River Conservancy; the Appalachian Mountain Club; the Audubon Society; Friends of Lynn Woods; Friends of Middlesex Fells; Friends of Hemlock Gorge; Friends of Manchester–Essex Woods; everyone behind the Bay Circuit Trail, the Wapack Trail, and the Mid-State Trail; The Trustees of Reservations; and the gutsy, huge-hearted members of every last conservation commission in the state. Gratitude to friends and family, whose sustained interest and support helped carry this book to fruition. Thanks to my brothers, Bobby and Alexander. Thanks to my father, Robert Weatherall, who gave me his strong legs, curiosity, love of trees, and propensity for taking the long, scenic route; thanks to my trusty and courageous hiking companion, Katy, my 14-pound terrier; and with my deepest respect, appreciation, and love, thanks to my husband, Christopher.

From Lafe Low: I wholeheartedly concur with Helen's acknowledgment of the myriad conservation organizations that preserve and protect some of the Bay State's finest wilderness areas. This would be a far less attractive world without the woods and trails to which we all love to retreat.

And while I hiked many of these fantastic journeys on my own, I was also joined by friends and family for several, most notably my intrepid son, Devin Low; his companion Ashley Squires; and my friends Peter Tamposi, Mark Grundstrom, Lisa Marshall, Scott Schultz, Brian Merritt, Jason Howell and son Liam, and Beth Phillips. Here's a list of who hiked with me and where:

- Devin Low: Beaver Brook, Middlesex Fells Reservation: Skyline Trail, Weir Hill
- Devin Low and Ashley Squires: Halibut Point State Park, Purgatory Chasm State Reservation, Indian Ridge Reservation, Goldsmith Reservation
- Lisa Marshall: Dogtown Common, Ravenswood Park, Mount Watatic
- Scott Shultz: Parker River National Wildlife Refuge: Hellcat Trail and Sandy Point State Reservation
- Jason and Liam Howell: Noanet Woodlands
- Beth Phillips: Borderland State Park, Elm Bank Reservation, Rocky Narrows
- Peter Tamposi and Mark Grundstrom: Cedar Hill and Sawink Farm, Mount Pisgah Conservation Area
- Brian Merritt: Mount Wachusett

# FOREWORD

Welcome to Menasha Ridge Press's 60 Hikes Within 60 Miles, a series designed to provide hikers with the information they need to find and hike the very best trails surrounding metropolitan areas.

Our strategy is simple: First, find a hiker who knows the area and loves to hike. Second, ask that person to spend a year researching the most popular and very best trails around. And third, have that person describe each trail in terms of difficulty, scenery, condition, elevation change, and other categories of information that are important to hikers. "Pretend you've just completed a hike and met up with other hikers at the trailhead," we told each author. "Imagine their questions; be clear in your answers."

Experienced hikers and writers Lafe Low and Helen Weatherall have selected 60 of the best hikes in and around the Boston metropolitan area. This second edition includes new hikes, as well as additional sections and new routes for some of the existing hikes. Lafe and Helen provide hikers (and walkers) with a great variety of hikes, all within roughly 60 miles of Boston—from urban strolls on city sidewalks to aerobic outings throughout the area surrounding the city.

You'll get more out of this book if you take a moment to read the Introduction, which explains how to read the trail listings. The "Maps" section will help you understand how useful topos are on a hike and will also tell you where to get them. And though this is a where-to, not a how-to, guide, readers who have not hiked extensively will find the Introduction of particular value.

As much for the opportunity to free the spirit as to free the body, let these hikes elevate you above the urban hurry.

*All the best,*
*The Editors at Menasha Ridge Press*

# PREFACE

There is nothing so restorative, so calming, so fulfilling as a walk in the woods. Whether a peaceful stroll through the trees, an aggressive hours-long hike up and over rocky crags, or something in between, you can't help but feel better after getting out into the woods. It is truly essential.

Everyone has different reasons for wanting to get out in the forest and go for a hike—to get in better shape, relax, get back to nature, take the dog for a walk, take your kids for a walk—and they're all good reasons. As long as you're getting out.

At the risk of sounding old, being out in the woods always takes me back to my childhood. I am reminded of the days when my friend Dan Quagliaroli and I would head out with overloaded backpacks, a huge sense of adventure, lofty ideals, and no idea where we wanted to go. Often we wouldn't even tell our moms where we were going because we truly made it up as we went along. Those were the days.

While this was not an original work for me, it still required that I retrace all the hikes in the original edition. I was chosen as the revising writer to update and expand on Helen Weatherall's excellent Boston-area hiking guidebook. As part of the update process, I also researched and wrote about five new hikes.

Boston is a remarkable area. You can truly get a sense of just how much green and wooded space is intermingled with the urban jungle when taking off from or landing at Logan International Airport during the day. It's quite a sight. There's the obvious density of the extended city but lots of green space as well. In fact, two of the largest reservations—the Blue Hills and Middlesex Fells Reservations—are so close you can still hear traffic on the highways when you first set out for a hike. Interestingly, those are also two of the more challenging hikes in this book. And both trails are called the Skyline Trail. Be prepared when you try them both. They will test your mettle.

The best part of writing these guidebooks is the pure process of exploration. I have also done *Best Tent Camping: New England* and *Best Hikes of the Appalachian Trail: New England* for Menasha Ridge Press, and each project has been a spiritual and emotional windfall. I can be somewhat of a creature of habit. I'll go to the same places over and over again. In writing this book and the others, my list of favorite places has grown by orders of magnitude. And for that I am grateful.

—*Lafe Low*

# 60 HIKES BY CATEGORY

| REGION<br>Hike Number/Hike Name | page | Mileage | Difficulty | Multiuse | Kid Friendly | Dog Friendly | Public Transport |
|---|---|---|---|---|---|---|---|
| **WITHIN BOSTON** | | | | | | | |
| 1 Charles River | 20 | 7.75 | E | ✓ | ✓ | ✓ | ✓ |
| 2 Jamaica Pond | 25 | 1.45 | E | ✓ | ✓ | ✓ | ✓ |
| 3 Spectacle Island: Boston Harbor Islands National & State Park | 29 | 2.5 | E | | ✓ | | ✓ |
| **SEASIDE HIKES** | | | | | | | |
| 4 Crane Beach | 36 | 6 | M | ✓ | ✓ | 10/1–3/31 | ✓ |
| 5 Halibut Point State Park | 41 | 2 | E | | ✓ | | |
| 6 Nasketucket Bay State Reservation | 46 | 2.75 | E | ✓ | ✓ | | |
| 7 Parker River National Wildlife Refuge: Hellcat Trail | 51 | 1.84 | E | | ✓ | ✓ | |
| 8 Sandy Point State Reservation | 56 | 2.5 | E–M | | ✓ | ✓ | |
| 9 World's End | 60 | 3.8 | E | | ✓ | ✓ | |
| **NORTH OF BOSTON** | | | | | | | |
| 10 Agassiz Rock Reservation | 66 | 0.75 | E–M | | ✓ | | |
| 11 Appleton Farms: Grass Rides | 70 | 2.6 | E | | ✓ | ✓ | |
| 12 Bald Hill Conservation Area | 74 | 6.53 | M | | | | |
| 13 Beaver Brook | 79 | 5.69 | M | ✓ | | | |
| 14 Dogtown Common | 84 | 5.25 | M | ✓ | | | |
| 15 Goldsmith Reservation | 89 | 3.67 | E–M | | ✓ | ✓ | |
| 16 Great Meadow–Gerrish's Rock | 93 | 0.8 | E | | ✓ | | |
| 17 Indian Ridge Reservation | 97 | 2.95 | E–M | | | | |
| 18 Lynn Woods | 102 | 5 | E–M | ✓ | | ✓ | |
| 19 Manchester–Essex Woodlands | 107 | 4.75 | E–M | | | | |
| 20 Maudslay State Park | 112 | 3.9 | M | ✓ | ✓ | ✓ | |
| 21 Middlesex Fells Reservation: Skyline Trail | 116 | 7.5 | S | ✓ | | | |
| 22 Old Town Hill Reservation | 121 | 2.6 | M | | ✓ | | |
| 23 Ravenswood Park | 125 | 4.5 | M | | ✓ | | |
| 24 Skug River Reservation | 130 | 3.05 | E–M | | ✓ | | |
| 25 Ward Reservation | 135 | 4.7 | M | | ✓ | | |
| 26 Weir Hill | 140 | 2.46 | E–M | | ✓ | | |
| 27 Willowdale State Forest | 145 | 7.6 | E–M | ✓ | ✓ | ✓ | |
| 28 Winnekenni Park | 150 | 5.6 | E | ✓ | ✓ | | |

| DIFFICULTY RATINGS | | |
|---|---|---|
| E = Easy | M = Moderate | S = Strenuous |

| REGION<br>Hike Number/Hike Name | page | Mileage | Difficulty | Multiuse | Kid Friendly | Dog Friendly | Public Transport |
|---|---|---|---|---|---|---|---|
| **SOUTH OF BOSTON** | | | | | | | |
| 29 Blue Hills Reservation: Hemenway Hill | 156 | 3.9 | M | ✓ | | | |
| 30 Blue Hills Reservation: Skyline Trail | 161 | 13 | S | ✓ | | | |
| 31 Borderland State Park | 166 | 6.25 | M | ✓ | ✓ | ✓ | |
| 32 Copicut Woods | 171 | 3.4 | E | | ✓ | | |
| 33 Destruction Brook Woods | 176 | 4.07 | E | | ✓ | | |
| 34 Noanet Woodlands | 181 | 5.11 | E–M | | ✓ | ✓ | |
| 35 Noon Hill | 186 | 4.6 | E | ✓ | ✓ | | |
| 36 Round Pond | 190 | 2.33 | E | | ✓ | ✓ | |
| 37 Slocum's River Reserve | 194 | 3.87 | E | | ✓ | ✓ | |
| 38 Wilson Mountain Reservation | 199 | 3.5 | E–M | | ✓ | | |
| 39 Whitney and Thayer Woods | 203 | 6.25 | E–M | | ✓ | | |
| **WEST OF BOSTON** | | | | | | | |
| 40 Ashland State Park | 210 | 3.5 | M | | | ✓ | |
| 41 Blackstone River and Canal Heritage State Park | 214 | 7.5 | E | ✓ | ✓ | | |
| 42 Callahan State Park | 218 | 7.37 | E–M | ✓ | ✓ | ✓ | |
| 43 Cedar Hill and Sawink Farm | 223 | 8 | E–M | | ✓ | | |
| 44 Centennial Reservation | 228 | 1.58 | E | | ✓ | | |
| 45 Douglas State Forest | 232 | 2.2 | E–M | | ✓ | | |
| 46 Elm Bank Reservation | 236 | 1.9 | E | | ✓ | | |
| 47 Foss Farm | 240 | 6.7 | M | | ✓ | | |
| 48 Franklin State Forest | 244 | 1.5 | E | ✓ | ✓ | ✓ | |
| 49 Great Brook Farm State Park | 248 | 6.82 | E–M | ✓ | ✓ | ✓ | |
| 50 Hammond Pond–Houghton Garden | 253 | 2.2 | E | ✓ | ✓ | ✓ | ✓ |
| 51 Hemlock Gorge Reservation | 258 | 1.3 | E | | ✓ | ✓ | ✓ |
| 52 Mount Pisgah Conservation Area | 262 | 4.75 | M | | ✓ | | |
| 53 Mount Wachusett | 267 | 5.74 | M–S | ✓ | | | |
| 54 Mount Watatic | 272 | 3.5 | M | | | | |
| 55 Ogilvie Town Forest | 276 | 3 | E–M | | ✓ | | |
| 56 Oxbow Meadows/Farrar Pond/Mount Misery:<br>In Thoreau's Footsteps | 281 | 8.67 | E–M | | ✓ | | |
| 57 Purgatory Chasm State Reservation | 286 | 2.25 | E–S | ✓ | ✓ | | |
| 58 Rocky Narrows | 290 | 3.8 | E–M | | ✓ | | |
| 59 Sudbury Memorial Forest | 294 | 5.75 | E–M | | ✓ | | |
| 60 Upton State Forest | 299 | 3.2 | M | ✓ | ✓ | ✓ | |

# More Hikes by Category

| REGION<br>Hike Number/Hike Name | | Wheelchair/ Stroller Friendly | Proximity to Water | Swimming | Bird-Watching | Historic Sites | Dramatic Views |
|---|---|---|---|---|---|---|---|
| **WITHIN BOSTON** | | | | | | | |
| 1 | Charles River | ✓ | ✓ | | | ✓ | ✓ |
| 2 | Jamaica Pond | ✓ | ✓ | | | | |
| 3 | Spectacle Island: Boston Harbor Islands National & State Park | ✓ | ✓ | ✓ | ✓ | | ✓ |
| **SEASIDE HIKES** | | | | | | | |
| 4 | Crane Beach | | ✓ | ✓ | ✓ | | ✓ |
| 5 | Halibut Point State Park | ✓ | ✓ | | ✓ | ✓ | ✓ |
| 6 | Nasketucket Bay State Reservation | ✓ | ✓ | ✓ | ✓ | | ✓ |
| 7 | Parker River National Wildlife Refuge: Hellcat Trail | | ✓ | | ✓ | | ✓ |
| 8 | Sandy Point State Reservation | ✓ | ✓ | ✓ | ✓ | | ✓ |
| 9 | World's End | ✓ | ✓ | ✓ | ✓ | | ✓ |
| **NORTH OF BOSTON** | | | | | | | |
| 10 | Agassiz Rock Reservation | | | | | | ✓ |
| 11 | Appleton Farms: Grass Rides | portions | | | ✓ | | |
| 12 | Bald Hill Conservation Area | | | | | | |
| 13 | Beaver Brook | | ✓ | | | | |
| 14 | Dogtown Common | | | | | ✓ | |
| 15 | Goldsmith Reservation | | ✓ | | ✓ | | ✓ |
| 16 | Great Meadow–Gerrish's Rock | | ✓ | ✓ | ✓ | | ✓ |
| 17 | Indian Ridge Reservation | | ✓ | | ✓ | | |
| 18 | Lynn Woods | portions | ✓ | | | ✓ | |
| 19 | Manchester-Essex Woodlands | | | | ✓ | | |
| 20 | Maudslay State Park | ✓ | ✓ | | ✓ | ✓ | ✓ |
| 21 | Middlesex Fells Reservation: Skyline Trail | | ✓ | | ✓ | | |
| 22 | Old Town Hill Reservation | | ✓ | ✓ | ✓ | | ✓ |
| 23 | Ravenswood Park | portions | | | ✓ | ✓ | |
| 24 | Skug River Reservation | | ✓ | | ✓ | | |
| 25 | Ward Reservation | | | | | | ✓ |
| 26 | Weir Hill | | ✓ | | | | ✓ |
| 27 | Willowdale State Forest | | ✓ | | ✓ | | |
| 28 | Winnekenni Park | ✓ | ✓ | | | ✓ | |

| REGION<br>Hike Number/Hike Name | Wheelchair/Stroller Friendly | Proximity to Water | Swimming | Bird-Watching | Historic Sites | Dramatic Views |
|---|---|---|---|---|---|---|
| **SOUTH OF BOSTON** | | | | | | |
| 29 Blue Hills Reservation: Hemenway Hill | | ✓ | | ✓ | | ✓ |
| 30 Blue Hills Reservation: Skyline Trail | | ✓ | | ✓ | | ✓ |
| 31 Borderland State Park | ✓ | ✓ | | ✓ | ✓ | |
| 32 Copicut Woods | | | | ✓ | | |
| 33 Destruction Brook Woods | | ✓ | | | | |
| 34 Noanet Woodlands | | | | | | ✓ |
| 35 Noon Hill | | ✓ | | | | |
| 36 Round Pond | | ✓ | | ✓ | | |
| 37 Slocum's River Reserve | | ✓ | | ✓ | | ✓ |
| 38 Wilson Mountain Reservation | | | | | | ✓ |
| 39 Whitney and Thayer Woods | | ✓ | | | | |
| **WEST OF BOSTON** | | | | | | |
| 40 Ashland State Park | | ✓ | ✓ | | | |
| 41 Blackstone River and Canal Heritage State Park | 0.6-mile portion | ✓ | | | ✓ | |
| 42 Callahan State Park | | | | | | |
| 43 Cedar Hill and Sawink Farm | | | | ✓ | | ✓ |
| 44 Centennial Reservation | | ✓ | | ✓ | | |
| 45 Douglas State Forest | | ✓ | ✓ | | | |
| 46 Elm Bank Reservation | ✓ | ✓ | | ✓ | | |
| 47 Foss Farm | | ✓ | | ✓ | | |
| 48 Franklin State Forest | | | | | | |
| 49 Great Brook Farm State Park | portions | ✓ | | | | |
| 50 Hammond Pond–Houghton Garden | portions | ✓ | | ✓ | ✓ | |
| 51 Hemlock Gorge Reservation | ✓ | ✓ | | | ✓ | |
| 52 Mount Pisgah Conservation Area | | | | ✓ | | ✓ |
| 53 Mount Wachusett | | | | ✓ | | ✓ |
| 54 Mount Watatic | | | | ✓ | | ✓ |
| 55 Ogilvie Town Forest | | | | | | |
| 56 Oxbow Meadows/Farrar Pond/Mount Misery: In Thoreau's Footsteps | | ✓ | | | ✓ | |
| 57 Purgatory Chasm State Reservation | | | | | | ✓ |
| 58 Rocky Narrows | | ✓ | | | | |
| 59 Sudbury Memorial Forest | | ✓ | | ✓ | | |
| 60 Upton State Forest | | ✓ | | | | |

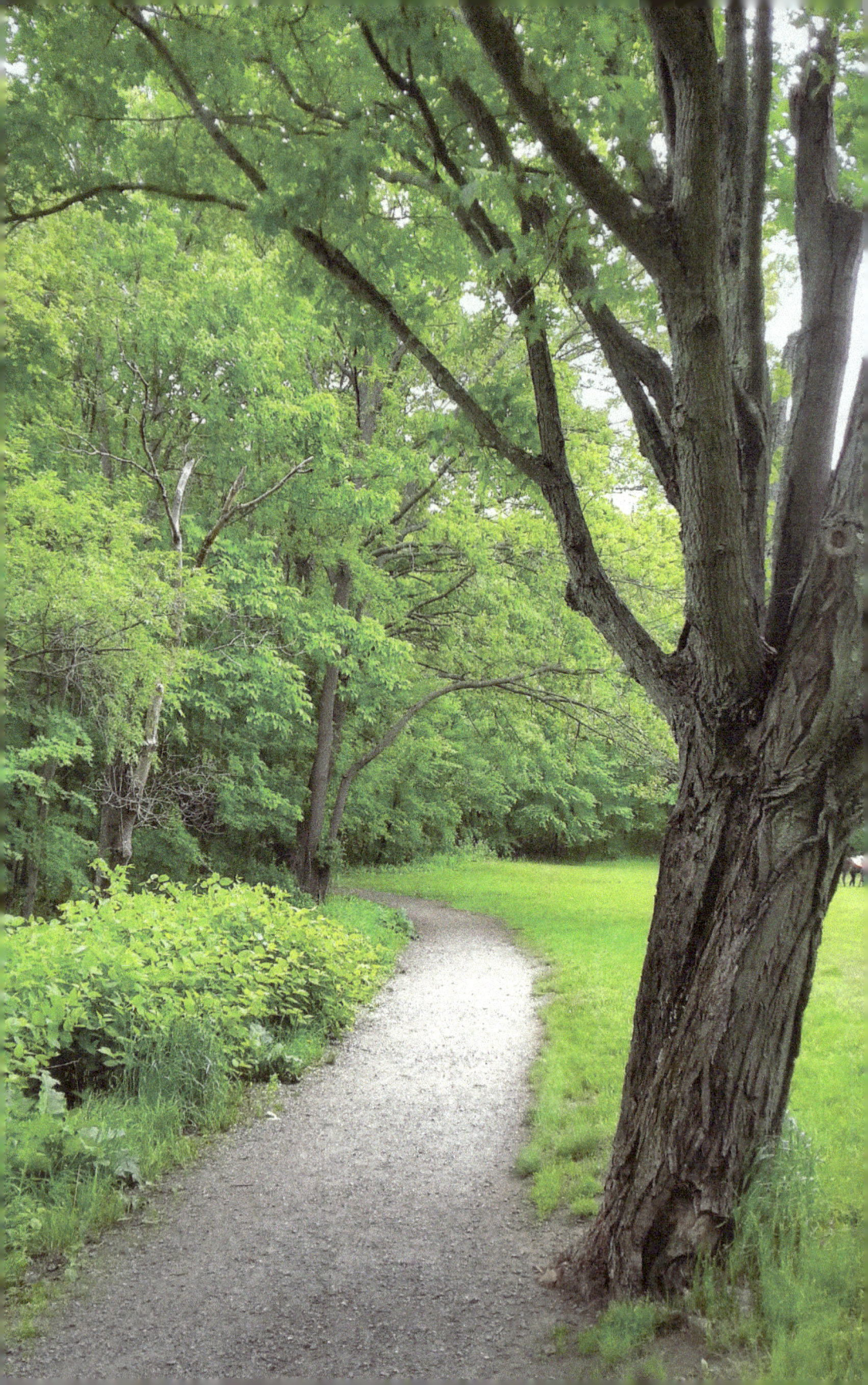

**Welcome to** *60 Hikes Within 60 Miles: Boston!* Whether you're new to hiking or a seasoned hiker, take a few minutes to read the following introduction. We'll explain how this book is organized and how to get the best use of it.

## *About This Book*

From the air, if you're coming into or leaving Logan International Airport, you can see the large amount of densely wooded green space around the Boston area—the Emerald Necklace, as envisioned by Fredrick Law Olmsted. So it was not a challenge to find 60 hikes within 60 miles of Boston Common. The challenge was narrowing down the list to the 60 best and striking a balance between the long, lung-pounding hikes, such as the two Skyline Trails (in Middlesex Fells and Blue Hills Reservation), and the shorter, more pastoral walks through the woods. Every hike presented here has something special to offer. Whether you live right in the thick of Boston or in the burbs, you won't have to drive far. Here's what the geographic sections encompass.

### WITHIN BOSTON

These hikes are, as the name implies, near downtown Boston. You can also reach these riding the T, which makes accessing them even easier.

### SEASIDE HIKES

There are many hikes along the circuitous coastline of Massachusetts. These hikes are all located on the shore of the mainland or even along the shores of some of the islands just off the coast.

### NORTH OF BOSTON

These hikes are to the north and east of Boston, including several as far up as Cape Ann and even one just over the border in New Hampshire.

### SOUTH OF BOSTON

This area includes the South Shore and many hikes near the coast of Buzzards Bay.

### WEST OF BOSTON

This section features some of the more remote-feeling hikes, even though they are still well within easy driving distance. The area west of Boston is the most widespread and includes many hikes just within or outside the course of I-495.

A 5.6-mile hike through Winnekenni Park (page 150), takes you on an old carriage trail through the woods, beside a lake, and to the grounds of a restored stone castle.

Each of these areas includes many hikes that are fairly easy, or that could be shortened to make them even easier, so they're great for families with young kids. You'll also find hikes that are a bit more moderate and will get your legs moving. Most of these treks can be made even longer or shorter depending on your preference. While each follows a prescribed path, equip yourself with a map and feel free to explore on your own. Most of these hikes happen within a network of trails that intersect and overlap and beg for further exploration.

## *How to Use This Guidebook*

### OVERVIEW MAP AND LEGEND

Use the overview map on page iv to assess the exact locations of each hike's primary trailhead. Each hike's number appears on the overview map and in the table of contents. As you flip through the book, a hike's full profile is easy to locate by watching for the hike number at the top of each page. The book is organized by region, as indicated in the table of contents. A map legend that details the symbols found on the trail maps appears on page viii.

### REGIONAL MAPS

The book is divided into regions, and prefacing each regional section is a regional map. These provide more detail than the overview map, bringing you closer to the hikes.

### TRAIL MAPS

A detailed map of each hike's route appears with its profile. On each of these maps, symbols indicate the trailhead, the complete route, significant features, facilities, and topographic landmarks such as creeks, overlooks, and peaks.

To produce the highly accurate maps in this book, the author used a handheld GPS unit to gather data while hiking each route, and then sent that data to the publisher's expert cartographers. However, your GPS is not a substitute for sound, sensible navigation that takes into account the conditions you observe while hiking.

Further, despite the high quality of the maps in this guidebook, the publisher and author strongly recommend you always carry an additional map, such as the ones noted in each entry's listing for "Maps."

### ELEVATION PROFILES

For trails with significant elevation changes, the hike description *will* include this profile graph. Entries for fairly flat routes will *not* display an elevation profile.

For hike descriptions where the elevation profile is included, this diagram represents the rises and falls of the trail as viewed from the side, over the complete distance (in miles) of that trail. On the diagram's vertical axis, or height scale, the number of feet indicated between each tick mark lets you visualize the climb. To avoid making flat hikes look steep and steep hikes appear flat, varying height scales provide an accurate image of each hike's climbing challenge. For example, one hike's scale might rise to more than 1,000 feet, such as Mount Wachusett, while another follows relatively flat riverbanks.

## THE HIKE PROFILE

Each profile contains a brief overview of the trail, a description of the route from start to finish, key at-a-glance information (such as the trail's distance and configuration and contacts for local information), GPS trailhead coordinates, and directions for driving to the trailhead area. Each profile also includes a map (see "Trail Maps" on previous page) and elevation profile (if the elevation gain is 100 feet or more). Many hike profiles also include notes on nearby activities.

### Key Information

The information in this box gives you a quick idea of the statistics and specifics of each hike.

DISTANCE & CONFIGURATION Distance notes the length of the hike round-trip, from start to finish. If the hike description includes options to shorten or extend the hike, those round-trip distances will also be noted here. Configuration defines the trail as a loop, an out-and-back (taking you in and out via the same route), a figure eight, or a point-to-point.

DIFFICULTY The degree of effort that a typical hiker should expect on a given route. For simplicity, the trails are rated as easy, moderate, or strenuous.

SCENERY A short summary of the attractions offered by the hike and what to expect in terms of plant life, wildlife, natural wonders, and historical features.

EXPOSURE A quick check of how much sun you can expect on your shoulders during the hike.

TRAFFIC Indicates how busy the trail might be on an average day. Trail traffic, of course, varies from day to day and season to season. Weekend days typically see the most visitors. Other trail users that may be encountered on the trail are also noted here.

TRAIL SURFACE Indicates whether the trail surface is paved, rocky, gravel, dirt, boardwalk, or a mixture of elements.

HIKING TIME  How long it takes to hike the trail. A slow but steady hiker will average 2–3 miles an hour, depending on the terrain.

DRIVING DISTANCE  Listed in miles from Boston Common. Even if you don't start there, the mileages should give you an estimate of travel times from where you live.

ELEVATION  Lists elevation at the trailhead and another figure for the highest or lowest altitude on the route. If there is no significant gain, that is also noted.

SEASON  Names the best time of year for doing the hike, in the authors' opinions.

ACCESS  Fees or permits required to hike the trail are detailed here—and noted if there are none. Trail-access hours are also shown here.

MAPS  Resources for maps, in addition to those in this guidebook, are listed here. (As previously noted, the publisher and author recommend that you carry more than one map—and that you consult those maps before heading out on the trail, to resolve any confusion or discrepancy.)

WHEELCHAIR ACCESS  At-a-glance, you'll see if there are paved sections or other areas for safely using a wheelchair.

FACILITIES  This item alerts you to restrooms, water, picnic tables, and other basics at or near the trailhead.

CONTACT  Listed here are phone numbers and website addresses for checking trail conditions and gleaning other day-to-day information.

LOCATION  The city (or nearby community) in which the trail is located.

COMMENTS  Here you will find assorted nuggets of information, such as whether or not dogs are allowed on the trails.

## In Brief

Think of this section as a taste of the trail, a snapshot focused on the historical land-marks, beautiful vistas, and other sights you may encounter on the hike.

## Description

The heart of each hike. Here the author provides a summary of the trail's essence and highlights any special traits the hike offers. The route is clearly outlined, including landmarks, side trips, and possible alternate routes along the way. Ultimately, the hike description will help you choose which hikes are best for you.

## Nearby Activities

Look here for information on things to do or points of interest: nearby parks, museums, restaurants, and the like. Note that not every hike has a listing.

## Directions

Used in conjunction with the GPS coordinates, the driving directions will help you locate each trailhead. Once at the trailhead, park only in designated areas.

## GPS Trailhead Coordinates

As noted in "Trail Maps," page 2, the author used a handheld GPS unit to obtain geographic data and sent the information to the publisher's cartographers. The trailhead coordinates—the intersection of the latitude (north) and longitude (west)—will orient you from the trailhead. In some cases, you can drive within viewing distance of a trailhead. Other hiking routes require a short walk to the trailhead from a parking area.

You will also note that this guidebook uses the degrees–decimal minute format for presenting the GPS coordinates.

**N42° 21.650'  W71° 04.250'**

The latitude and longitude grid system is likely quite familiar to you, but here is a refresher, pertinent to visualizing the GPS coordinates:

Imaginary lines of latitude—called parallels and approximately 69 miles apart from each other—run horizontally around the globe. The equator is established to be 0°, and each parallel is indicated by degrees from the equator: up to 90°N at the North Pole and down to 90°S at the South Pole.

Imaginary lines of longitude—called meridians—run perpendicular to latitude lines and are likewise indicated by degrees. Starting from 0° at the Prime Meridian in Greenwich, England, they continue to the east and west until they meet 180° later at the International Date Line in the Pacific Ocean. At the equator, longitude lines are also approximately 69 miles apart, but that distance narrows as the meridians converge toward the North and South Poles.

For more on GPS technology, visit usgs.gov.

## TOPOGRAPHIC MAPS

The maps in this book have been produced with great care and, used with the hike text, will direct you to the trail and help you stay on course. However, you'll find superior detail and valuable information in the U.S. Geological Survey's 7.5-minute-series topographic maps. At mytopo.com, for example, you can view and print free USGS topos of the entire United States. Online services such as Trails.com charge annual fees for additional features such as shaded relief, which makes the topography stand out more. If you expect to print out many topo maps each year, it might be worth paying for such extras. The downside to USGS maps is that most are outdated, having been created 20–30 years ago; nevertheless, they provide excellent topographic detail. Of course, Google Earth (earth.google.com) does away with topo maps and their inaccuracies, replacing them with satellite imagery and its own inaccuracies. Regardless, what one lacks, the other augments. Google Earth is an excellent tool whether you have difficulty with topos or not.

If you're new to hiking, you might be wondering, "What's a topo map?" In short, it indicates not only linear distance but also elevation, using contour lines. These lines spread across the map like dozens of intricate spider webs. Each line represents a particular elevation, and at the base of each topo a contour's interval designation is given. For example, if the contour interval is 20 feet, then the distance between each contour line is 20 feet. Follow five contour lines up on the same map, and the elevation has increased by 100 feet. In addition to the sources listed previously and in Appendix B, you'll find topos at major universities, outdoor gear shops, and some public libraries, as well as online at nationalmap.gov and store.usgs.gov.

## *Weather*

It has been said there is no such thing as bad weather, only inappropriate clothing. Bostonians and New Englanders as a whole pay close attention to forecasts, while simultaneously regarding them with stubborn disdain and skepticism. This is due both to disposition and to the weather's high degree of variability, not just season to season but minute by minute. A 20° drop or upward lurch in temperature is not unheard of either on a sultry summer evening or on a silvery afternoon in winter. Often the most reliable weather predictor is a stiff wind, for it likely signals a shift from humid to dry, hot to cool, or vice versa.

| | JAN | FEB | MARCH | APRIL | MAY | JUNE |
|---|---|---|---|---|---|---|
| Hi Temp | 36°F | 39°F | 46°F | 56°F | 67°F | 77°F |
| Lo Temp | 22°F | 24°F | 31°F | 41°F | 50°F | 59°F |
| Precipitation | 3.35" | 3.27" | 4.33" | 3.74" | 3.5" | 3.66" |
| | JULY | AUG | SEPT | OCT | NOV | DEC |
| Hi Temp | 82°F | 80°F | 73°F | 62°F | 52°F | 42°F |
| Lo Temp | 64°F | 64°F | 57°F | 46°F | 38°F | 28°F |
| Precipitation | 3.43" | 3.35" | 3.43" | 3.94" | 3.98" | 3.78" |

*Source:* USClimateData.com

Boston's proximity to the sea and all that travels along the Gulf Stream from the Gulf of Mexico to Newfoundland and on across the Atlantic Ocean largely explains its fickle weather. In summer, the soggy winds of occasional Caribbean-born hurricanes add muscle and heft to the otherwise modest surf that smacks at the shore. These winds are known to drag in heat and humidity that settles on Boston's neighborhoods like a soggy blanket. Other storms, such as Canada-bred nor'easters, deftly carve out the heat and replace perspiration with goose bumps.

Bear in mind, too, that on any given day, the temperature at the shore is well below that of inland locations.

While there is no disagreement that a brilliant sunny day with the temperature between 65° F and 70° F is ideal for a hike in the hills, in today's age of synthetic performance fabrics, you can have a pleasant hiking experience in almost all conditions. Indeed, facing the elements when properly dressed is a distinctly satisfying pleasure. To ensure you are in league with the weather when you set out on a hike, be sure to pack extra clothing. Having a windbreaker or dry T-shirt to change into after a sweaty climb or cloudburst can make all the difference. Remember, there's no bad weather, only bad clothing.

## Water

How much is enough? Well, one simple physiological fact should convince you to err on the side of excess when deciding how much water to pack: a hiker walking steadily in 90° heat needs approximately 10 quarts of fluid per day. That's 2.5 gallons. A good rule of thumb is to hydrate prior to your hike, carry (and drink) 6 ounces of water for every mile you plan to hike, and hydrate again after the hike. For most people, the pleasures of hiking make carrying water a relatively minor price to pay to remain safe and healthy. So pack more water than you anticipate needing, even for short hikes.

If you are tempted to drink found water, do so with extreme caution. Many ponds and lakes encountered by hikers are fairly stagnant, and the water tastes terrible. Drinking such water presents inherent risks for thirsty trekkers. Giardia parasites contaminate many water sources and cause the dreaded intestinal giardiasis that can last for weeks after ingestion. For information, visit the Centers for Disease Control website at cdc.gov/parasites/giardia.

In any case, effective treatment is essential before using any water source found along the trail. Boiling water for two to three minutes is always a safe measure for camping, but day hikers can consider iodine tablets, approved chemical mixes, filtration units rated for giardia, and UV filtration. Some of these methods (for example, filtration with an added carbon filter) remove bad tastes typical in stagnant water, while others add their own taste. As a precaution, carry a means of water purification to help in a pinch or if you realize you have underestimated your consumption needs.

## Clothing

Nothing about the weather in and around Boston is certain but its variability. It is not a question of if the weather will change, but when. Even if it is a brilliant blue-sky morning when you prepare to head for the hiking trail, grab a fleece jacket or vest for later in the day when temperatures dip, especially in the deep shade of the woods. Taking along a waterproof, all-weather jacket made of a performance fabric is always an excellent idea. A lightweight jacket—a mood and possibly lifesaver, when weather conditions take a turn for the worse—also offers excellent protection against voracious bugs. Cotton is great for lounging around the house but not so great for outdoor activities during which you may be sweating one moment and getting chills the next. Choose your clothing wisely.

The person who packs a hat and mittens may suffer some teasing, but he or she may also wind up the envy of all when icy winds blow down from Canada, catching your hiking party unprepared. The same can be said of the one who thinks to bring wind and rain pants. Hypothermia can set in even when thermometers register temperatures above freezing.

And anyone who has gotten a blister or stubbed a toe knows the importance of wearing appropriate footwear. The best shoes for hiking are boots with solid ankle support. The sneakers or sandals you wear every day may feel more comfortable, but their flimsy soles mean more work for your feet and ankles when hiking over rough terrain.

Weather, unexpected trail conditions, fatigue, extended hiking duration, and wrong turns can individually or collectively turn a great outing into a very uncomfortable one at best—and a life-threatening one at worst. Thus, proper attire plays a key role in staying comfortable and, sometimes, in staying alive. Here are some helpful guidelines:

➤ **Choose silk, wool, or synthetic fabrics for maximum comfort in all of your hiking attire—including hats, socks, and everything in between.** Cotton is fine if the weather remains dry and stable, but you won't be happy if that material gets wet.

➤ **Always have a hat tucked into your day pack or hitched to your belt.** Hats offer all-weather sun and wind protection as well as warmth if it turns cold.

➤ **Be ready to layer up or down as the day progresses and the mercury rises or falls.** Today's outdoor wear makes layering easy, with such designs as jackets that convert to vests and zip-off or button-up legs.

➤ **Wear hiking boots or sturdy hiking sandals with toe protection.** Flip-flopping along a paved urban greenway is one thing, but never hike a trail in open sandals or casual sneakers. Your bones and arches need support, and your skin needs protection.

➤ **Pair that footwear with good socks.** If you prefer not to sheathe your feet when wearing hiking sandals, tuck the socks into your day pack. You may need them if the weather plummets or if you hit rocky turf and pebbles begin to irritate your feet. And, in an emergency, if you have lost your gloves, you can use your socks as mittens.

➤ **Don't leave rainwear behind, even if the day dawns clear and sunny.**
Tuck into your day pack, or tie around your waist, a jacket that is breathable
and either water-resistant or waterproof. Investigate different choices at your
local outdoors retailer. If you are a frequent hiker, ideally you'll have more
than one rainwear weight, material, and style in your closet to protect you in
all seasons in your regional climate and hiking microclimates.

## Essential Gear

Today you can buy outdoor vests that have up to 20 pockets shaped and sized to carry
everything from toothpicks to binoculars. Or, if you don't aspire to feel like a burro,
you can neatly stow all of these items in your day pack or backpack. The following list
showcases never-hike-without-them items, in alphabetical order, as all are important:

➤ **Extra clothes** Raingear, warm hat, gloves, and change of socks and shirt

➤ **Extra food** Trail mix, granola bars, or other high-energy foods

➤ **Flashlight or headlamp** with extra bulb and batteries

➤ **Insect repellent** In some areas and seasons, this is vital.

➤ **Maps and a high-quality compass** Even if you know the terrain from previous
hikes, don't leave home without these tools. And, as previously noted, bring
maps in addition to those in this guidebook, and consult your maps prior to
the hike. If you are versed in GPS usage, bring that device too, but don't rely
on it as your sole navigational tool, as battery life can dwindle or die. And be
sure to compare its guidance with that of your maps.

➤ **Pocketknife and/or multitool,** such as a Leatherman or Victorinox

➤ **Sunscreen** Note the expiration date on the tube or bottle; it's usually
embossed on the top.

➤ **Water** As emphasized more than once in this book, bring more than you think
you will drink. Depending on your destination, you may want to bring a con-
tainer and iodine or a filter for purifying water in case you run out.

➤ **Whistle** This little gadget will be your best friend in an emergency.

➤ **Windproof matches and/or a lighter,** as well as a fire starter

### FIRST AID KIT

Besides all the aforementioned items, those below may appear overwhelming for a
day hike. But any paramedic will tell you that the products listed here—in alphabetical order because all are important—are just the basics. The reality of hiking is that
you can be out for a week of backpacking and acquire only a mosquito bite. Or you
can hike for an hour, slip, and suffer a bleeding abrasion or broken bone. Fortunately,
these items will collapse into a very small space. You may also purchase convenient,
prepackaged kits at your pharmacy or on the Internet.

➤ **Adhesive bandages**

➤ **Antibiotic ointment** Neosporin or the generic equivalent

➤ **Athletic tape**

➤ **Benadryl or the generic equivalent, diphenhydramine** In case of allergic reactions

➤ **Blister kit**, such as Moleskin/Spenco 2nd Skin

➤ **Butterfly-closure bandages**

➤ **Elastic bandages or joint wraps**

➤ **Epinephrine in a prefilled syringe** Typically by prescription only, for people known to have severe allergic reactions to hiking occurrences such as bee stings

➤ **Gauze** One roll and a half dozen 4-by-4-inch pads

➤ **Hydrogen peroxide or iodine**

➤ **Ibuprofen or acetaminophen**

*Note:* Consider your intended terrain and the number of hikers in your party before you exclude any article cited above. A botanical garden stroll may not inspire you to carry a complete kit, but anything beyond that warrants precaution. When hiking alone, you should always be prepared for a medical need. And if you are a twosome or with a group, one or more people in your party should be equipped with first aid materials.

## General Safety

The following tips may have the familiar ring of your mother's voice as you take note of them.

➤ **Always let someone know where you will be hiking and how long you expect to be gone.** It's a good idea to give that person a copy of your route, particularly if you are headed into any isolated area. Let them know when you return.

➤ **Always sign in and out of any trail registers provided.** Don't hesitate to comment on the trail condition if space is provided; that's your opportunity to alert others to any problems you encounter.

➤ **Do not count on a cell phone for your safety.** Reception may be spotty or nonexistent on the trail, even on an urban walk—especially if it is surrounded by towering trees.

➤ **Always carry food and water, even for a short hike.** And bring more water than you think you will need. (That cannot be said often enough!)

➤ **Ask questions.** State forest and park employees are there to help. It's a lot easier to solicit advice before a problem occurs, and it will help you avoid a mishap away from civilization when it's too late to amend an error.

➤ **Stay on designated trails.** Even on the most clearly marked trails, there is usually a point where you have to stop and consider which way to go. If you become disoriented, don't panic. As soon as you think you may be off track, stop, assess your current direction, and then retrace your steps to the point where you went astray. Using a map, a compass, and this book, and keeping in mind what you have passed thus far, reorient yourself, and trust your judgment on which way to head. If you become absolutely unsure of how to continue, return to your vehicle the way you came in. Should you become completely lost and have no idea how to find the trailhead, remaining in place along the trail and waiting for help is most often the best option for adults and always the best option for children.

➤ **Always carry a whistle, another precaution that cannot be overemphasized.** It may be a lifesaver if you do become lost or sustain an injury.

➤ **Be especially careful when crossing streams.** Whether you are fording the stream or crossing on a log, make every step count. If you have any doubt about maintaining your balance on a log, ford the stream instead: use a trekking pole or stout stick for balance *and face upstream as you cross.* If a stream seems too deep to ford, turn back. Whatever is on the other side is not worth risking your life.

➤ **Be careful at overlooks.** While these areas may provide spectacular views, they are potentially hazardous. Stay back from the edge of outcrops, and make absolutely sure of your footing; a misstep can mean a nasty and possibly fatal fall.

➤ **Standing dead trees and storm-damaged living trees pose a significant hazard to hikers.** These trees may have loose or broken limbs that could fall at any time. While walking beneath trees, and when choosing a spot to rest or enjoy your snack, look up!

➤ **Know the symptoms of subnormal body temperature, known as hypothermia.** Shivering and forgetfulness are the two most common indicators of this stealthy killer. Hypothermia can occur at any elevation, even in the summer, especially when the hiker is wearing lightweight cotton clothing. If symptoms present themselves, get to shelter, hot liquids, and dry clothes as soon as possible.

➤ **Know the symptoms of heat exhaustion (hyperthermia).** Light-headedness and loss of energy are the first two indicators. If you feel these symptoms, find some shade, drink your water, remove as many layers of clothing as practical, and stay put until you cool down. Marching through heat exhaustion leads to heatstroke, which can be fatal. If you should be sweating and you're not, that's the signature warning sign. Your hike is over at that point—heatstroke is a life-threatening condition that can cause seizures, convulsions, and eventually death. If you or a companion reaches that point, do whatever can be done to cool the victim down, and seek medical attention immediately.

➤ **Most important of all, take along your brain.** A cool, calculating mind is the single-most important asset on the trail. It allows you to think before you act.

➤ **In summary: Plan ahead.** Watch your step. Avoid accidents before they happen. Enjoy a rewarding and relaxing hike.

## *Watchwords for Flora and Fauna*

Hikers should remain aware of the following concerns regarding plant- and wildlife, described in alphabetical order.

### BLACK BEARS

Though attacks by black bears are uncommon, the sight or approach of a bear can give anyone a start. If you encounter a bear while hiking, remain calm and avoid running in any direction. Make loud noises to scare off the bear, and back away slowly. In primitive and remote areas, assume bears are present. In more-developed sites, check on the current bear situation prior to hiking.

Every now and then, you'll see stories on the Boston news of a black bear wandering around a suburban neighborhood. It's rare, but not impossible. Most encounters are motivated by food, as bears have an exceptional sense of smell and not particularly discriminating tastes. While this is of greater concern to backpackers and campers, on a day hike, you may plan a lunchtime picnic or munch on an energy bar or other snack from time to time. If you see a black bear approaching as you're having lunch, it's best to leave your lunch and be on your way. Remain aware and alert, and you should be fine.

### BLACK FLIES

Black flies are not dangerous, but they are certainly pests and a maddening annoyance. The worst a black fly will cause is an itchy welt. They are most active mid-May–June, during the day, and especially before thunderstorms, as well as during the morning and evening hours. Insect repellent has some effect (especially if it contains DEET), though the only way to keep out of their swarming midst is to keep moving.

### MOSQUITOES

One of the advantages of hiking in fall, winter, or early spring is the absence of biting insects. The greater Boston area certainly has its share of winged tormentors. As a rule, conditions that suppress bugs include stiff breezes, dry air, and frost.

Conversely, these airborne pests love windless, humid air. When preparing for a hike, approach the bug issue as you would the weather: dress appropriately. Wearing a long-sleeved cotton shirt and loose cotton pants gives excellent protection from the swarms of mosquitoes that materialize around wetlands and elsewhere when the heat of the sun subsides in the later afternoon. Unlike mosquitoes and black flies, greenheads—a fierce variety of horsefly—pose a threat only in areas near the salt marshes where they breed. Greenhead season on Crane Beach and Plum Island usually runs from mid-July through the first week of August.

In some areas, mosquitoes are known to carry the West Nile or Triple E (eastern equine encephalitis) virus, so take precautions to avoid their bites. Ward them off with insect repellent and/or repellent-impregnated clothing. A note about DEET: Though the EPA deems this repellent to be safe, the agency also advises limiting its use and washing it off when protection is no longer needed. Before you reach for insect repellent, strike out on the trail just to see what you'll need. Have it handy, but know that you won't necessarily need to use it.

## POISON IVY, OAK, AND SUMAC

Recognizing poison ivy, oak, and sumac and avoiding contact with them is the most effective way to prevent the painful, itchy rashes associated with these plants. In the Northeast, poison ivy ranges from a thick, tree-hugging vine to a shaded ground cover, three leaflets to a leaf; poison oak occurs as either a vine or a shrub, with three

leaflets as well; and poison sumac flourishes in swampland, each leaf containing 7–13 leaflets. Urushiol, the oil in the sap of these plants, is responsible for the rash. Usually within 12–14 hours of exposure (but sometimes much later), raised lines and/or blisters will appear, accompanied by a terrible itch. Refrain from scratching because bacteria under the fingernails can cause infection. Wash and dry the rash thoroughly, applying a calamine lotion to help dry it out. If itching or blistering is severe, seek medical attention. Remember to wash not only any exposed parts of your body but also clothes, gear, and pets, as they can transmit the oil to you or someone else.

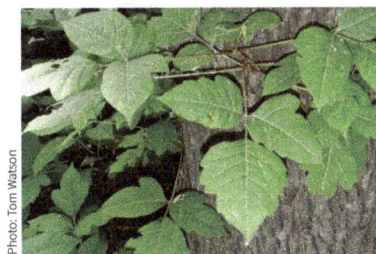

Photo: Tom Watson

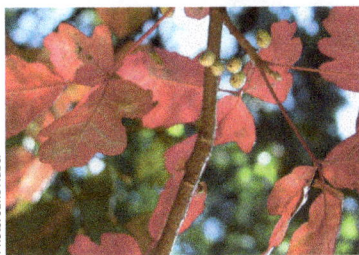

Photo: Jane Huber

## SNAKES

Spend some time hiking in and around Boston and you may be surprised by the variety of snakes you encounter. Most snakes sighted will be garter snakes, black racers, brown

snakes, harmless water snakes, and perhaps the flashy, slender eastern ribbon
snake. All but two of Massachusetts's
14 native snake species are harmless. The
state's two venomous species, the timber
rattlesnake and the copperhead, are not
only shy and reclusive but also woefully
rare. The most likely place you'll see a
timber rattler sunning itself is in the Blue
Hills Reservation. Despite great efforts
to protect them, both snakes are listed as
endangered, and therefore it is illegal to harass, kill, collect, or possess them. To
calm your fears or add interest to your hiking experience, consider spending a few
minutes studying snakes before heading into the woods. If you do have the good
fortune of spotting a snake while hiking, treat it with respect: give it a wide berth,
and let it go its way.

The best rule is to leave all snakes alone, giving them plenty of space as you
hike past and making sure any hiking companions (including dogs) do the same.
When hiking, stick to well-used trails, and wear over-the-ankle boots and loose-
fitting long pants. Do not step or put your hands beyond your range of detailed
visibility, and avoid wandering around in the dark. Step *onto* logs and rocks, never
*over* them, and be especially careful when climbing rocks. Always avoid walking
through dense brush or willow thickets.

## TICKS

Ticks are often found on brush and tall grass, where they seem to be waiting to hitch
a ride on a warm-blooded passerby. Adult ticks are most active April–May and again
October–November. Among the varieties of ticks, the black-legged tick, commonly
called the deer tick, is the primary carrier of Lyme disease. Wear light-colored clothing
to make it easier for you to spot ticks before they migrate to your skin. At the end of
the hike, visually check your hair, the back of your neck, your armpits, and your socks.
During your posthike shower, take a moment to do a more complete body check.

For ticks that are already embedded, removal with tweezers is best. Grasp the
tick close to your skin, and remove it by pulling straight out firmly. Do your best to
remove the head, but do not twist. Use disinfectant solution on the wound. Don't
panic if you are bit by a tick, but do respond quickly. Ticks need to be embedded
for 24–48 hours to transmit any toxins. And even after that, you have about a week
to begin an antibiotic regimen to ward off infection. If you see the telltale bull's-eye
rash around the bite, contact your doctor. Try to save the tick itself in a plastic bag
for identification if you can.

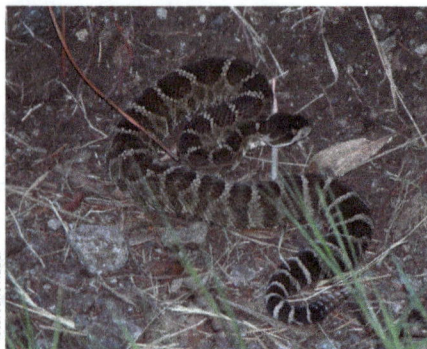

# *Hunting*

Separate rules, regulations, and licenses govern the various types of hunting (bow, shotgun, and black powder) and related seasons. Though there are generally no problems, hikers may wish to forgo trips during late fall, when the woods suddenly seem filled with orange and camouflage. At the very least, be cautious, wear hunter orange, and stay on the trails. Hunting is allowed in many state forests and parks throughout Massachusetts, including the following that are profiled in this book:

- ➤ Blackstone River and Canal Heritage State Park
- ➤ Franklin State Forest
- ➤ Douglas State Forest
- ➤ Sandy Point State Reservation
- ➤ Wachusett Mountain State Reservation
- ➤ Willowdale State Forest

## HUNTING REGULATIONS

Here are the official hunting rules and regulations as spelled out on the Department of Conservation and Recreation (DCR) website:

Hunting is allowed in many state forests and parks, as well as DCR watershed properties. It is good practice to contact the individual park or forest to learn about special regulations before you arrive.

Hunters must comply with all relevant hunting laws and regulations. Additional hunting regulations specific to DCR properties include:

- ➤ **You can't hunt, trap, or discharge a firearm within 500 feet of the border of a DCR-designated campsite or camping structure,** including those along the Appalachian Trail.
- ➤ **You can't hunt within 500 feet of any DCR-designated picnic area, camping area, residence, service building, parking lot, camping structure, or designated swimming area.**
- ➤ **You can't install a permanent tree stand on DCR property.** A permanent tree stand is a hunting platform or structure attached to a tree by nails, bolts, wire, or other fasteners that go through the bark into the wood. The tree stand may not be in place longer than 30 days.

## HUNTING HOURS

Hunting hours are generally 30 minutes before sunrise to 30 minutes after sunset, with the following exceptions:

- ➤ **Pheasant hunting hours for properties stocked with pheasants are sunrise–sunset.**

➤ Waterfowl hunting hours end at sunset.

➤ Coyote and fox hunting hours end at midnight.

➤ Hunting waterfowl on the coast is permitted on DCR property in the inter-tidal zone. This is the land between the high- and low-water marks.

Here are a couple of helpful links with Massachusetts hunting rules and regulations that are updated fairly regularly:

➤ mass.gov/hunting-regulations

➤ mass.gov/topics/hunting-fishing

➤ eregulations.com/massachusetts/huntingandfishing

## Trail Etiquette

Always treat the trail, wildlife, and fellow hikers with respect. Here are some guidelines to remember.

➤ **Plan ahead in order to be self-sufficient at all times.** For example, carry necessary supplies for changes in weather or other conditions. A well-planned trip brings satisfaction to you and to others.

➤ **Hike on open trails only.** In seasons or construction areas where road or trail closures may be a possibility, use the website addresses or phone numbers shown in the "Contact" line for each hike to check conditions prior to heading out. Do not attempt to circumvent such closures.

➤ **Avoid trespassing on private land,** and obtain all permits and authorization as required. Leave gates as you find them or as directed by signage.

➤ **Be courteous** to other hikers, bikers, equestrians, and anyone else you encounter on the trails.

➤ **Never spook wild animals or pets.** An unannounced approach, a sudden movement, or a loud noise startles most critters, and a surprised animal can be dangerous to you, to others, and to itself. Give animals plenty of space.

➤ **Observe the yield signs around the region's trailheads and backcountry.** Typically, they advise hikers to yield to horses, and bikers to yield to both horses and hikers. On hills, hikers and bikers should yield to any uphill traffic. When encountering mounted riders, hikers can courteously step off the trail, on the downhill side if possible. So the horse can see and hear you, calmly greet the riders before they reach you, and do not dart behind trees. Resist the urge to pet horses unless you are invited to do so.

➤ **Stay on the existing trail,** and do not blaze any new trails.

➤ **Be sure to pack out what you pack in, leaving only your footprints.** No one likes to see the trash someone else has left behind.

## Tips on Enjoying Hiking in Boston

The Boston area is rich with history, dramatic scenery, beautiful forests, impressive rock formations, pristine lakes and rivers, spectacular shorelines, and plenty of places where you can find a bit of wilderness to call your own for an afternoon. And it's all quite close. This guide profiles 60 of what we feel are some of the nicer hikes within the immediate Boston area, but there are certainly others. Grab a DeLorme *Massachusetts Atlas & Gazetteer,* this book, and any maps you may have of the area, and go exploring. In short order, you can feel like you are miles from anywhere and anyone.

I am always a big fan of combining two activities, and there is ample opportunity to do that with many of these hikes. Many are near one of the state park campgrounds, such as Harold Parker State Forest or Wompatuck State Park, so you could combine a camping trip with a hike or two.

If you're more ambitious, you can also do a bit of rock climbing while hiking and exploring Purgatory Chasm or the Hammond Pond hike. Any of the hikes on or near water, such as Spectacle Island, Ashland State Park, or Blackstone River and Canal Heritage State Park, can also involve some kayaking, canoeing, or fishing. And most of these hikes are in state forests or parks that also permit mountain biking.

Or if you'd just like to relax on the beach after a hike, Crane Beach, Sandy Point State Reservation, or Douglas State Forest would be perfect. Check the 60 Hikes by Category table on page xii to see what hikes might fit in with the other activities you have in mind. And enjoy your adventure.

It's well worth spending some time on the beach at Nasketucket Bay State Reservation.

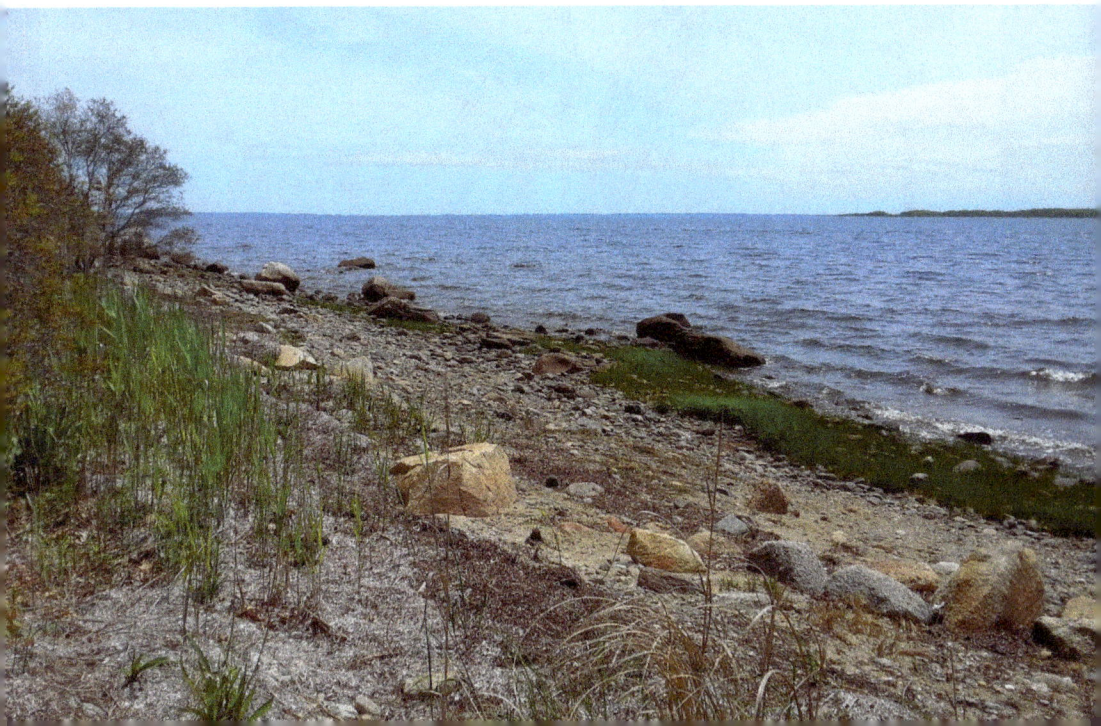

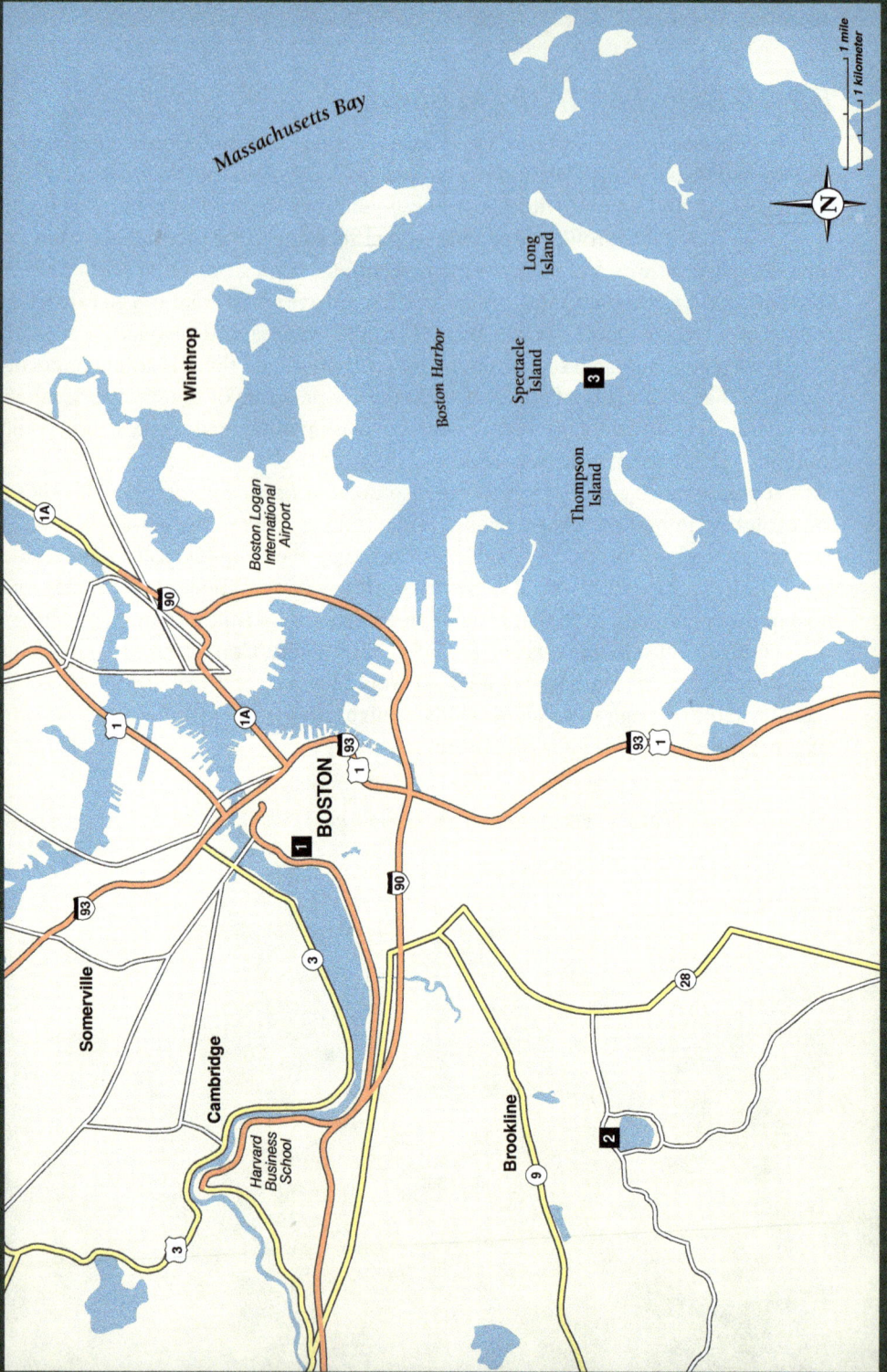

Massachusetts Bay

Winthrop

Long Island

Boston Logan International Airport

Boston Harbor

Spectacle Island

Thompson Island

1A

90

1

1A

93

1

93

1

BOSTON

1

90

93

3

28

Somerville

Cambridge

Harvard Business School

Brookline

9

2

3

1 mile
1 kilometer

N

# WITHIN BOSTON

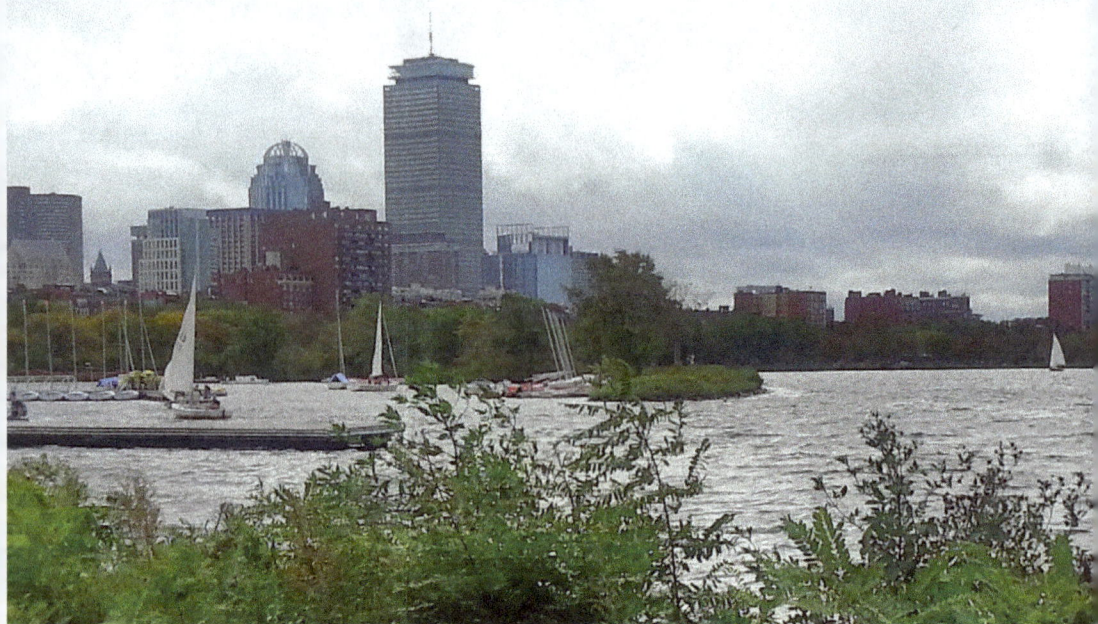

The views from along the banks of the Charles River are all classic Boston.

**TO REALLY GET TO KNOW** Boston, one of the best places to start is the Charles River basin. Once a sprawling tidal river with winding estuaries and thousands of acres of salt marsh, the lower Charles today takes you on a tour of the Esplanade and Cambridge on the other side of the river. You'll pass Harvard University and loop back to Boston over a scenic footbridge.

## DESCRIPTION

The Charles River is an urban oasis—a true treasure. To start this tour of the lower Charles, cross at the foot of the Charles Street MBTA station onto Charles Street. Cross over to the south bank of the Charles River via the pedestrian footbridge ahead. As you rise above the rush of traffic, the pace of the city eases.

You come to the rippling waters of the Charles and, to the right, the silhouette of the Longfellow Bridge, renamed in 1927 to honor poet Henry Wadsworth Longfellow, who professed his love for the river in his poem "To the River Charles." At the foot of the pedestrian bridge, head left on the paved walkway in the shade of willows and Norway maples, past the Community Boating center to a cove protected by a breakwater. Immediately after the cove, the path arrives at the Hatch Shell, made famous by Arthur Fiedler and the Boston Pops orchestra. Bear right to cross an impressively sculpted footbridge guarded by snarling granite lions.

**DISTANCE & CONFIGURATION:** 7.75-mile loop

**DIFFICULTY:** Easy

**SCENERY:** The Charles River, with historic Boston on the south and Cambridge on the north

**EXPOSURE:** Mix of sun and shade

**TRAFFIC:** Light–heavy, depending on time and day

**TRAIL SURFACE:** Pavement with stretches of grass or packed earth

**HIKING TIME:** 2.5–3 hours

**DRIVING DISTANCE FROM BOSTON COMMON:** Driving is not recommended. However, if you do drive, look for parking at Boston Common, where there are plenty of meters and a parking garage, or at the Government Center garage.

**ELEVATION:** 350' at trailhead, no significant gain

**SEASON:** Year-round

**ACCESS:** Open sunrise–sunset; free

**MAPS:** Available at tinyurl.com/charlesrivermap

**WHEELCHAIR ACCESS:** Yes

**FACILITIES:** Public restrooms, snacks, soft drinks, sandwiches, hot dogs, pretzels, and coffee available at various locations around the Charles

**CONTACT:** Charles River Reservation, mass.gov /locations/charles-river-reservation, 617-727-4708

**LOCATION:** Charles River at the Charles/MGH MBTA station, Boston, MA

**COMMENTS:** Memorial Drive from Western Avenue to Mount Auburn Street in Cambridge is off-limits to cars 11 a.m.–7 p.m. on Sundays from the last Sunday in April to the second Sunday in November.

This is downtown Boston. You will not be alone as you walk along the Charles. You'll be joined by runners, walkers, bicyclists, skateboarders, parents pushing strollers, and all manner of humanity enjoying the serene banks of the river. As you move along, out in the inlet to the right you'll be able to spot a couple of dragon boats resting at their mooring in between races. Arching around two more lagoons, the path crosses another picturesque footbridge and arrives at a junction. To keep clear of bicyclists and others on wheels, stay with the path beside the water.

A thick grove of trees shades a playground gracefully integrated into the park. Looking diagonally west across the water, you can see the dome of Massachusetts Institute of Technology (MIT) resting on the horizon, looking like the bald head of a scientist pondering some obscure concept of theoretical physics.

Mount the stairs of the Harvard Bridge directly ahead and, once at the top, bear right to cross the river to Cambridge. Familiar sights on the skyline include the famous Citgo sign lighting the sky above Kenmore Square and Fenway Park.

As you move along the bridge, you'll be able to note your distance in "Smoots." The distance between each Smoot is exactly 5 feet 7 inches—the height of Oliver Smoot, MIT class of 1962. In 1958, MIT's Lambda Chi Alpha fraternity conceived a prank, or hack, as they call it, to determine the distance from the MIT dorms in Boston to the MIT campus. To serve as a measuring unit, Lambda Chi Alpha's pledge master chose Smoot, who was a handy height and carried a name that "sounded scientific." So they laid Smoot down end-to-end again and again from Boston to Cambridge and found the distance to be 364.4 Smoots and one ear. And so it was that Oliver Smoot found his calling, for he went on to become president of the International Organization for Standardization (ISO) and chairman of the American National Standards Institute (ANSI).

## Charles River

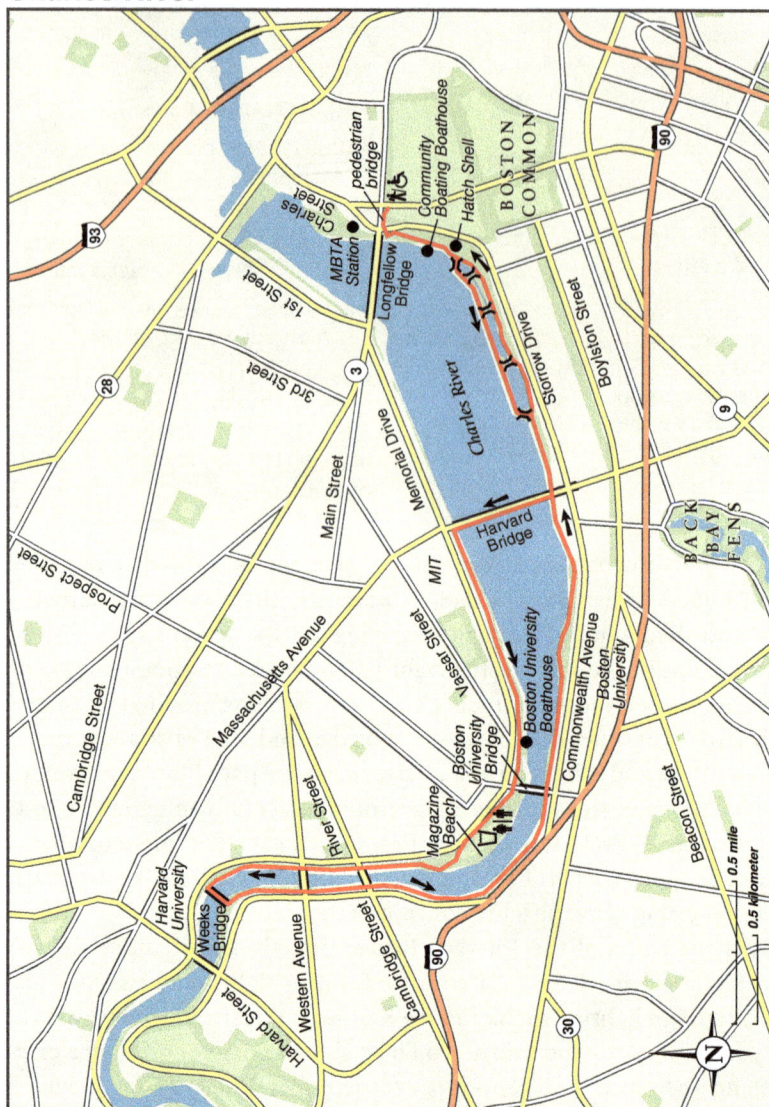

On the Charles's northern bank, bear left to hike west toward Harvard University, either on the paved bicycle route or on the winding footpath closer to the water. Across traffic whooshing by on Memorial Drive sits the MIT campus. This mile-long stretch to the Boston University (BU) Bridge is quiet and focused, with few distractions besides the teams of rowers skimming up and down the river. After passing the BU boathouse on the left and the funky architecture of the Hyatt, stay close to the river to navigate the BU Bridge.

Once past the soccer field and fitness station, bear left on a paved drive to enter the park and reunite with the riverbank, following the path as it curves back to meet Memorial Drive. Bending north, the path crosses into Cambridgeport. Before the first bridge to Cambridge was built, this tract of land was a marshy tidal zone with Pelham's Island at its epicenter. Once made accessible, the marsh was drained and filled, and in 1805 the port was officially opened.

Approaching Harvard, the path along the embankment crosses streets at two more bridges, River Street and Western Avenue. Piebald-trunked sycamore trees planted in 1900 by landscape architect Charles Eliot lend grace and shade to Memorial Drive from here on up the river.

In 1974, a Cambridge woman named Isabella Halsted struck upon the idea of a riverfront park that would see Memorial Drive closed to cars. Halsted garnered popular support then sealed victory by attending a charity auction and placing the winning bid for a lunch date with Senator Edward Kennedy. To this day, the road is closed on Sundays April–November.

Shortly after Western Avenue, where the river winds west opposite Harvard's handsome redbrick campus, the path leads to the lovely John W. Weeks footbridge. Built in 1926 for the benefit of students at Harvard Business School, it is the only footbridge across the Charles. Having reached the hike's halfway point, bear left to make the river crossing.

On arriving at the Charles's south side, on the edge of a Boston neighborhood named for the 19th-century painter Washington Allston, turn left to loop back east. For approximately 1.2 miles, the path is quite narrow and exposed to the rush of traffic on Storrow Drive, but in a dramatic return to peace, the path swings away from the riverbank at the BU Bridge. A boardwalk runs under a railroad trestle, taking the path through the realm of nursery-tale ogres before reemerging at the BU boathouse.

Stay left when the path splits to hike beside the river. Over the past few decades, efforts by the Charles River Watershed Association and other groups have restored the health of the Charles to such an extent that the 20-member Charles River Swimming Club held its first 1-mile race on the Charles on July 21, 2007.

On arriving back at the Harvard Bridge, continue east and bear left at the first footbridge to retrace your steps to the chain of lagoons. Then, to vary the return route, turn off at the next footbridge to switch to the south side of the Esplanade, and make your way to the inner lagoon adorned with an exuberant fountain. On a summer evening with the moon rising in the warm light of the setting sun, there is no place more transcendently beautiful. Beyond this poetic pool is another lagoon of equal charm and intrigue. The Hatch Shell lies directly ahead, and farther south, the docks and boathouse of Community Boating Boston. Follow the path past these familiar sites, meandering on whim to reach the pedestrian bridge that leads back to Charles Street.

## NEARBY ATTRACTIONS

Besides the countless things to do and places to see in Boston, Cambridge, and Charlestown, the Charles River itself offers several notable attractions, especially for those itching to get out on the water. Arrange canoe and kayak rentals with Charles River Canoe and Kayak (open Thursday–Sunday; 617-965-5110), riverboat sightseeing tours with the Charles Riverboat Company (100 Cambridgeside Place, Ste. 320, Cambridge; 617-621-3001), and romantic gondola cruises courtesy of Gondola di Venezia (Tuesday–Friday, 7–11 a.m., and Wednesday–Sunday, 2 p.m.–midnight; 800-979-3370; bostongondolas.com).

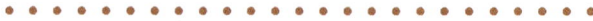

• • • • • • • • • • • • • • • • • • • • • • • • •

**GPS TRAILHEAD COORDINATES**  N42° 21.650'  W71° 04.250'

**DIRECTIONS**  The Charles River is best reached by foot, bicycle, or public transportation. To ride the T, take the Red line to the Charles Street station. Exit the station, cross onto Charles Street via the crosswalk, then cross over the pedestrian bridge to the banks of the Charles River.

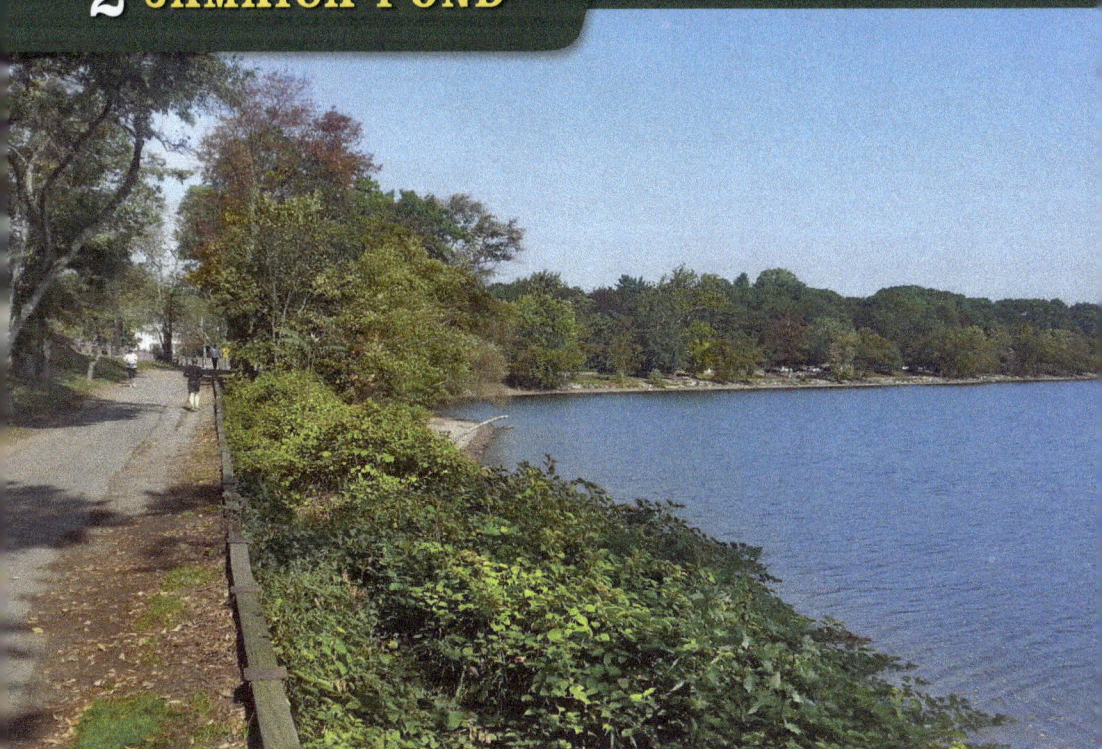

Jamaica Pond is more of a walk than a hike, but a very pleasant walk nonetheless.

**THIS WONDERFUL WALK** for all ages and abilities is located in a historic neighborhood right in the heart of Boston.

## DESCRIPTION

The question of how Jamaica Pond and the surrounding Jamaica Plain neighborhood got its name may never be resolved. Some say it's an anglicized pronunciation of Kuchamakin, a chief of the Massachusett tribe. Others say it comes from the involvement of some of its founding citizens in the rum trade with Jamaica. It has also been suggested it was so named in 1677 to commemorate Oliver Cromwell's success at wresting control of Jamaica from Spain. Others state the shape of the pond simply resembles the outline of the island of Jamaica.

The largest freshwater pond in Boston at 68 acres, Jamaica Pond was Boston's primary source of drinking water until the mid-1880s. The Jamaica Plain Aqueduct Company, incorporated in 1795, laid 45 miles of pipes to convey the water. The frozen pond provided households the ice needed to keep food from spoiling. The Jamaica Pond Ice Company supplied Boston nearly all its ice for more than half a century.

Landscape architect Frederick Law Olmsted was largely responsible for turning Jamaica Pond into a public park. With the construction of Franklin Park, the Arnold

**DISTANCE & CONFIGURATION:** 1.45-mile loop

**DIFFICULTY:** Easy

**SCENERY:** Views from the banks of a kettle pond, spectacular trees, 1912 boathouse designed by Dorchester architect William Downer Austin

**EXPOSURE:** Mixed sun and shade

**TRAFFIC:** Can vary greatly from light to heavy, depending on time of day and weather

**TRAIL SURFACE:** Choice of clay or pavement

**HIKING TIME:** 30–45 minutes

**DRIVING DISTANCE FROM BOSTON COMMON:** 4.5 miles

**ELEVATION:** 59' at trailhead, no significant gain

**SEASON:** Year-round

**ACCESS:** Open sunrise–sunset; free

**MAPS:** Not needed, as it's one large loop around the pond

**WHEELCHAIR ACCESS:** Yes

**FACILITIES:** Restrooms, drinking fountain, community boathouse offering rowboat and sailboat rentals and youth programs

**CONTACT:** Boston Parks and Recreation, boston.gov/parks/jamaica-pond, 617-635-4505

**LOCATION:** 507 Jamaicaway, Jamaica Plain, Boston, MA

**COMMENTS:** Festivals and events are held at the pond throughout the year. Concerts are held at the pavilion next to the boathouse all summer long.

Arboretum, and the Muddy River Improvement Project in progress, Olmsted's concept of a "green ribbon" around Boston was well under way. This greenbelt around the city is now called the Emerald Necklace.

Jamaica Pond looks much as it has since the retreat of the Wisconsin Glacier. Olmsted's aim was to have the landscape look as natural and poetic as possible. As stated in his own words, he saw the pond as "a natural sheet of water, with quiet, graceful shores, rear banks of varied elevation and contour, for the most part shaded by a fine natural forest-growth to be brought out over-hanging, darkening the water's edge and favoring great beauty in reflections and flickering half-lights."

Where you start your hike around Jamaica Pond is often dictated by parking opportunities. Most begin on its northwestern side, near parking along Perkins Street. Where a crosswalk meets the path, bear right and walk counterclockwise, passing a sandy beach dotted with fishermen. Rounding a turn, the path runs beside a stone wall bordering Francis Parkman Drive to the right and the shore of the pond.

A hundred yards or so farther, Shea's Island obstructs the view across the water. Neither entirely natural nor entirely man-made, this island is said to have begun as a bump formed from the edges of two conjoined kettle holes that make up Jamaica Pond. Local lore has it the island was first improved by Indians, who built it up with stones to create a fish trap. Today flocks of Canada geese, mallard ducks, and American coot congregate around the hummock.

Halfway along the bank and partway up a gentle slope, the path passes an enormous tree. This and the tremendous beeches growing to the right of the path ahead are likely among the few trees remaining from Olmsted's time. Beyond the beeches, the path approaches the junction of Prince Street and Parkman Drive, the original site of historian Francis Parkman's house.

## Jamaica Pond

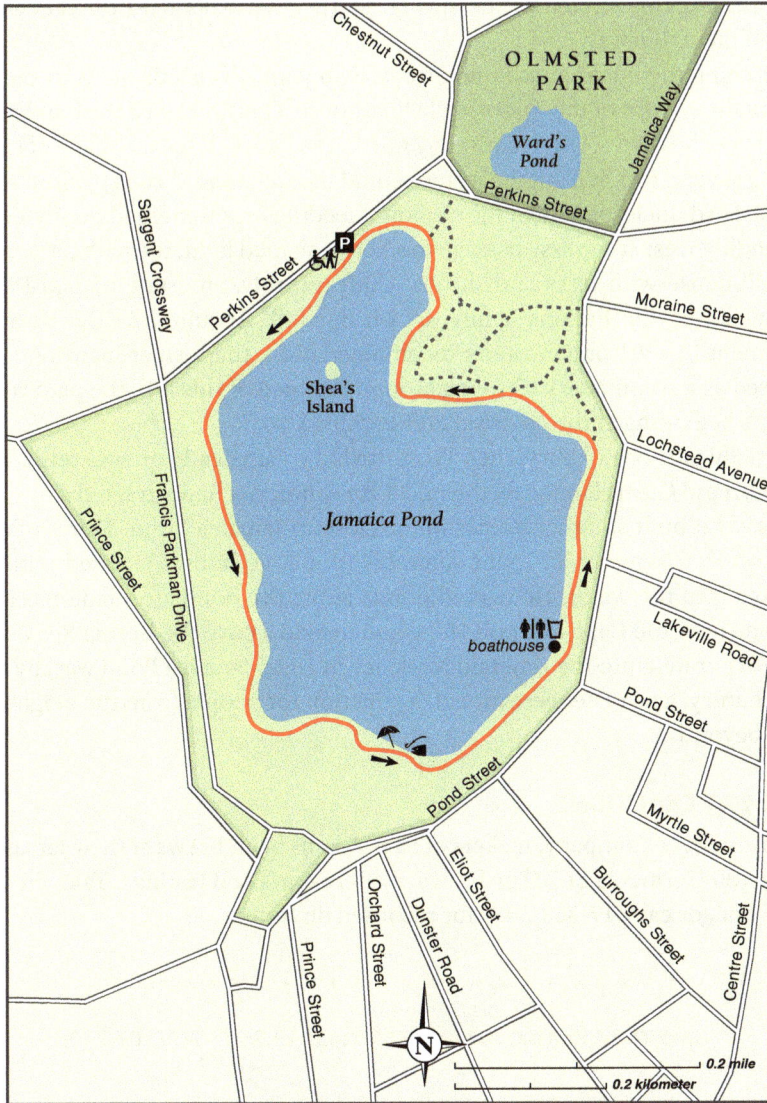

**OLMSTED PARK**

Ward's Pond

Chestnut Street

Jamaica Way

Perkins Street

Sargent Crossway

Moraine Street

Perkins Street

P

Shea's Island

Lochstead Avenue

Francis Parkman Drive

*Jamaica Pond*

Prince Street

boathouse

Lakeville Road

Pond Street

Prince Street

Orchard Street

Dunster Road

Eliot Street

Burroughs Street

Myrtle Street

Centre Street

Pond Street

N

0.2 mile

0.2 kilometer

Rounding the pond's southern bank, recessed between the water and the land that defines the banks of the shore, the path climbs past the spot where the Jamaica Pond Ice Company icehouse once stood. Head away from the path here to walk along the water. This wide beach is a favorite for fishermen practicing fly-casting. Looking north on a summer's day, you will likely see sailboats tacking lazily across the water.

From the beach, climb the granite stairs back to the path, and turn left to walk toward the boathouse. Stout fruit trees, planted to replace Olmsted's originals, blossom along this stretch in the spring. Mighty red oaks fend off cars along the length of the Arborway.

Reaching the junction at Pond Street, help yourself to a drink from the spring-fed fountain in front of the Tudor-style boathouse. Continue past the bandstand and a row of benches to the left. Continuing north, the path echoes the shape of the pond, traveling several feet in from the water behind the trees and shrubs planted along the bank. Mallard ducks paddle in the shallows, feeding on submerged pondweed.

Bending west at a grassy passage to a kettle-shaped field, the path passes a short, steep hill dense with trees and shrubs. Until recently, an estate named Pinebank, once owned by the Perkins family, sat on this hill. Acquired by the Boston Park Department in 1891 on Olmsted's recommendation, the former mansion has since been used as a commissary. Curving around the base of this hill, the path returns to the hike's beginning at the crosswalk off Perkins Street.

Initially part of Roxbury, then West Roxbury, Jamaica Plain was settled in 1640 by the intrepid Curtis family. By the mid-19th century, it had attracted many wealthy families, who built summer homes on or close to Jamaica Pond. Francis Parkman, author of *The Oregon Trail,* spent summers in a large house outfitted with a dock extending into the water. He named points along the pond after famous capes. He called one jetty the Cape of Good Hope and named a cove the Bering Sea.

Incorporated into the Emerald Necklace in 1892, Jamaica Pond was, by the turn of the century, a favorite recreational destination for people from the neighborhood and far beyond.

## NEARBY ATTRACTIONS

The Boston Beer Company, makers of Sam Adams beer, brews at their Jamaica Plain location (30 Germania St.). The brewery offers tours and tastings. Take the MBTA's Orange line, or call 617-368-5080 for recorded directions.

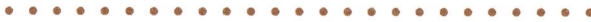

• • • • • • • • • • • • • • • • • • • • • • • • •

**GPS TRAILHEAD COORDINATES** N42° 19.250'  W71° 07.270'

**DIRECTIONS** Jamaica Pond is located on the Arborway across from Pond Street in the Jamaica Plain neighborhood of Boston. Parking and trailhead are on Perkins Street.

# 3 SPECTACLE ISLAND: Boston Harbor Islands National & State Park

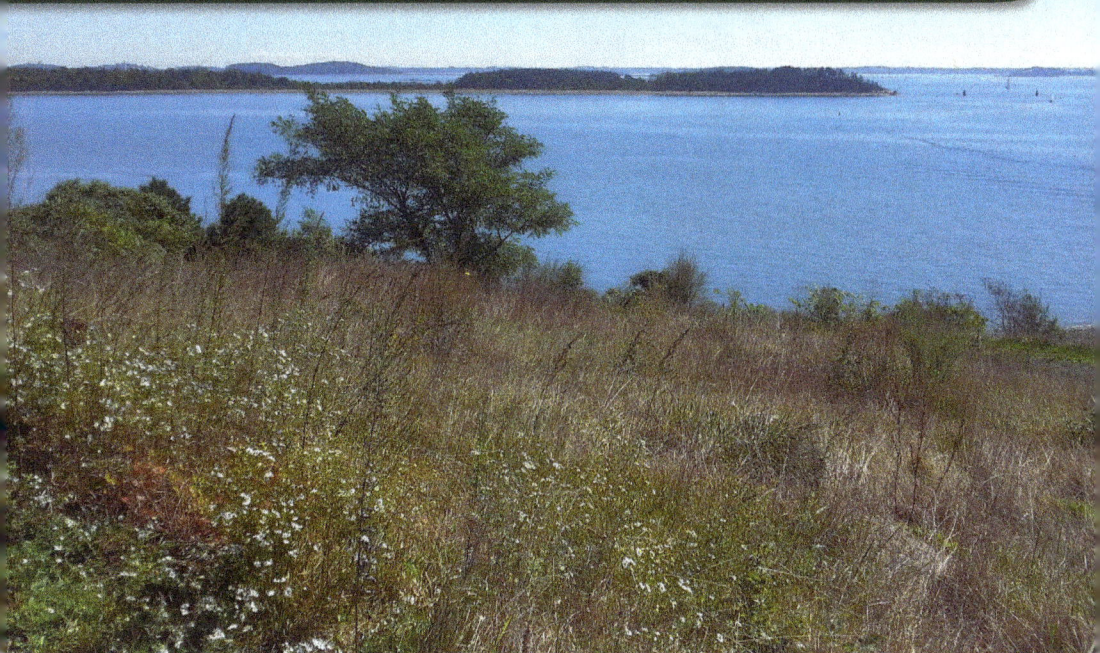

You can easily get lost in the dramatic views from Spectacle Island.

**ONCE A LANDFILL** for the city of Boston, the beautiful, windswept Spectacle Island is now a true gem. The trail circumnavigating it offers dramatic views of Boston Harbor and the Boston skyline.

## DESCRIPTION

The Boston Harbor Islands are a spectacular resource, almost hiding in plain sight. Most of the islands are clearly visible from Boston, and the ferries and the islands themselves are often bustling with people eager to escape the city heat for ocean breezes, but it seems surprising the islands aren't even more popular. Spectacle Island is one of several open to the public free of charge (save for the ferry ticket). The others are Peddocks, Lovells, Grape, Bumpkin, and Georges, which is home to the historic Fort Warren. You can also camp in a yurt on Peddocks Island or go tent camping with a permit on Grape, Bumpkin, and Lovells.

Getting to Spectacle Island couldn't be easier, but you can't drive or hike there. Catch a ferry at Marriott Long Wharf. The ferry ticket office and dock are on the left side of the hotel when looking out to the harbor. Be sure to check the schedule, as there is a summer schedule and a spring/fall schedule. There are far fewer ferries

**DISTANCE & CONFIGURATION:** 2.5-mile loop

**DIFFICULTY:** Easy

**SCENERY:** Views of the other Boston Harbor islands and Boston skyline

**EXPOSURE:** Full sun

**TRAFFIC:** Light–heavy, depending on time of year and weather

**TRAIL SURFACE:** Firmly packed gravel

**HIKING TIME:** 45-minute outer loop

**DRIVING DISTANCE FROM BOSTON COMMON:** 4.5 miles, although you can't drive

**ELEVATION:** 157' at trailhead, no significant gain

**SEASON:** Late June–Labor Day

**ACCESS:** Open 9 a.m.–sunset. Park access is free, but getting there requires a ferry trip. Check bostonharborislands.org/ferry-schedule for current schedule and ticket prices.

**MAPS:** Available at visitor center

**WHEELCHAIR ACCESS:** Yes

**FACILITIES:** Restrooms, drinking fountain, snack bar

**CONTACT:** Boston Harbor Islands, bostonharbor islands.org/spectacle-island, 617-223-8666

**LOCATION:** Boston Harbor, Boston, MA

during the spring and fall, so plan accordingly. (If you do try to drive, please be sure to roll up your windows!)

After the 25-minute or so ferry ride, you'll pull up to the massive dock on the west side of the island. After you step off the boat and walk down the dock, look for the interpretive trail that circumnavigates the island. The trail heads north directly from the ferry dock and visitor center. As you set off, you'll pass an outdoor shower for those hardy souls who decided to take a dip in Boston Harbor.

The trail leading away from the beach is a wide, carriage road–like path. The surface is firmly packed dirt, sand, and gravel. While there are two small drumlins (they are in fact called North Drumlin and South Drumlin) toward the center of the island, the trail around the outer perimeter is relatively flat. It is also extremely well defined and virtually impossible to miss or get off-trail. The trail initially follows a beach fence along some dense beach growth. There's a gentle rise here as the trail nears the north end of the island and follows around North Drumlin. As you come around the northeast corner of the island, there is a fascinating sculpture commemorating the island signal lights.

North and South Drumlin provide panoramic views of Boston Harbor and the skyline. Both are well worth a visit while hiking around Spectacle Island. There are trails leading up to the center of the island and the tops of the drumlins, but stay on the outer interpretive trail for now. After curving around the north end of the island and passing the signal lights sculpture, you'll have a straight shot down the eastern, seaward side of the island.

As you come around the southern end of the island, you can see the southern flank of Long Island to the east, Moon Island to the south, and Thompson Island to the west. The walk around the island has a similar feel—and certainly similar scenery—to World's End (which is also part of Boston Harbor Island National Park—see Hike 9, page 60). As you round the southwestern tip of the island, you're faced with a dramatic

## Spectacle Island: Boston Harbor Islands National & State Park

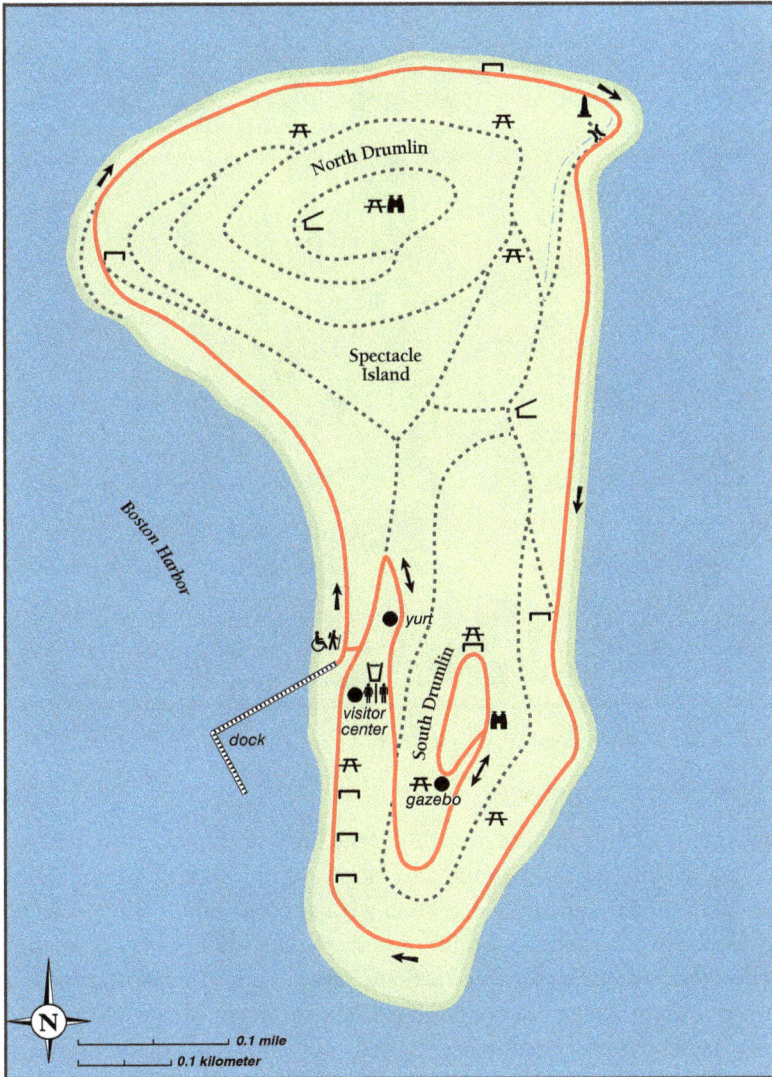

view of the Boston skyline. Then it's a short, straight shot back to the visitor center. The loop around the island is about 45 minutes, not accounting for any time spent on a bench or two admiring the view and the action in Boston Harbor.

From here, if you have the time before the next ferry, it's well worth the short hike up to the top of South Drumlin. North Drumlin is also fantastic, but you're more likely to find a moment of solitude on South Drumlin. The trail extends from the visitor center then takes a hairpin turn south (right). After passing the yurt that

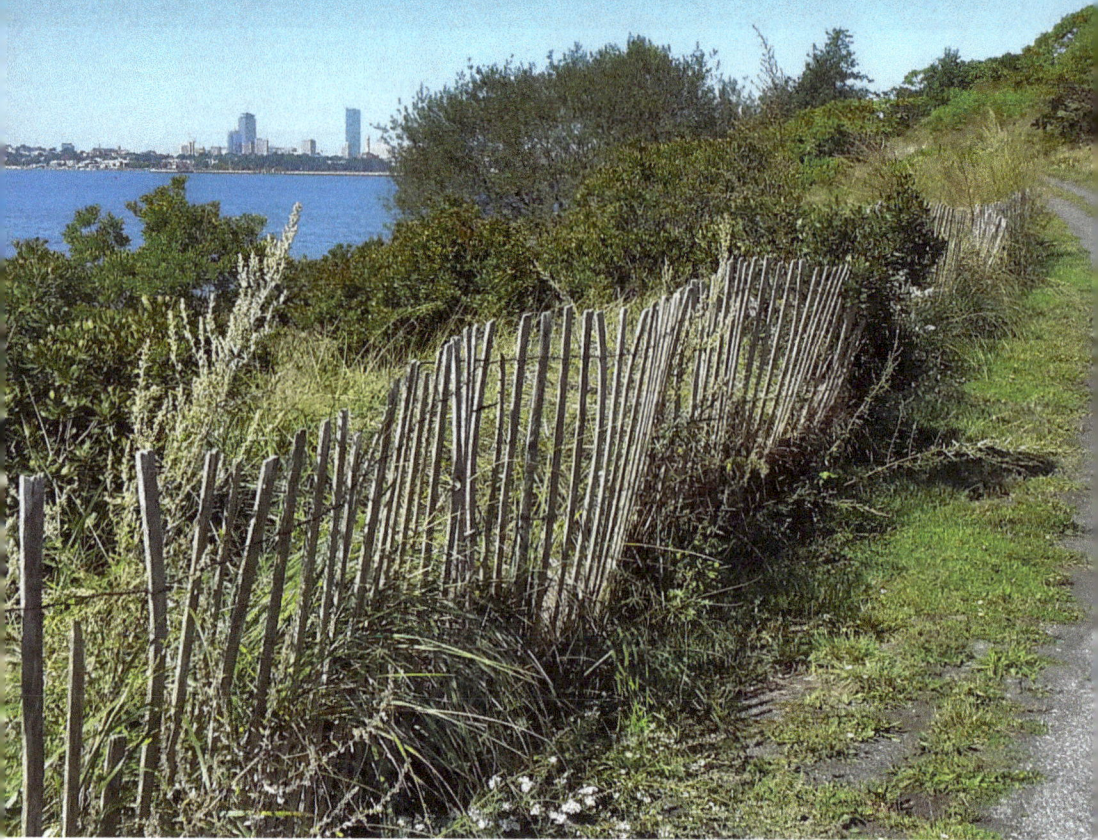

Glimpses of the Boston skyline mix with views of the rustic beach grasses.

is home to some of the park rangers during the busy summer season, the trail climbs gently along the side of the drumlin and loops around. Near the top of the drumlin are a bench, a picnic table, and a gazebo with another table—all spectacular spots to enjoy the view. It's a short, 15-minute jaunt to the gazebo from the visitor center.

Boston Harbor Islands National & State Park is a popular spot, so you will almost certainly have company on the trails—especially on warm, clear summer days. There are several benches perched along the path to stop and watch the boat traffic moving through Boston Harbor and the air traffic coming in and out of Logan. The sounds of island life, the waves washing against the rocky shore, and the sound of birds and insects mix with the sounds of the marine and air traffic.

Stay on the defined trails to preserve the fragile, windswept island vegetation. It's no challenge staying on the trail, as it is quite well defined and maintained. The only problem as you walk along may be tripping and losing your footing as you get distracted by the spectacular views. It's curious to note Spectacle Island was once a landfill for the city of Boston. After dumping stopped, the continued natural forces of the tides filled in the spaces between the northern and southern parts of the island

and actually expanded the island's footprint. Today, Spectacle Island is truly a spectacle among the archipelago of the Boston Harbor Islands.

## NEARBY ATTRACTIONS

When you return to land, if you're hungry or thirsty, you're in the right place. It's downtown Boston, so your options are virtually limitless. There's a Legal Sea Foods (617-742-5300, legalseafoods.com) right near the Marriott. Walk a bit farther down Atlantic Avenue to Trade (617-451-1234, trade-boston.com), which offers all sorts of food and drink. Head in closer to town and you can find just about any variety of cuisine that suits your mood. Exploring a bit and finding something unexpected is at least half the fun.

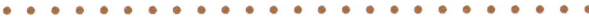

• • • • • • • • • • • • • • • • • • • • • • • • • •

**GPS TRAILHEAD COORDINATES** N42° 19.250' W71° 07.270'

**DIRECTIONS** Take the ferry from the ferry dock located next to the Marriott Long Wharf. The ferry dock is on the north side of the hotel, to the left as you look out to the harbor.

Spectacle Island is not far from Boston, but you'll feel as if you're a million miles away.

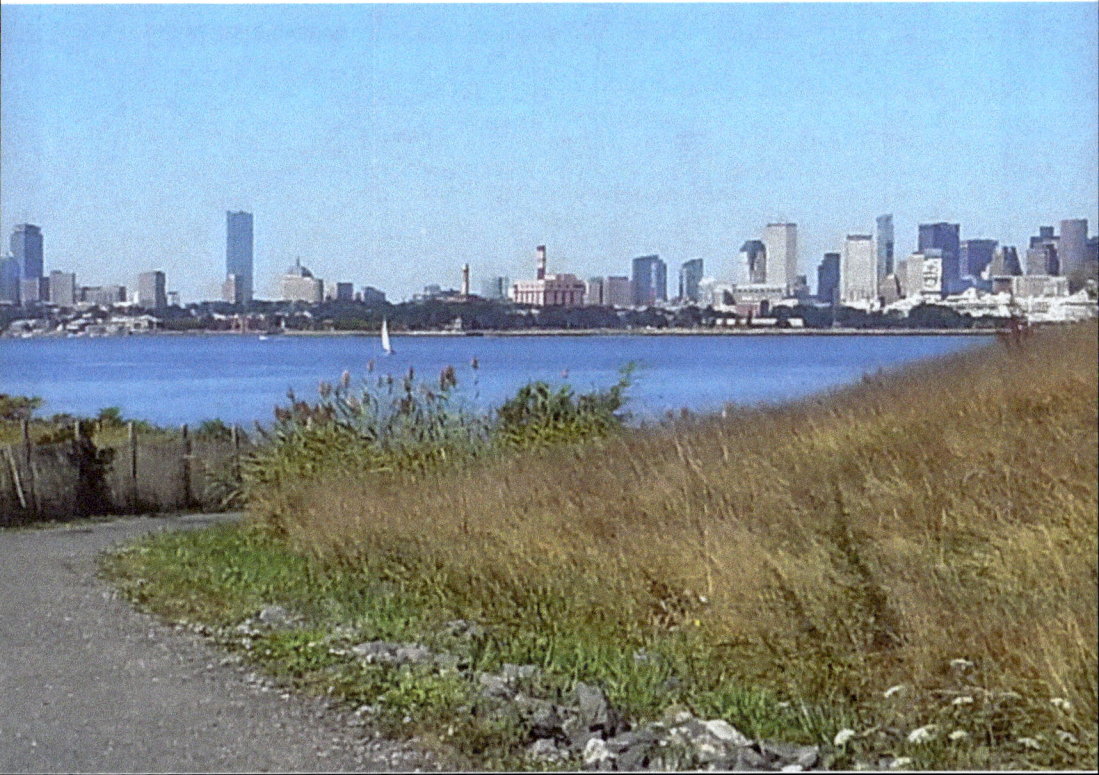

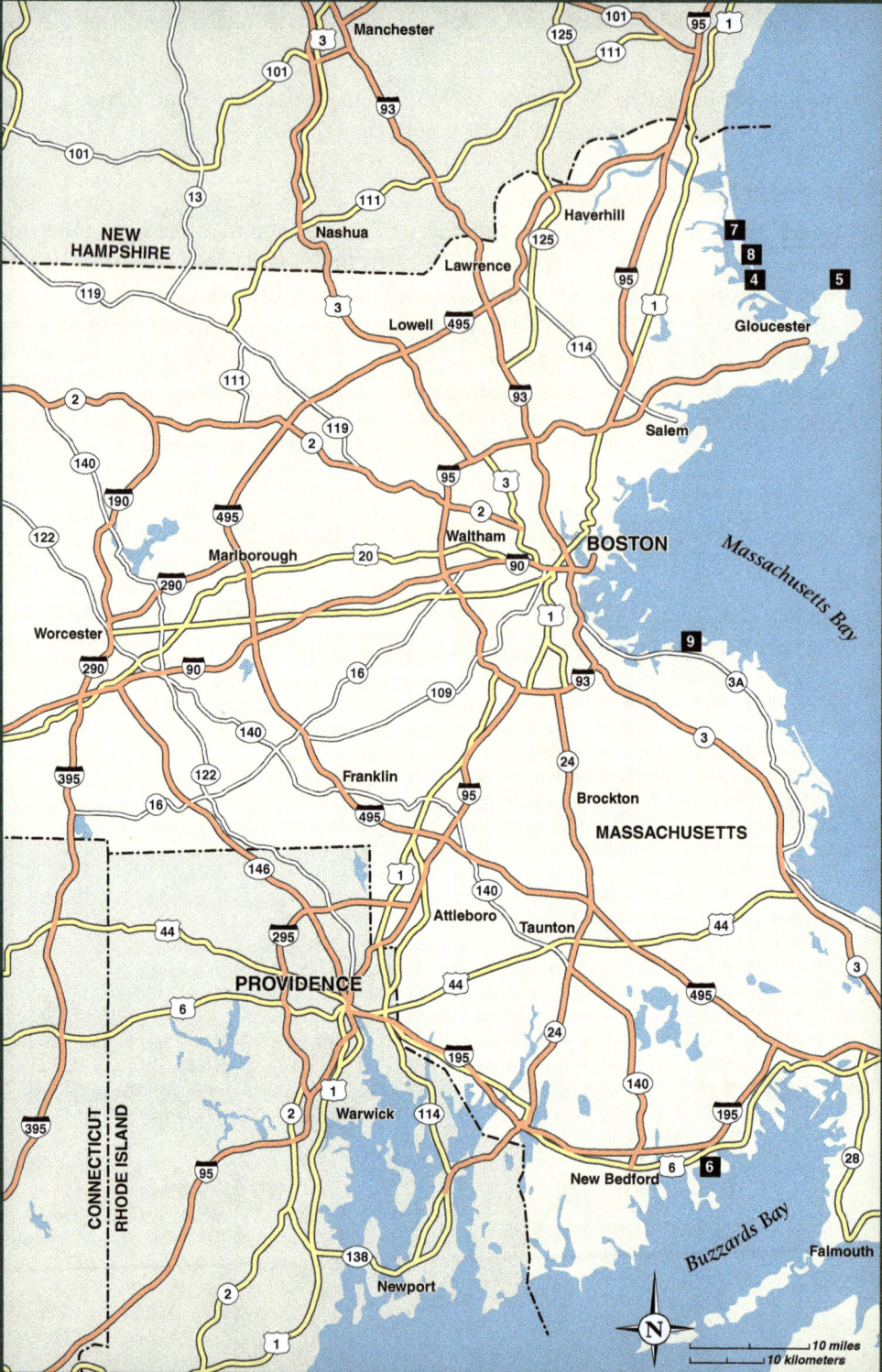

# SEASIDE HIKES

# 4 CRANE BEACH

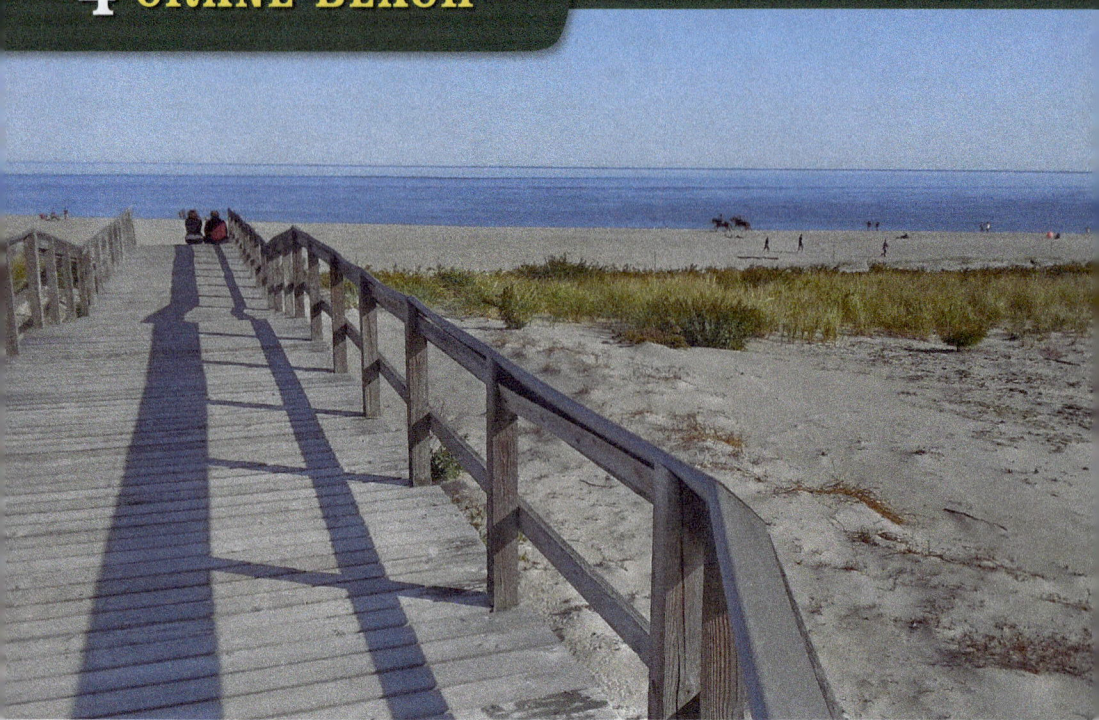

Plan to spend the whole day at Crane Beach, and even then you won't want to leave.

**ON THIS HIKE** you will follow the shoreline of one of Massachusetts's most immaculate beaches. Approaching the marshes of Essex and the coast of Gloucester, you'll cross into the high dunes of the inner beach and hike back along where the waves meet the beach.

## DESCRIPTION

One of the few hikes in this book that you could do barefoot, this trip along the shores and through the dune sea of Crane Beach is quite an experience. From the parking lot to the right of the entrance, take the southernmost boardwalk to the beach. If it is a warm, clear day, you will want to free your feet from your shoes, sink your toes in the sand, and feast your eyes on the cobalt-blue sea.

When the air is dry and free of haze and fog, you can sometimes see the Isles of Shoals off the coast of Portsmouth, New Hampshire, as dark slivers on the horizon. On most days, you'll also see Newburyport's Plum Island stretching close to Ipswich's densely populated Great Neck; Little Neck on the left across from the mouth of Fox Creek; and the grand estate at Castle Hill. On a beach as pristine as Crane, just wandering about as your spirit wills makes more sense than following a prescribed route. This hike therefore invites—even encourages—improvisation as it leads from the water-lapped tide line to the deep sands of Crane's highest inner dunes and back.

**DISTANCE & CONFIGURATION:** 6-mile balloon

**DIFFICULTY:** Moderate

**SCENERY:** Miles of pristine beach; dunes; views of Plum Island, Cape Ann, and acres of salt marsh

**EXPOSURE:** Full sun

**TRAFFIC:** Light–moderate

**TRAIL SURFACE:** Beach sand

**HIKING TIME:** 3 hours

**DRIVING DISTANCE FROM BOSTON COMMON:** 31 miles

**ELEVATION:** 7' at trailhead, no significant gain

**SEASON:** Year-round

**ACCESS:** Open 8 a.m.–sunset. You can purchase an annual parking permit for $75, or the following day parking fees apply: Memorial Day–Labor Day: $15/weekday, $20/weekend day for Trustees members; $25/weekday, $30/weekend day for nonmembers. Labor Day–Columbus Day: $5/weekday, $15/weekend day for Trustees members; $10/weekday, $20/weekend day for nonmembers. Off-season (Columbus Day–Memorial Day): $5/day for Trustees members, $10/day for nonmembers.

**MAPS:** Posted at spots on trails and entry on boardwalks

**WHEELCHAIR ACCESS:** No

**FACILITIES:** Restrooms and snack bar open Memorial Day–Labor Day; only outhouses open in off-season

**CONTACT:** The Trustees of Reservations, thetrustees.org/places-to-visit, 617-542-7696

**LOCATION:** 310 Argilla Road, Ipswich, MA

**COMMENTS:** Leashed dogs permitted October 1–March 31 but restricted to below high-tide line

To start your exploration, turn right and lay down some footprints in the sand as you head southeast. Though New England's beach season is understood to run from the first day of summer through Labor Day, a good many New Englanders know the beach is at its most sublime in autumn. It even has a dramatic appeal during the winter months. Though the water at Crane Beach is often warmer than at nearby Plum Island, it can still be numbingly cold all year. It's most tolerable (least painful?) in August, particularly at low tide, after sizzling sands have passed the sun's energy on to the retreating sea.

If the tide is high or coming in fast, follow a course closer to the dunes across the loose, finely ground, whitish granite sand sparkling with mica. In places, veins of feldspar color the sand a hard, heat-absorbing purple. Keep an eye out for piping plovers as you head down the beach. Crane's is one of three locations in North America where these birds—classified as threatened by the U.S. Fish & Wildlife service—are known to rear young. They lay their eggs directly on the sand, so they need undisturbed stretches of beach. For this reason, The Trustees of Reservations ask beach visitors to help them protect their resident plovers by staying out of sensitive nesting areas.

Like any beach or natural coastal area, the contours of Crane Beach are constantly changing. Hurricane forces and even gentle afternoon breezes act to reshape the beach. Generations ago, the dunes cast deep shadows all along the peninsula. Today the sands are much flatter, spreading east in a long peninsula. Crosscurrents furrow the flats in a wet, sandy corduroy, concealing razor clams and sea clams.

Following a trajectory of your own choosing, look to the dunes gaining in magnitude to the right, and you will find a passage to the inner beach. Until this point, wire

## Crane Beach

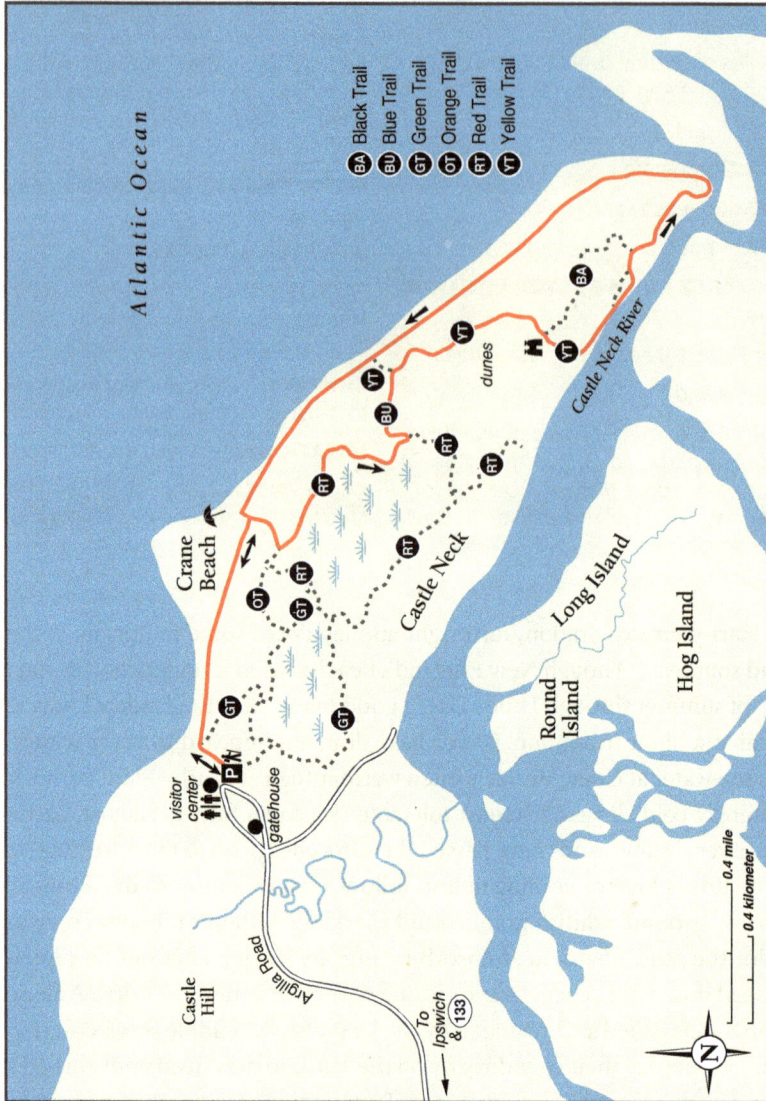

Crane Beach

Black Trail  **BA**
Blue Trail  **BU**
Green Trail  **GT**
Orange Trail  **OT**
Red Trail  **RT**
Yellow Trail  **YT**

Atlantic Ocean

Castle Neck River

dunes

Crane Beach

Castle Neck

Long Island

Hog Island

Round Island

visitor center

gatehouse

Argilla Road

Castle Hill

To Ipswich & (133)

0.4 mile
0.4 kilometer

fencing restricts foot traffic to the seaweed-laced high-water mark and sands lying to the east. Turn here and follow this wide, wire-bordered avenue west into the muffled sands beyond. Knife-sharp blades of beach grass fall in wind-tousled waves over the banks alongside. Without this grass and its binding roots, there would be no dunes.

The grade of the soft, sandy trails steepens to crest a dune down the path several hundred feet. Striding down the other side in the loose sand, you'll come to a level junction. Bear left to take the yellow trail south. The air in the still valleys is warmer and softer than the biting salt air blowing off the sea. In this unique microclimate, intriguing plants, such as hardy mushrooms and bayberry bushes, take root.

After winding along the rim of a bog on the right, the trail takes a serpentine tack southeast, funneling through dune clefts before climbing to a sandy pinnacle overlooking the beach's southernmost tip. From here you can see Gloucester's Wingaersheek Beach on the opposite shore, the channel flowing past Conomo Point to Essex Harbor, and the lands surrounding the Crane family's Great House to the northwest.

Continue following numbered yellow trail markers as they lead across Castle Neck and deliver you to a spot directly across from Choate Island, or Hog Island, as it is informally known. This beautiful island with a humble name has the distinction of being the birthplace of Senator Rufus Choate, the burial place of Cornelius Crane, and the setting for much of Nicholas Hytner's film *The Crucible.* This stretch of beach on a secluded cove receives more visitors by boat than by foot. Occasionally, harbor seals swim ashore here to enjoy some sun or respite from life at sea.

Leave the yellow trail, and make your own track southeast along the neck's thin fringe of beach. As you round the peninsula's tip, the wind will catch you at a different angle. Heading west, you'll see the beach broaden again. Across from Gloucester's Halibut Point, mixed flocks of gulls congregate where a foamy seam marks a crosscurrent. As your course bends northwest, Plum Island comes into view, followed by the cottages and the water tower on Great Neck, and finally Crane's Castle nestled regally on its hill. When fading light or foul weather sends you back to your car, cut back into the loose sand of the seaweed-strewn upland to find the first of the two boardwalks.

In 1908, amid a rumor that the brother of President Taft had bought "Castle Hill Farm," Crane Plumbing heir Richard T. Crane purchased the 250 acres made up of bald drumlins and picturesque meadows flush to salt marsh for $125,000. Years later in 1945, 14 years after her husband's death on his 58th birthday, Florence Crane gave 1,000 acres, including most of Crane Beach and Castle Neck, to The Trustees of Reservations. When she died only four years later, she bequeathed also the Great House and an additional 300 surrounding acres.

## NEARBY ATTRACTIONS

Any trip to Crane Beach should include a stop at Russell Orchards (143 Argilla Road, 978-356-5366, russellorchards.com). From April 28 through November 25, this family-run business sells fresh fruits, vegetables, baked goods (including scrumptious cider donuts and delectable pies), hot and cold beverages, and fine fruit wines made on-site. Those looking for a hearty meal of local seafood might like to try one of the many restaurants located on MA 133 between Ipswich and Essex. To reach MA 133 from Crane Beach, drive approximately 0.5 mile on Argilla Road, bear left onto Northgate Road, and continue to the end. At the intersection of Northgate Road and MA 133, turn left and continue 3 miles to Main Street in Essex.

• • • • • • • • • • • • • • • • • • • • • • • • • •

**GPS TRAILHEAD COORDINATES** N42° 41.050'  W70° 45.950'

**DIRECTIONS** From MA 128 N (also called Yankee Division Highway), toward Gloucester, take Exit 20A and follow US 1A N 8 miles to Ipswich. Turn right onto MA 133 east and follow it 1.5 miles. Turn left onto Northgate Road and follow it 0.5 mile. Turn right onto Argilla Road and travel 2.5 miles to the Crane Beach gatehouse at the end of the paved road.

Deep in the dune sea at Crane Beach

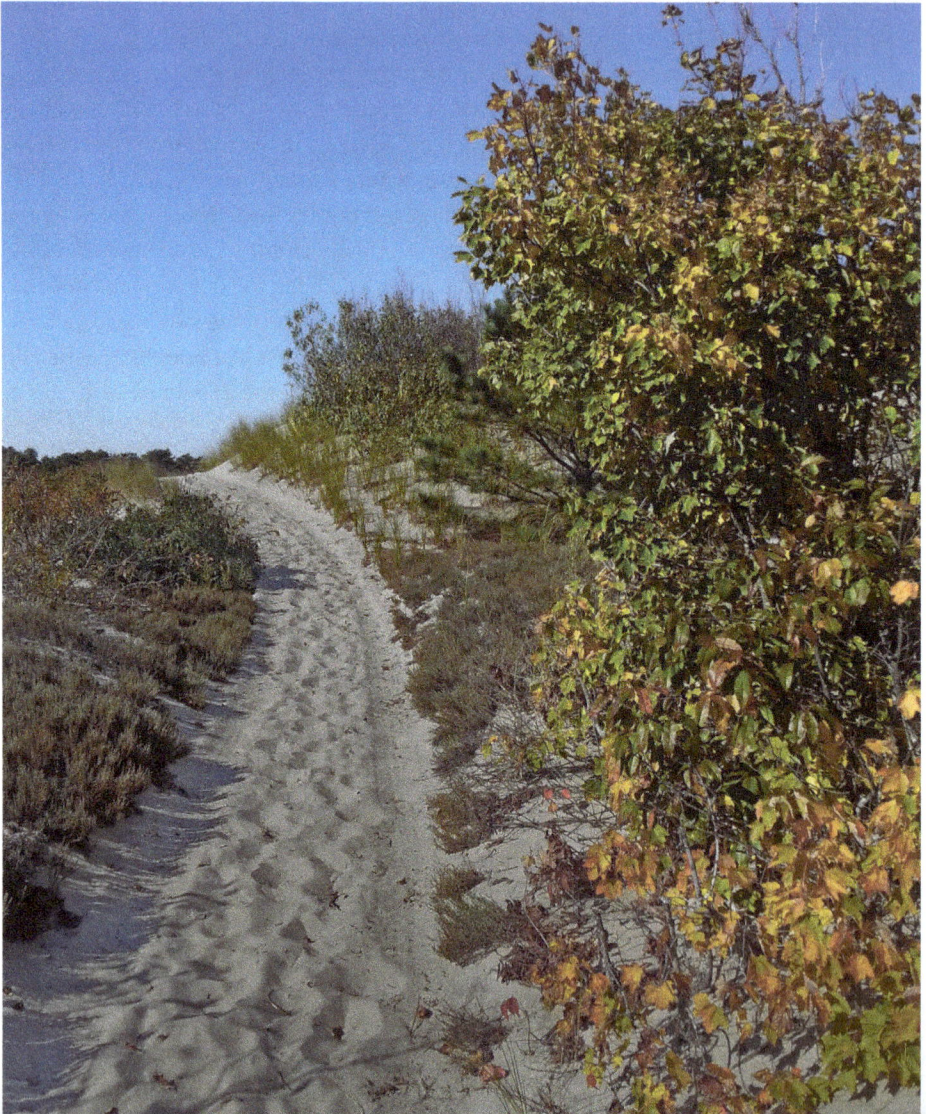

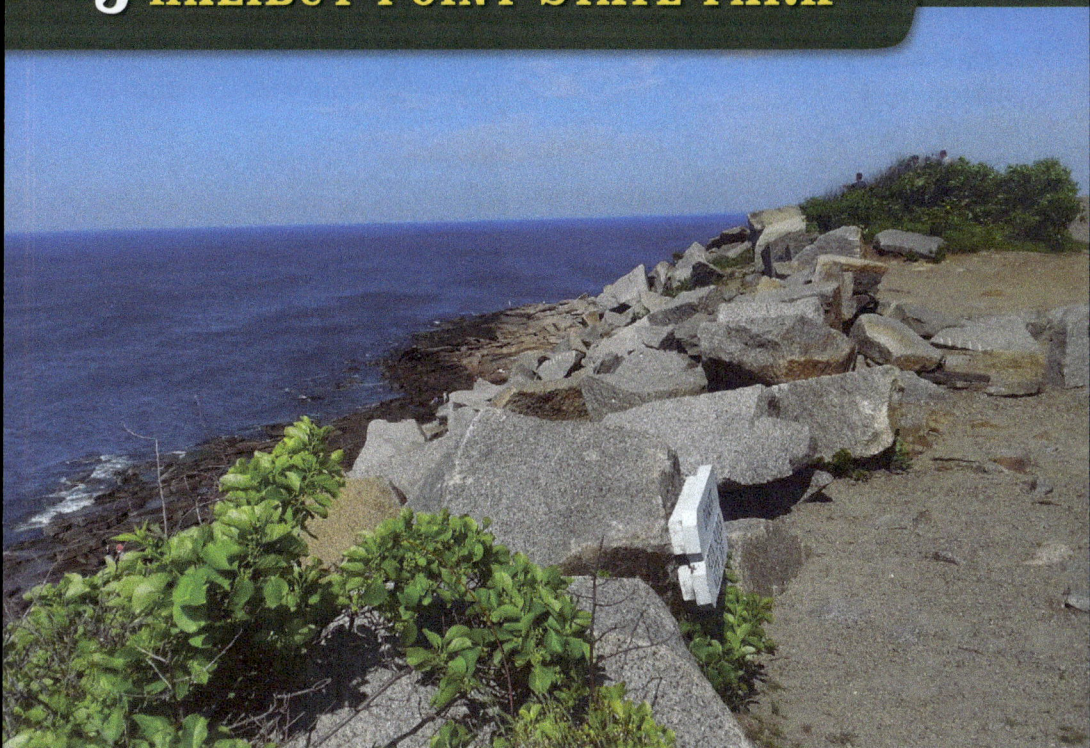

# 5 HALIBUT POINT STATE PARK

The Atlantic comes crashing in against the rocks at Halibut Point State Park.

**SHAPED BY GEOLOGICAL FORCES,** glacial ice sheets, the labor of quarrymen, and crashing waves off the Atlantic, Halibut Point presents a variety of scenery. On warm summer days, this knuckle of granite facing the sea offers a pleasant place to sunbathe and picnic. When the weather turns, the point is a terrific place to observe the raw power of the Atlantic Ocean crashing on the rocks.

## DESCRIPTION

For nearly a century, men equipped with hand tools, steam-powered tools, and dynamite cut stone from Babson Farm Quarry at Halibut Point. The crash of 1929 and the emergence of concrete finally closed the industry down. The chiseled borders of the quarry remain as a dramatic reminder of the area's history.

Cross Gott Avenue at the northwest corner of the parking lot to pick up the wooded path to the visitor center. Halfway along, you will pass two small quarries, with narrow trails leading to them to the right. These days they are filled with rainwater and camouflaged by vines and scrub, smaller companions to the massive quarry you're approaching.

Arriving at a broad T intersection—you will feel the onshore breeze and catch a view of the sea. Shifting your focus from the distant waves to the foreground, you'll

41

**DISTANCE & CONFIGURATION:** 2-mile loop

**DIFFICULTY:** Easy

**SCENERY:** Views of granite quarries and rocky coastline of Cape Ann

**EXPOSURE:** Mostly sunny with some shade

**TRAFFIC:** Moderate

**TRAIL SURFACE:** Packed dirt and gravel leading to coast, large granite slabs and boulders along tidal zone

**HIKING TIME:** 1.5 hours; may vary depending on weather conditions

**DRIVING DISTANCE FROM BOSTON COMMON:** 42 miles

**ELEVATION:** 24' at trailhead, no significant gain

**SEASON:** Year-round

**ACCESS:** Summer, 8 a.m.–9 p.m.; off-season, sunrise–sunset. Parking $5 MA resident, $10 nonresident

**MAPS:** Available at kiosk in parking lot

**WHEELCHAIR ACCESS:** Yes, on paths to visitor center and around main quarry.

**FACILITIES:** Restrooms and picnic tables

**CONTACT:** Massachusetts Dept. of Conservation and Resources, mass.gov/locations /halibut-point-state-park, 617-626-1250

**LOCATION:** Gott Avenue, Rockport, MA

**COMMENTS:** Halibut Point is an excellent spot for bird-watching and exploring the rocks down by the shoreline.

see the enormous water-filled quarry before you. Herring gulls and ducks now bob on thin ripples raised by wind gusting across this old work site where men cut great slabs of rock, producing this enormous void.

Take the trail to the left to find the visitor center, or continue walking along the edge of the quarry on the gravel path past sparse woods of cherry, sumac, and blackberries. Markers along the quarry coordinate with a self-guided tour. It's always advisable to grab a map when one is available, but the trails here are quite obvious, well defined, and well marked.

Heading northeast, pass the quarry to your left as you turn toward the ocean. After walking a short distance downhill, you will find a narrow, packed-earth path leading to the right. Leave the gravel trail and pick up this new path, traveling northeast. At the next fork, take the right-hand path to continue east. The trail winds gently along the quarry border. There's not much elevation gain or loss, as the plateau surrounding the quarry is fairly flat.

Closer to the shore now, you will see wild beach roses that, when blooming in the heat of summer, give off a heady scent. Keep right at each of the next splits to reach the easternmost end of the reservation. At the border, the trail turns toward the sea.

Down on the rocky shoreline, you'll see sheets of granite mixed with irregular boulders tossed into heaps by quarrymen and the thunderous surf. The coast here is a dramatic setting for picnicking, sunbathing, surf-casting, tidal-pool gazing, and rock-hopping. If your inclination is to do nothing at all, there is always plenty to watch, from day sailors cruising around the point to migrating birds. And watching the ocean meet the barrier of the rocky coast is spectacular in all weather and in all seasons.

After spending some time pondering the coast, make your way northwest, keeping the breaking waves to your right. No walk along here is ever the same, as

## Halibut Point State Park

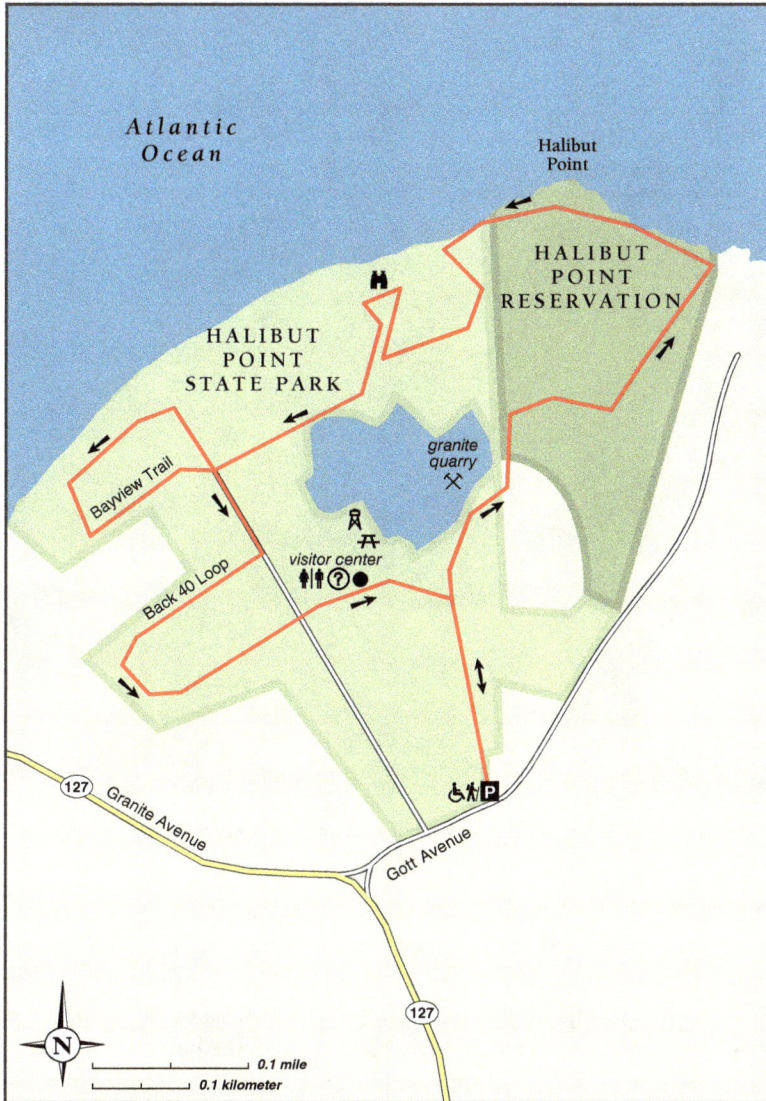

the tide level determines your route and your ability or inclination to leap across chasms. Beware of low tide, when kelp and sea moss clinging to rocks can make for treacherous footing.

Looking ahead, you will see a mountain of granite blocks tapering steeply to the sea. Walk along the base of this granite behemoth for a good look to appreciate the hours of sweat and strain represented by this pile of castoffs. Though forces of nature have reshaped the pile, it was quarrymen who heaved the stone here.

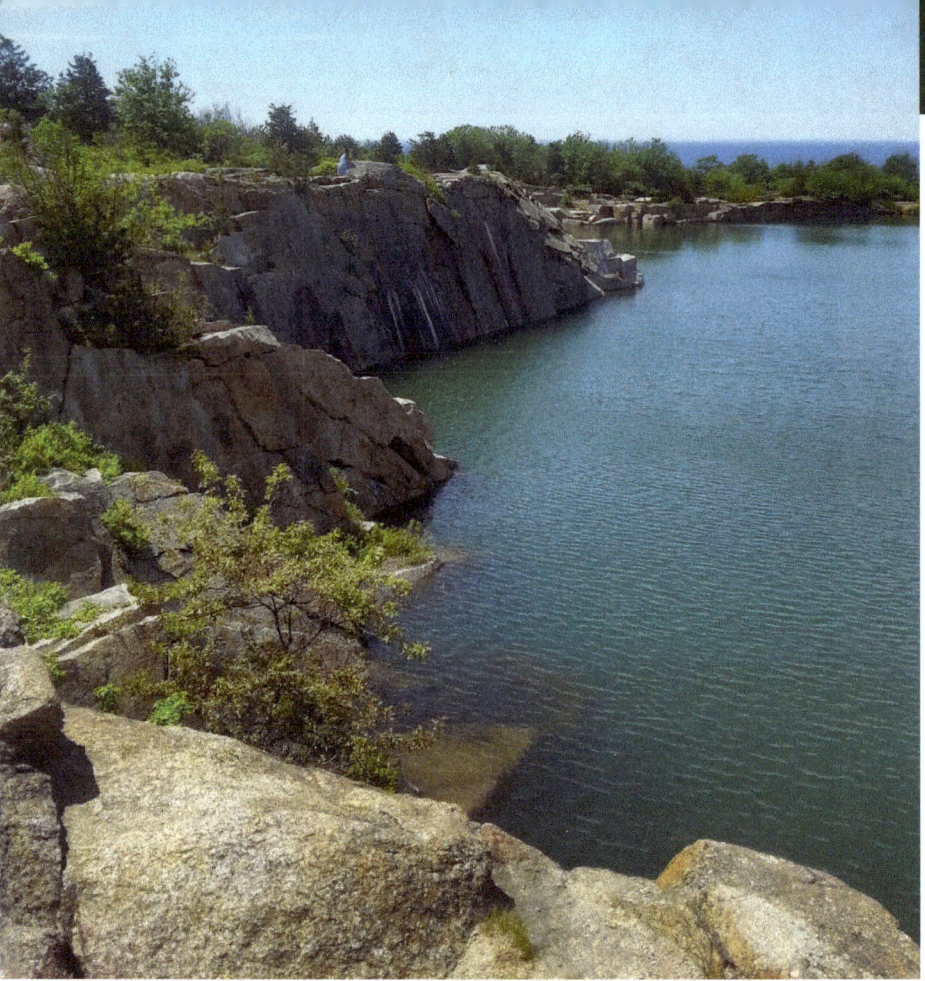

The land at Halibut Point State Park was once home to an active granite quarry.

Once you have taken in this impressive sight, backtrack to a broad, sandy trail leading right. The trailhead is not formally marked, but a sign warning of the dangers of swimming off the point alerts you to the turn, as does the miniature Stonehenge just inside the bend. Impromptu artists have arranged palm-sized quarry remnants into intriguing sculptures in a sandy enclosure just off the path.

Follow the gravel trail back uphill; once at the top, bear right to continue to the lookout on the peak of the mountain of quarry debris. The trail here remains firmly packed dirt and gravel, and the ascent is quite gentle. From this point, on a clear day, you can see as far north as Maine's Mount Agamenticus and the Isles of Shoals off the coast of New Hampshire, and Plum Island and Newburyport in the nearer distance. If you really want a sweeping view of the surrounding ocean and up into the mountains of southern Maine, visit the observation tower, which was used as a lookout post during World War II.

Leaving the peak, walk back toward the visitor center and the observation tower. To tour the grounds, turn right and follow the wide path west past birch, sumac, and cedar trees. A short way farther, turn onto the Bayview Trail to head back toward the sea. This trail descends steeply and then rises again as it curves west. Looking up, you're likely to see a flock of cormorants fly by, traveling from rookery to fishing grounds.

Curving back uphill, the Bayview Trail loops southwest past a grassy overlook. A small trail to the right leads to another lookout. Returning to the Bayview Trail, follow it to its end, then continue straight ahead on a wide gravel path.

Look for a sign for the Back 40 Loop, and take this grassy route west, walking downhill before swinging left to head south once more on this peaceful lane.

Closing the loop, you find yourself back at the clearing where you began. From this junction, continue straight to join the trail that leads to the rear of the visitor center. Keep left to pass in front of the visitor center and rejoin the path that leads back to the parking lot.

Legend has it that the first house built on Rockport's hardscrabble turf was erected around the bend from Halibut Point in 1692. The "Old House," as it is known locally, was built by two young men from Salem for their mother, who had been condemned at the Salem Witch Trials. Spared death because she was pregnant, the woman was expelled from the community and exiled to the wilderness of Cape Ann. Bears, wolves, and Agawam Indians lived there as well, and a handful of hunting shanties built by settlers of Ipswich accented the landscape.

Soon after building himself a cabin at the spot, resident John Babson discovered a bear living nearby. Not interested in having such a neighbor, he hunted it down, skinned it, and strung its hide over a rock by the sea to dry. Passing fishermen saw the bear's shaggy remains and dubbed the rough spit of land Bearskin Neck.

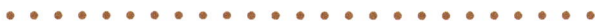

• • • • • • • • • • • • • • • • • • • • • • • • • • • •

**GPS TRAILHEAD COORDINATES** N42° 41.200' W70° 37.883'

**DIRECTIONS** From Boston, take US 1 to MA 128 N (toward Gloucester). At the first traffic circle in Gloucester, go three quarters of the way around and take MA 127 toward Pigeon Cove. Continue approximately 5 miles, passing through Annesquam and Lanesville into Rockport. Turn left onto Gott Avenue; the parking lot is on the right.

# 6 NASKETUCKET BAY STATE RESERVATION

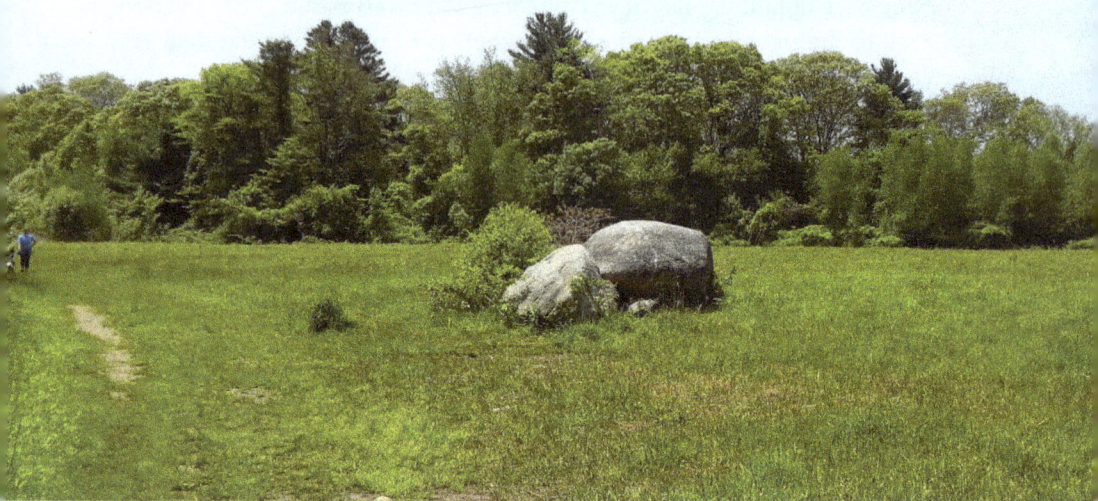

Nasketucket Bay State Reservation is a unique mix of grasslands, woods, and shoreline.

**ONCE OPEN FARMLAND,** this reservation now offers wooded trails, open fields, and access to a classic rocky New England beach on the waters of historic Buzzards Bay.

## DESCRIPTION

Once you arrive at Nasketucket Bay State Reservation, from the kiosk at the head of the parking lot you can follow a short connector path to the start of the Bridle Trail. Rolling wide and flat over a swath cut through woods and weeds, the trail bends farther west to meet the Meadow Trail just ahead.

If you would like to make a slight diversion, just before the Meadow Trail is an unmarked (as of researching this edition) trail to the right. This is the relatively new Shaw Farm Trail and bike path. It takes you on an excursion of slightly more than a mile through an open field along a majestic column of massive oak and maple trees, through some densely forested swamp, and along the far edge of the Shaw Farm. A simple out-and-back about a mile each way from the Bridle Trail, it's quite a scenic hike if you'd like to add this into your plans.

If your plan is to proceed directly to the Meadow Trail, then keep your eyes open off to the right; the sign was fairly worn and difficult to see, much less read, when I researched this edition. Once you arrive at the trail, bear right and follow

**DISTANCE & CONFIGURATION:** 2.75-mile double loop

**DIFFICULTY:** Easy

**SCENERY:** Woods, former farmlands, views of Nasketucket and Buzzards Bay

**EXPOSURE:** A mix of sun and shade

**TRAFFIC:** Light

**TRAIL SURFACE:** Flat packed dirt, grass, beach sand, rocks

**HIKING TIME:** 1–2 hours, depending how much time you want to spend on the beach

**DRIVING DISTANCE FROM BOSTON COMMON:** 60 miles

**ELEVATION:** 21' at trailhead, no significant elevation gain

**SEASON:** Year-round

**ACCESS:** Open sunrise–sunset; free

**MAPS:** On a kiosk in the parking lot and at tinyurl.com/nasketucketmap

**WHEELCHAIR ACCESS:** Wheelchair users can access the full length of smooth, firm Bridle Trail (although it can get a bit wet if there has been a lot of rain).

**FACILITIES:** None

**CONTACT:** Massachusetts Dept. of Conservation and Resources, mass.gov/locations/nasketucket -bay-state-reservation, 617-626-1250

**LOCATION:** 94 Brandt Island Road, Mattapoisett, MA

**COMMENTS:** This is a great family hike that ends up on a rocky beach where you can hike and hang out.

---

this narrower, somewhat overgrown path a few hundred yards behind wetland to another split. Keep left to step out from the dense thicket of blueberry bushes and tangled shrubs, and proceed across the open grassland toward the needle-thin tower at the center. Because of light traffic, this path can be difficult to discern, so feel free to improvise. You really can't get too turned around here; all the loops here at Nasketucket Bay State Reservation eventually connect with each other, and the Bridle Trail cuts right through the middle.

This area was once part of a farm. Now this open meadow is a refuge for all manner of flora and fauna, birds, and insects. The tower topped with propellers was erected by the state to collect wind data as part of an alternative-energy initiative. If those work out, there may eventually be more wind turbines installed.

South of the tower, the trail becomes more defined and easier to follow. Hike along the meadow as it tapers to a point along the edge of the woods to the right. If you're out there at the right time of the year, you'll find some blackberries growing close to the ground as the trail filters into the Bridle Trail by a posted marker. Continue southeast several feet to where you meet the Holly Trail. Leave this sandy belt, and turn left into the woods. Passing by white pines and short scrubby ground cover, the path curves east. On the right, a stone wall fades away behind tree limbs.

There are plenty of maple, oak, and basswood trees growing along the trail. You'll also start seeing several holly trees. As the trail continues south toward the seashore, you'll enter the holly grove and start seeing the angular trees with elephant-gray limbs and tough, crinkled leaves. Beyond a stretch where the trail dips and mud puddles form even in dry months, past a grove of beech trees, the trail emerges from the woods to cross the sun-bleached tail of the Bridle Trail.

## Nasketucket Bay State Reservation

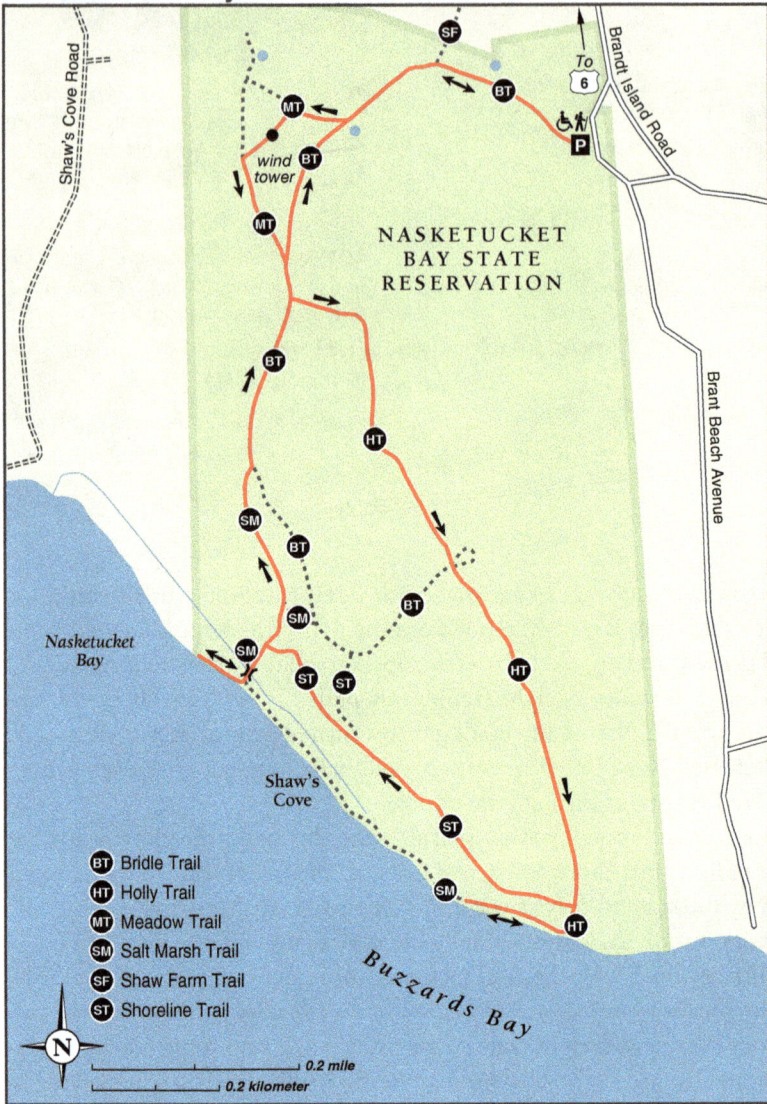

NASKETUCKET BAY STATE RESERVATION

Shaw's Cove Road

Brandt Island Road

To 6

P

wind tower

Nasketucket Bay

Shaw's Cove

Brant Beach Avenue

Buzzards Bay

BT  Bridle Trail
HT  Holly Trail
MT  Meadow Trail
SM  Salt Marsh Trail
SF  Shaw Farm Trail
ST  Shoreline Trail

N

0.2 mile
0.2 kilometer

Beyond this junction, the Holly Trail continues to Buzzards Bay. Silvery birch and oak mix in the forest with increasingly impressive-looking holly trees. Glance to the right here over the stone wall running alongside the trail, and you'll catch a sharp sliver of light flashing off the water less than a mile away. The trail passes several minor side trails cut by human, or perhaps animal, bushwhackers.

Sloping gently downhill, the trail soon arrives at a rocky beach. Just before that you'll see a right turn to the Shoreline Trail. Unless the weather is nasty, take a break and head for the rocky beach and the soothing waters of the ocean. From your vantage point on the rocks along the shore, the fist of land at the end of a scrawny arm of rocks to the east is Brandt Island. Mattapoisett Neck and Antassawamock reach beyond to Buzzards Bay; Woods Hole lies approximately 11 miles farther south as the crow flies; and 6 miles farther out is Vineyard Haven of Martha's Vineyard. Once you're done on the beach, backtrack to the head of the Shoreline Trail.

As you travel west 0.4 mile along the edge of land nibbled by storm surges, you'll pass over a wetland with some muddy patches where logs laid flat improve footing. After brushing past a boggy meadow, the trail snakes past an uncommonly large sassafras tree and a pine grove. You'll see another grove of holly trees of varying sizes as well. After swinging left and then right, the trail spills into a grassy clearing. At this three-way junction, bear left to take the Salt Marsh Trail, and head southwest back to the seashore.

Approaching the beach, this former cart road encounters a substantial stone bridge built over a channel. The view straight on is of Nasketucket Bay, with Sconticut Neck lying prone on the horizon. The tidal zone of the Nasketucket River lies to the

Extensive boardwalks traverse the otherwise swampy areas of the forest.

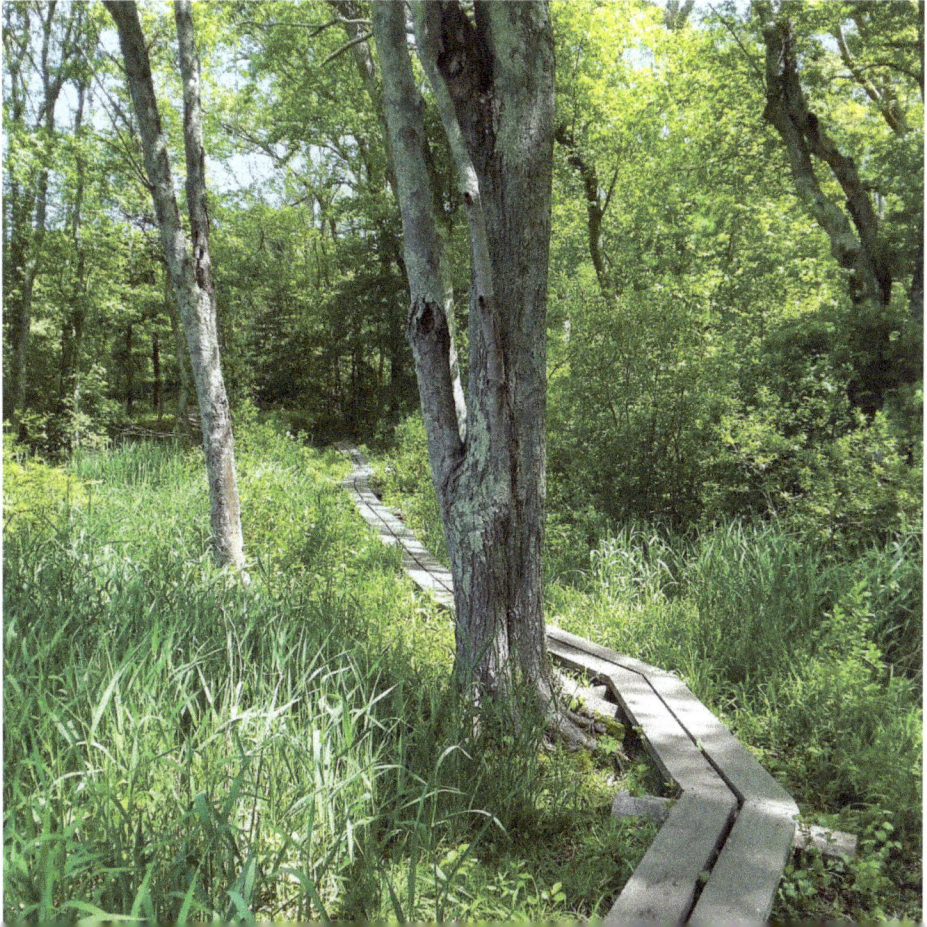

right, and just before it is Shaw's Cove. The shallows behind the strip of sand left in a glacier's wake have filled in over the ages to form salt marsh, which is home to a variety of endangered species. In fact, the marsh to the west is part of the South Shore Marshes Wildlife Management Area. If you'd like to spend some more time on a rocky beach, hike right, toward Shaw's Cove. A 5-foot granite spike jutting from the sand 100 yards along serves as a handy destination point. After looping around this odd protuberance, head back to the Salt Marsh Trail.

Passing blackberry bushes and beach roses, return to the grassy junction you passed through before, and continue straight on the Salt Marsh Trail, heading northeast. Starting wide and becoming narrower, the trail travels through woods, climbing a subtle incline as it nears the Bridle Trail. At this split, keep left, beside the salt marsh. The Salt Marsh Trail soon turns to upland and once more crosses the Bridle Trail. Bear left onto the tried-and-true Bridle Trail, and follow it back to the parking lot.

## NEARBY ATTRACTIONS

Immerse yourself in the rich maritime heritage of the area with a visit to the New Bedford Whaling Museum (18 Johnny Cake Hill, New Bedford; 508-997-0046). Admission is free for members, $17 for adults, $15 for senior citizens (65 and older), $10 for students (19 and over), $7 for children ages 4–14, and free for children under 3. The museum is fully wheelchair accessible.

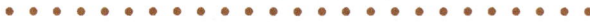

• • • • • • • • • • • • • • • • • • • • • • • • • •

**GPS TRAILHEAD COORDINATES**  N41° 38.133'  W70° 50.217'

**DIRECTIONS**  From Boston take I-93 S. At Exit 4, merge left onto MA 24 S. After 18.3 miles, take Exit 14A onto I-495 S toward Cape Cod. Continue 19.7 miles, and at Exit 1 merge onto I-195 W. After 9.1 miles, take Exit 19A toward Mattapoisett, and at 0.3 mile merge onto North Street. After 0.9 mile, turn right onto US 6. Continue 1.7 miles to a left turn onto Brandt Island Road. Follow Brandt Island Road, bearing left at the fork, then bear right when you see the sign for Brandt Beach Road. You can park in the small gravel lot on the right, tucked behind the Massachusetts Department of Environmental Management (DEM) sign. There is room for approximately 15–20 cars.

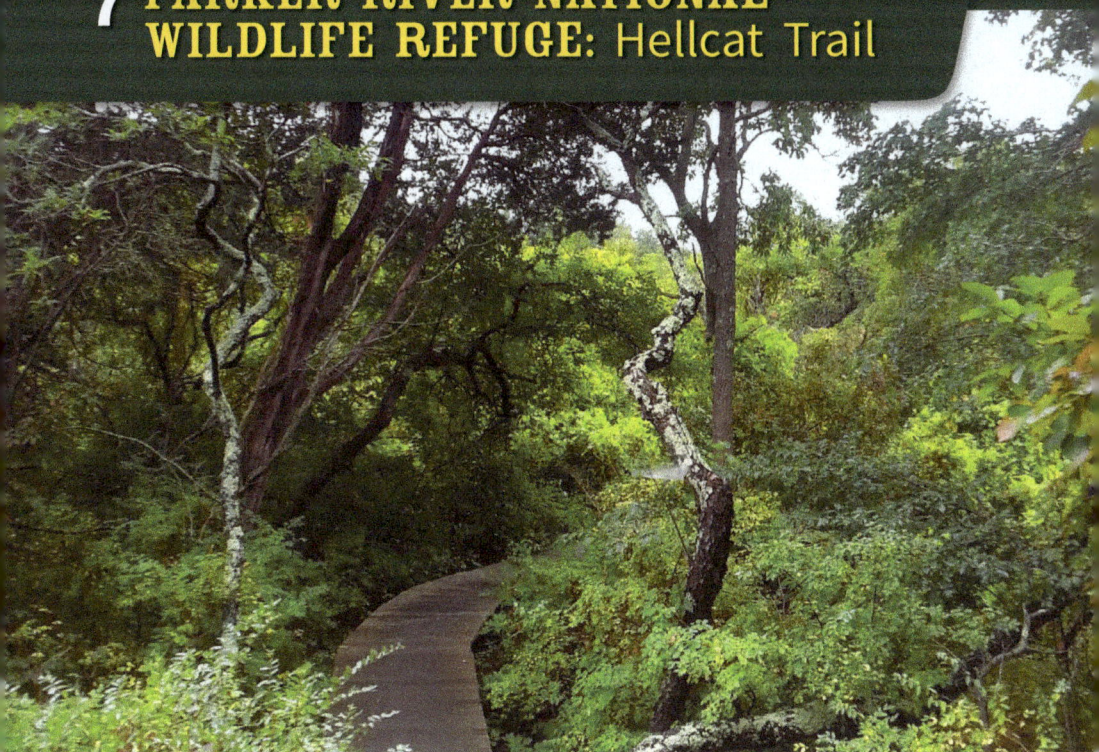

The Hellcat Trail is made up entirely of an extensive series of boardwalks to preserve the landscape.

**TRAVELING OVER AN** elevated boardwalk, this hike surveys the freshwater marsh of the Parker River Wildlife Refuge, passes through Plum Island's inner beach, and then crests enormous dunes to reach a lookout over the Atlantic Ocean. Those interested in increasing their hiking time can add the Pine Wood Trail, located south of the Hellcat Trail, and/or the Sandy Point State Reservation hike (page 56) that loops around the southern end of the island opposite Ipswich Bay.

## DESCRIPTION

In days long past, there was not a more remote and forbidding place on Plum Island than the Hellcat Swamp. Today, thanks to an elevated boardwalk, nearly anyone can venture into the farthest reaches of the swamp and the inner beach that insulates the swamp from the sea.

Begin at the trailhead located north of the parking lot beside the path that leads northwest to a wildlife lookout tower. Step up onto the boardwalk and follow it south through bayberry bushes to a junction where the trail divides in two. To start the hike with a tour of Plum Island's dunes, bear right, and continue east. As it's an extended boardwalk, it is virtually impossible to lose the trail. Even the steps are

**DISTANCE & CONFIGURATION:** 1.84-mile double loop

**DIFFICULTY:** Easy

**SCENERY:** Salt marshes, sand dunes, Atlantic Ocean

**EXPOSURE:** Mostly shaded, with some exposed areas

**TRAFFIC:** Moderate

**TRAIL SURFACE:** Boardwalks traverse the dunes and marsh along the entire length of the trail

**HIKING TIME:** 30–45 minutes

**DRIVING DISTANCE FROM BOSTON COMMON:** 53 miles

**ELEVATION:** 5' at trailhead, no significant gain

**SEASON:** Year-round

**ACCESS:** Open sunrise–sunset. Daily entrance fee is $5 per car and $2 for people on foot or bicycle; annual pass is $20 (credit cards not accepted).

**MAPS:** Available at the Parker River National Wildlife Refuge headquarters and visitor center (6 Plum Island Turnpike, Newburyport, MA), the gatehouse, and the trailhead while supplies last. Also available at tinyurl.com/parkerrivermap.

**WHEELCHAIR ACCESS:** A small section of trail off the southernmost parking area (7) is designed for wheelchair users. In addition, Pines Trail (at parking area 5) and many of the wildlife-observation areas are wheelchair accessible.

**FACILITIES:** There are no concession stands on the refuge; however, there are several restaurants and shops where the Plum Island Turnpike ends just outside the refuge entrance. Facilities at Hellcat Swamp include restrooms, an information center, a public boat launch, and many wildlife observation areas.

**CONTACT:** U.S. Fish and Wildlife Service, fws.gov /refuge/parker_river, 978-465-5753

**LOCATION:** Plum Island, Newburyport, MA

**COMMENTS:** Although Plum Island's 6.3-mile beach is closed April 1–August 31 for piping plovers to nest and rear their chicks, the Hellcat Trail remains open all year. Also, as an interpretive trail that's entirely boardwalk, it is convenient for families with small children or less mobile hikers.

painted yellow to help you avoid tripping or losing your footing. This is accessible to anyone who can walk.

Ahead, where the boardwalk bends north to cross the island, the trail passes through woodland where black oaks and red maples grow in an oasis created by the weather-shielding dunes and marsh. Farther along, the boardwalk reaches an area where freshwater vernal pools form when hard-hitting storms bore craters in the sand. As sources of rain-fed freshwater, these pools are critical to the island's wildlife.

After bearing east once more, the trail cuts across the access road. Cross carefully, then take up the boardwalk again as it climbs into the beach's back dunes. You'll pass through a grove of tenacious black cherry (*Prunus serotina*) and cedar trees.

Continue left at the split beyond the road to loop around the Dunes Trail. As the trail emerges from the shelter of the inner dunes and proceeds through the more exposed territory of secondary dunes, you can't help but notice the botanical changes. Where fierce wind and salt spray are able to penetrate, only the hardiest plants, such as beach heather (*Hudsonia tomentosa*), manage to survive. Their root system provides a modicum of stability for the shifting sand dunes. On the western slopes of the next set of dunes, you'll see bayberries and beach plums (*Prunus maritima*) growing in sheltered niches.

An incongruous stand of black pine (*Pinus nigra*) lies ahead to the northeast. These trees were planted as part of a dune-stabilization effort during the 1950s. Although the

## Parker River National Wildlife Refuge: Hellcat Trail

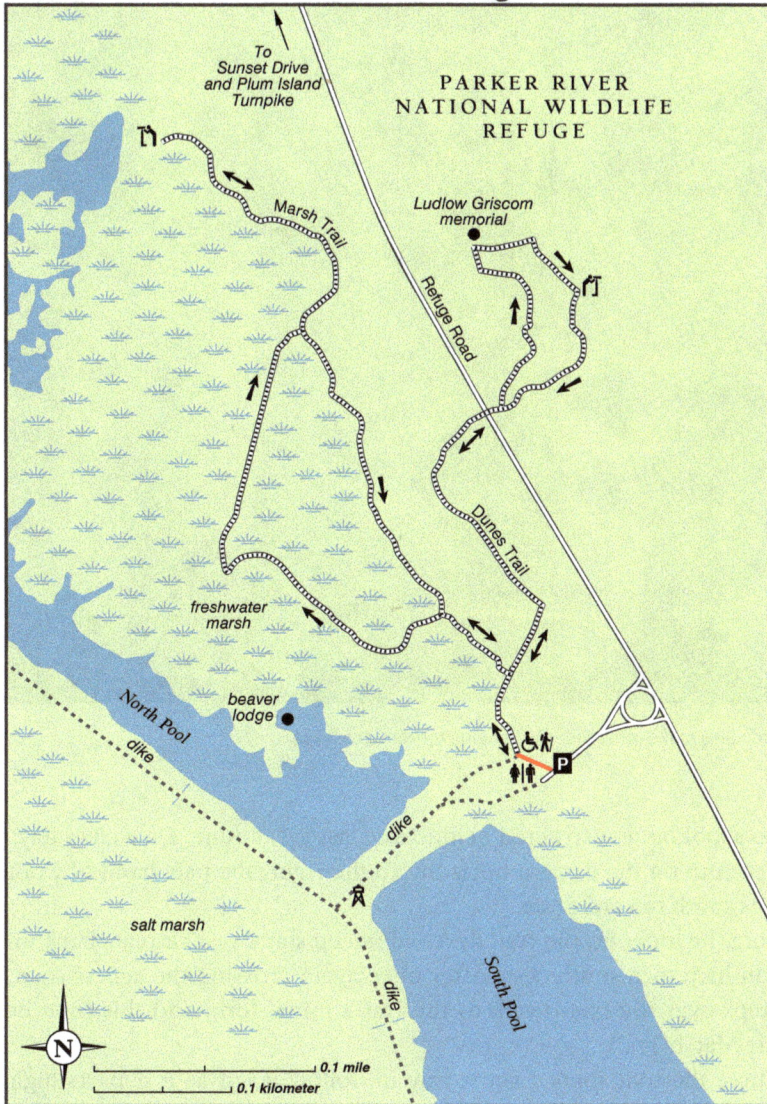

To
Sunset Drive
and Plum Island
Turnpike

PARKER RIVER
NATIONAL WILDLIFE
REFUGE

Marsh Trail

Ludlow Griscom
memorial

Refuge Road

Dunes Trail

freshwater
marsh

North Pool

dike

beaver
lodge

P

salt marsh

dike

South Pool

dike

N

0.1 mile

0.1 kilometer

black pine took hold successfully, the project was of dubious merit. What scientists understand now but didn't then is that barrier islands quell forces—such as hurricane winds—by deadening them with the drag of sand and waterlogged marsh peat.

Bear right at a memorial to conservationist Ludlow Griscom, and follow the boardwalk trail to the east. You'll be able to see the Joppa Flats and Merrimack River to the left. The walls of sand block sight of all but a sliver of the Atlantic to the east. Sloping uphill toward the primary dunes, the boardwalk scales a set of

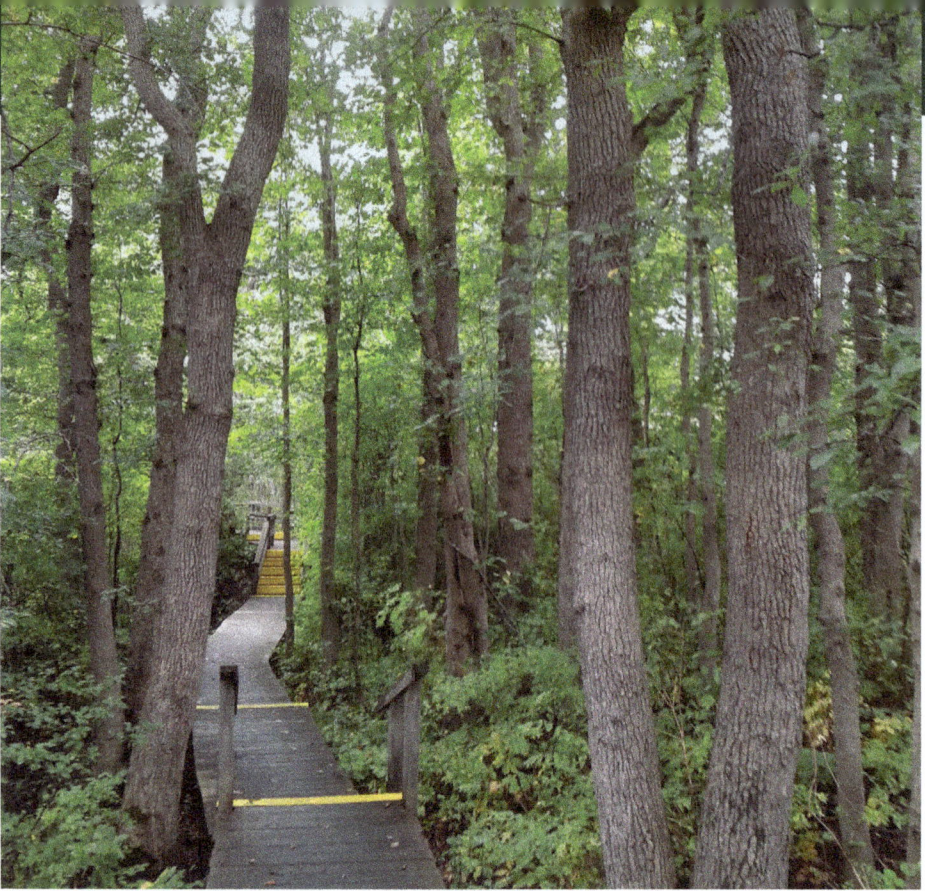

The boardwalks make otherwise challenging terrain accessible.

stairs to a lookout constructed behind one last great dune. On a clear day, you can see Cape Ann on the eastern horizon. To the right, the pale band of Crane Beach stretches south toward Essex.

From the lookout, the trail descends steep stairs as it retreats back under tree cover on its return southwest. After once again crossing the access road, retrace your steps over the boardwalk to the trail's initial fork, and this time bear right onto the Marsh Trail.

Where the trail splits a short way in, follow it left as it departs high ground dense with bayberry and beach plum for open marsh thick with cattails. Elevated above the marsh floodplain, the boardwalk bears west and bends north. If you're out on this boardwalk as early as March, you'll be treated to the sights and sounds of migratory birds arriving and filling the air with a symphony of honks, screeches, and chirps. Upwards of 350 species have been sighted on the island, and Hellcat Swamp is a favorite viewing location. Purple martins arrive in mid-April, as do hundreds of American kestrels, sharp-shinned hawks, and other raptor species. As spring eases into summer, you'll see waves of warblers, thrushes, vireos, fly-catchers, and other songbirds arrive and settle to rejuvenate and nest.

After arching out to a lookout station that provides a view over the northern freshwater pool and the town of Newbury beyond, the trail aims east and returns to high ground. Upon reaching a junction, bear left to access a wildlife lookout.

Returning by the same path, bear left at the next fork in the boardwalk, and continue south through the shrub land that borders the marsh. Sharp white birches lean into the breeze above an otherwise tangled thicket. Continue straight at the next fork, then bear right at the last to arrive back at the trailhead. If you'd like, you can extend the hike by following the trail to the right of Hellcat Trail to a lookout tower positioned beside the dike and the freshwater pools.

The ocean tides, terrain, and weather have long conspired to make Hellcat Swamp inaccessible at best. Before 1942, when the Audubon Society turned over its Annie H. Brown Wildlife Sanctuary to the federal government, allowing it to become part of the Parker River National Wildlife Refuge, there was no way to reach it other than by boat or by foot. After acquiring the land, the government constructed the access road that now runs the entire length of the island, increasing access to this dramatic landscape.

## NEARBY ATTRACTIONS

Newburyport boasts an assortment of attractions, including many historic homes listed on the National Register of Historic Places. A locale of unique appeal to boat lovers is Lowell's Boat Shop (978-388-0162), located in nearby Amesbury. The boat shop opened for business in 1793 and has been producing dories ever since.

For information, schedules, and listings of special events, visit Historic New England's website, historicnewengland.org. Though steeped in history, Newburyport is a vibrant commercial and cultural center with many excellent restaurants.

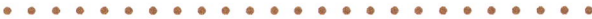

• • • • • • • • • • • • • • • • • • • • • • • • • • •

**GPS TRAILHEAD COORDINATES** N42° 44.483' W70° 47.733'

**DIRECTIONS** From Boston, take Storrow Drive E, following signs for US 1 N. Merge onto US 1 N toward Tobin Bridge/Revere. At 15.1 miles, merge onto I-95 N. From I-95, take Exit 57 and travel east on MA 113 to MA 1A S. At the intersection with Rolfe's Lane, turn left, and continue 0.5 mile to its end. Turn right onto Plum Island Turnpike and travel 2 miles, crossing Sergeant Donald Wilkinson Bridge to Plum Island. Take the first right onto Sunset Drive and travel 0.5 mile to the refuge entrance. Continue 3.5 miles to the Hellcat Wildlife Observation area, on the left.

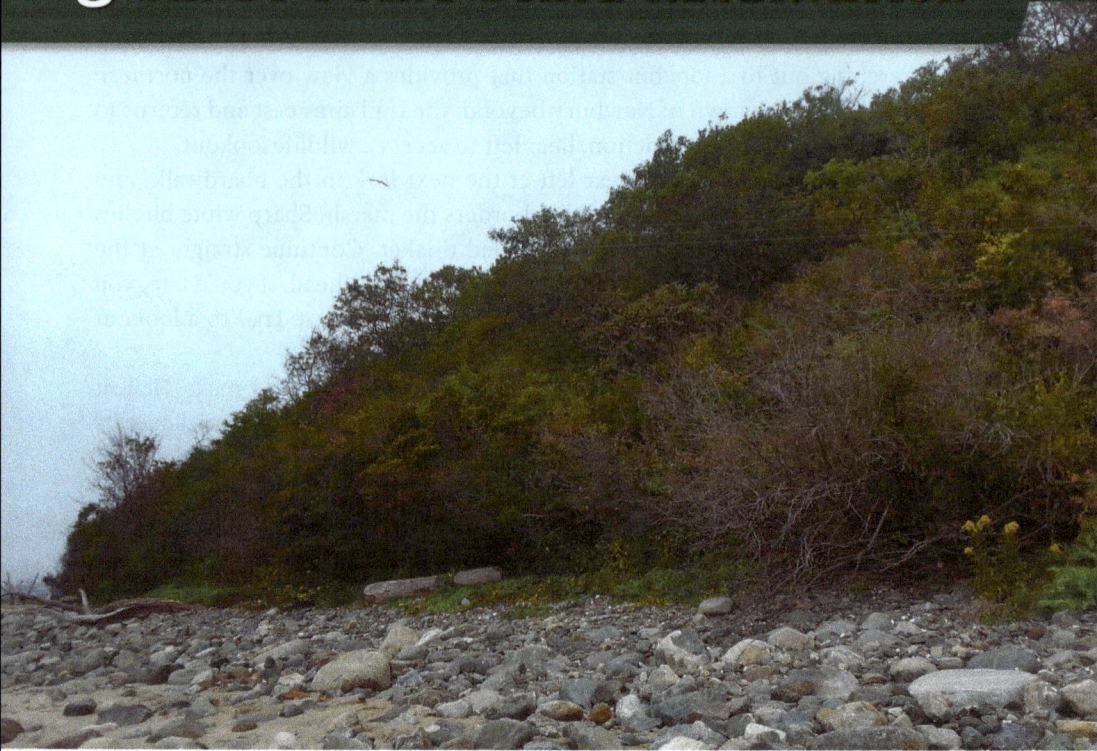

The beach at Sandy Point State Reservation will keep you there long after your hike is over.

**ON THIS EXPLORATION** of the southernmost tip of Plum Island, you will forge your own trail around a drumlin known as Bar Head to reach Ipswich Bluffs (Stage Island). From there, the Sandy Point Trail leads into the shelter of dunes and salt marsh to complete the loop.

## DESCRIPTION

Plum Island would not be the 8-mile barrier beach it is today without this drumlin poised at its southern tip. Planetary forces conspired to shape Plum Island 6,000–7,000 years ago. Along with earthquakes down the Parker River fault line and unrelenting wind and waves, subsiding earth and a rising sea level contributed to the island's creation. Once the beach materialized, the growing gap between the belt of sand and shore gradually filled to form freshwater marsh. Three thousand years ago, the sea level stabilized and, for the most part, the island and its beach looked much like it does today—despite occasional rearranging by ferocious coastal storms.

From the Sandy Point State Reservation parking area behind Bar Head, set out hiking east on the wide path that leads through the dunes to the beach. With the ocean in full view, bear right and, choosing a course through the many boulders, tree trunks, and other often curious tidal detritus, hike south toward the drumlin of

**DISTANCE & CONFIGURATION:** 2.5-mile loop

**DIFFICULTY:** Easy–moderate

**SCENERY:** Beach; views of the Atlantic Ocean, Ipswich Bay, and salt marshes adjoining Plum Island Sound and the Parker River

**EXPOSURE:** Full sun

**TRAFFIC:** Moderate

**TRAIL SURFACE:** Sand, packed dirt, and a short section of paved road

**HIKING TIME:** 1 hour

**DRIVING DISTANCE FROM BOSTON COMMON:** 48 miles

**ELEVATION:** 11' at trailhead, no significant gain

**SEASON:** Year-round

**ACCESS:** Open sunrise–sunset. Entrance fee is $5 per car and $2 for people on foot or bicycle.

**MAPS:** Available at the information center located at the gatehouse; more information and resources are also available at the refuge headquarters, located on Rolfe's Lane just off Plum Island Turnpike, or at tinyurl.com/sandypointmap

**WHEELCHAIR ACCESS:** A small section of trail off the southernmost parking area (7) is designed for wheelchair users. In addition, Pines Trail (at parking area 5) and many of the wildlife-observation areas are wheelchair accessible.

**FACILITIES:** Restrooms, information center, public boat launch, many wildlife-observation areas. There are no concession stands on the reservation. However, there are several restaurants and shops located where Plum Island Turnpike meets the northern end of the island.

**CONTACT:** Massachusetts Dept. of Conservation and Resources, tinyurl.com/sandypointres, 617-626-1250

**LOCATION:** Plum Island, Ipswich, MA

**COMMENTS:** Due to efforts to save the piping plover from extinction, nearly all of Plum Island's beach is closed every year April 1–August 31, but Sandy Point State Reservation is open year-round. A hike on Sandy Point begins with the 8-mile drive from the entrance gate to the trailhead. Though slow and dusty during dry summer months, the drive can be something of a safari—you are likely to spot a good deal of wildlife, some of it quite rare, such as the snowy owls that sometimes stop by in the spring, fall, and winter.

Castle Hill, across the bay. You will basically follow the shoreline around here. This is not as much a defined trail as following the land along the shoreline.

The boulders protruding from the sand and sea on the beach east of Bar Head are called Emerson's Rocks. Encrusted with barnacles and slick with seaweed, the exposed rocks are menacing enough. When hidden by surf at high tide, they have been positively murderous to ships. Between 1772 and 1936, no fewer than 55 ships wrecked off Plum Island. Of these, 10 were dashed to pieces at Emerson Rocks. At least 27 more vessels—schooners, trawlers, and steamers—went down near the mouth of the Merrimack River. The treacherous waters, rocks, and shoals of Ipswich Bay channel claimed at least eight ships as they tried to enter Plum Island Sound from Ipswich Bay over the years.

When bearing west around the end of Sandy Point, take care not to get trapped on the wrong side of a channel as the tide pours in—otherwise, be resigned to getting wet feet and possibly a drenching. You'll be heading toward the spit of land known as Ipswich Bluffs. Documented finds along this stretch where the wind howls over the finger of upland called Ipswich Bluffs add credence to legends that pirates buried treasure in these parts.

## Sandy Point State Reservation

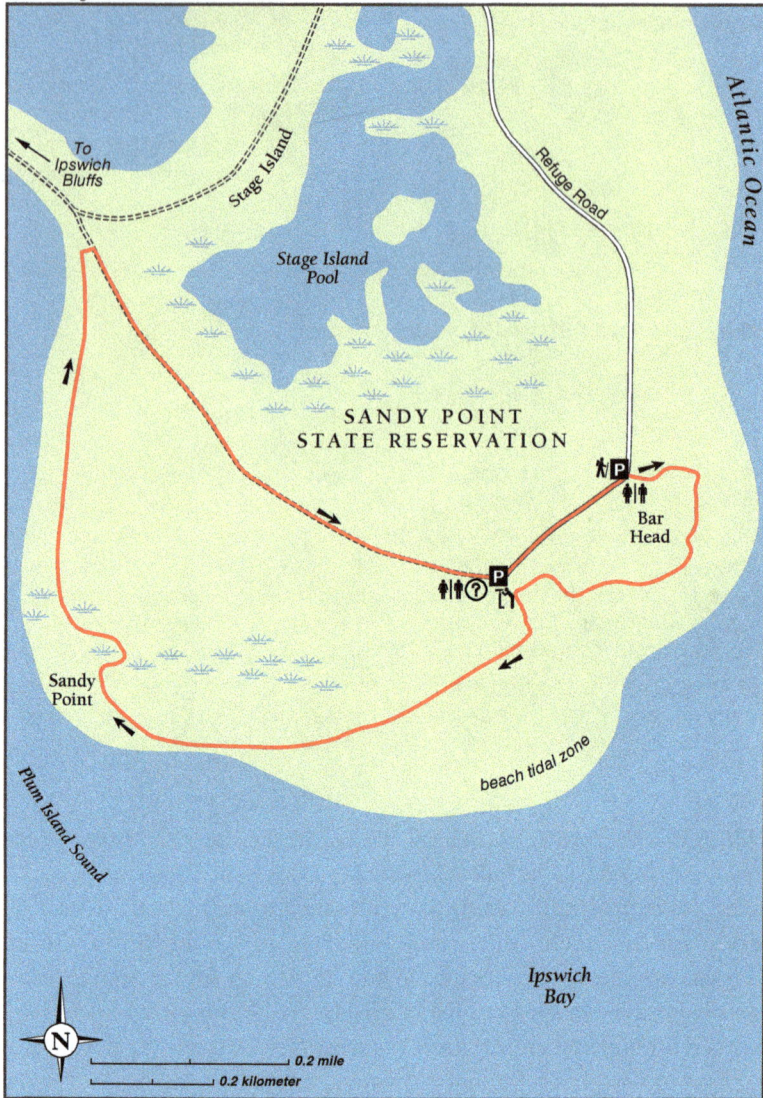

When you reach the tree-covered stretch where the bluffs begin, you should see a sign directing you north, away from the beach, to Stage Island. Take this turn to the right and follow the lightly worn footpath into the shelter of brush. The trail is vague in places but generally cuts a line between the Stage Island estuary and dunes drifted against the western side of the Bar Head drumlin. Even after all manner of human intervention over the years, this area remains wilderness.

Where the Sandy Point Trail reaches the iron gate by a parking area beside upland and beach, cross the pavement, bearing left to follow the drive back to the entrance of the Sandy Point State Reservation.

This area was first populated in the mid-1600s, following the arrival of Reverend Thomas Parker (namesake of the Parker River) and company. Besides good grazing, thatch for roofs, and teeming waterfowl, it contained enormous quantities of beach plums. Soon after, this sliver of land became known as Plum Island. Thankfully, instead of being developed as a resort or residential community, the bulk of the island was conserved as a wildlife refuge and park. In 1943, the Massachusetts Audubon Society sold the 1,600-acre Annie H. Brown Wildlife Sanctuary to the federal government, allowing it to merge with the Parker River National Wildlife Refuge.

## NEARBY ATTRACTIONS

Newburyport is steeped in history and remains a vibrant commercial and cultural center with many excellent restaurants and many historic homes listed on the National Register of Historic Places. A locale of unique appeal to boat lovers is Lowell's Boat Shop (978-388-0162), located in nearby Amesbury. The boat shop opened for business in 1793 and has been producing dories ever since.

For information, schedules, and listings of special events, visit historicnew england.org.

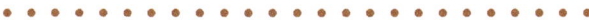

• • • • • • • • • • • • • • • • • • • • • • • • • •

**GPS TRAILHEAD COORDINATES** N42° 44.483' W70° 47.733'

**DIRECTIONS** From Boston, take Storrow Drive east, following signs for US 1 N. Merge onto US 1 N toward Tobin Bridge/Revere. At 15.1 miles, merge onto I-95 N. From I-95, take Exit 57 and travel east on MA 113 to MA 1A S. At the intersection with Rolfe's Lane, turn left and continue 0.5 mile to the end of that road. Turn right onto Plum Island Turnpike and travel 2 miles, crossing the Sargent Donald Wilkinson Bridge to Plum Island. Take the first right onto Sunset Drive and travel 0.5 mile to the refuge entrance.

# 9 WORLD'S END

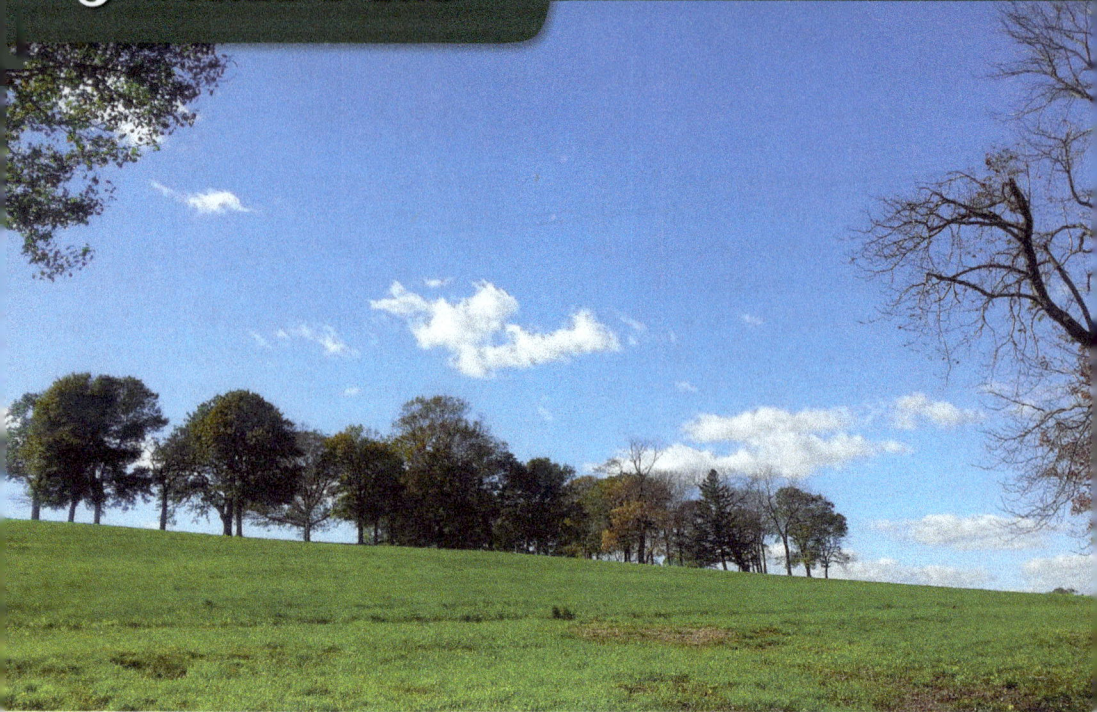

The scenery at World's End is breathtakingly beautiful.

**EXPLORE A SCENIC PENINSULA,** following a trail along the outer rim. The landscaping touches of Frederick Law Olmsted are still apparent, as are signs of the peninsula's agricultural past.

## DESCRIPTION

It's a good thing the trail surface is primarily hard packed and fairly smooth throughout World's End because your attention will be captivated by the scenery. The open fields, sweeping hillside, and statuesque trees lining much of the trail are impressive. It feels a bit like A. A. Milne's Hundred Acre Wood combined with Treasure Island.

The trails are also well-defined and easy to follow. While there are several overlapping loops that all beg exploration, the trail specified here begins at the northeast end of the upper parking lot. This path, the width of a carriage, heads directly into an increasingly dense forest of oak and pine. While most of the trails passing through World's End are wider carriage roads, these trails are more like true hiking trails. Down a rocky slope to the left, you will catch a glimpse of a marshy bog and an open meadow. Farther along on the right, the trail opens to a marshy shore and a waterway called Porter's Cove.

The path bends left after the water view and meets a trail splitting to the right. Take this narrower trail to the right and, looking through the eastern-side underbrush,

**DISTANCE & CONFIGURATION:** 3.8-mile double loop

**DIFFICULTY:** Easy

**SCENERY:** Spectacular views of the Boston skyline, Hingham Harbor, and the Weir River

**EXPOSURE:** Partially shaded most of the way, except for parts of the carriage road and the causeway linking the twin drumlins of World's End

**TRAFFIC:** Trails are popular but never crowded

**TRAIL SURFACE:** Packed dirt, mowed grassland, gravel

**HIKING TIME:** 1.3 hours

**ELEVATION:** 140' at trailhead, no significant gain

**SEASON:** Year-round

**DRIVING DISTANCE FROM BOSTON COMMON:** 15 miles

**ACCESS:** Sunrise–sunset; free for members of The Trustees of Reservations and children

under age 12, $6 for nonmembers. World's End is managed by The Trustees of Reservations but is also considered part of the Boston Harbor Islands National Park.

**MAPS:** Available in office at entrance or at tinyurl.com/worldsendmap

**WHEELCHAIR ACCESS:** Much of World's End is accessible by wheelchair, but the Rocky Neck area is not.

**FACILITIES:** Well-maintained outhouses near parking lot, picnic tables on a hill beside entrance

**CONTACT:** The Trustees of Reservations, thetrustees.org/places-to-visit, 617-542-7696

**LOCATION:** Martin's Lane, Hingham, MA

**COMMENTS:** The Trustees of Reservations organizes occasional special events, such as evening owl watches. Horseback riding is allowed; the annual permit costs $100. Leashed dogs are welcome.

you will see waves lapping at the rocky coast. On the left, pass a freshwater bog populated by ducks. Another fork and a small pond lie just beyond. Stay right, keeping with the water.

There's never too much elevation gain on these trails. As you come around to face north, you get a clear view of the Weir River and the town of Hull on the opposite bank. Looking west, you will see the great hourglass-shaped peninsula of World's End stretching toward Boston. You may also see a smattering of eider ducks and seagulls populating the water.

The trail comes back around, heading southeast as it reaches the base of Rocky Neck. At each of three forks, bear right to head south. Dipping through a cedar thicket, the trail soon opens to meadowland. Leave the woods behind and walk uphill to rejoin the carriage road that forms the primary loop around World's End. Stepping onto this level, gravel path, head north (right), keeping the Weir River over your right shoulder. The carriage path here is frequently punctuated with majestic ash trees.

The fields at World's End are regularly mowed to keep them level. Majestic elm trees once dominated the landscape, but most were lost to Dutch Elm disease decades ago. Ash trees now stand in their place. Raptors, bluebirds, and bobolinks fill the forest. Follow the carriage road as it eases downhill around the right of Planter's Hill and arrives at sea level. The trail here is still firm, hard-packed gravel. Ahead, look for the glacial isthmus linking Planter's Hill to the northern tip of World's End. This spit of gravel and ground shells serves as a causeway to the outer peninsula. On a clear day, you can catch dramatic glimpses of the Boston skyline to the northwest.

## World's End

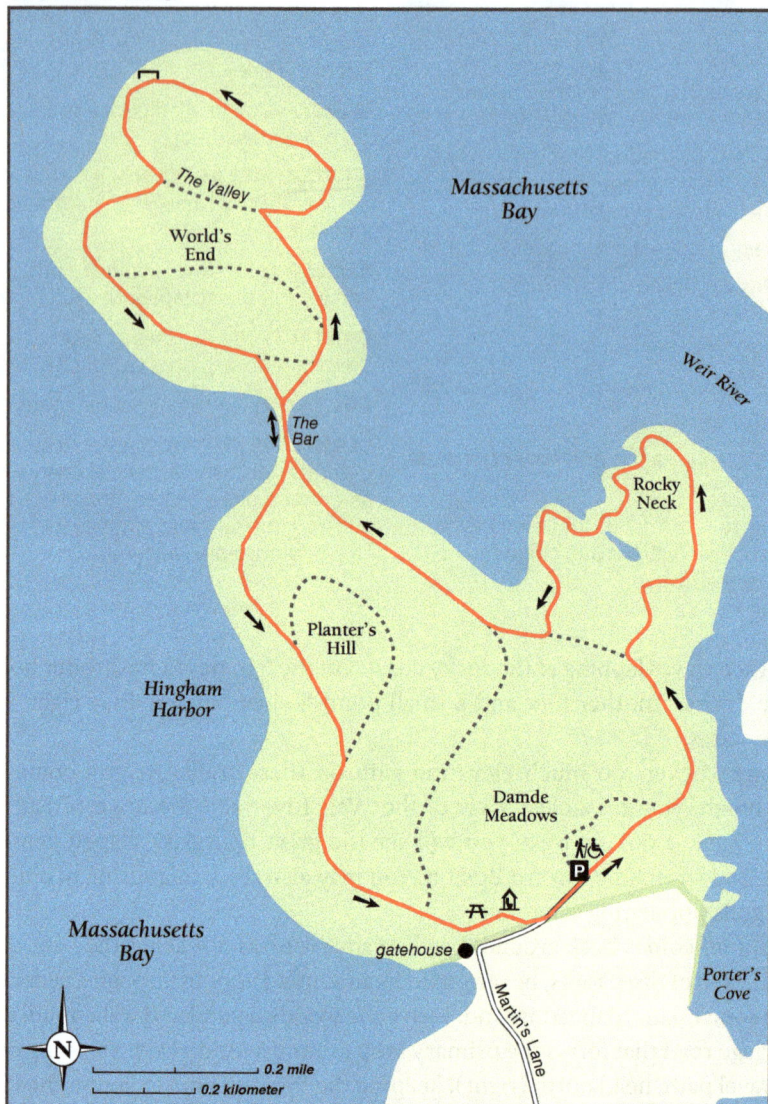

Massachusetts
Bay

The Valley

World's
End

Weir River

The
Bar

Rocky
Neck

Planter's
Hill

Hingham
Harbor

Damde
Meadows

Massachusetts
Bay

gatehouse ●

Porter's
Cove

Martin's Lane

N

0.2 mile
0.2 kilometer

Cross over the causeway and follow the carriage road uphill, bearing right. Continuing north, the road soon reaches a split. Follow the straighter path, which takes you into what's referred to as the Valley. Shortly you reach another junction. Turn sharply right and follow the trail as it circles the land counterclockwise. The road rises out of the dark woods of the Valley to lead back to a domed meadow. From here you'll see the waterfront homes of Hull.

Upon reaching the end of the island, the road curves sharply south. This point affords a clear view of Boston. A wedge cut into the treeline and a waiting bench invite hikers to sit for a moment to look at the city's skyline.

Continue down the road as it heads south along the western side of the reservation. Hingham Harbor lies to the right through the trees, at the bottom of a steep embankment. Keep walking beside the harbor when the trail merges with each of two routes coming from the east. Sitting well below the top of a meadow to your left, the trail gradually climbs as it approaches a northern lookout above the causeway.

Having completed the loop around World's End, make your way downhill to "The Bar," and cross back over to Planter's Hill. Unless the footpath etched into the face of this steep hill lures you, stay with the carriage road as it continues right.

Approaching the mainland, the road again eases downhill. Soon you will see a stone wall on the left, paralleling your path. A little farther along, another stone wall picks up on the right, delineating fields that once held livestock. Martin's Cove bends in around Pine Hill to the left, and to the right you will see Damde Meadows. As you walk downhill to a causeway, notice the tide spilling through from one side to the other.

Straight ahead up a rise, you can spot the reservation's entrance. After the trail splits to the left, leave the cove and climb the granite steps. At the top, you'll find picnic tables set in a clearing overlooking the salt marsh estuary. Not far beyond, you will pass two outhouses before again reaching the lower parking area.

World's End has a rich history. In a near brush with global fame in 1945, officials from the town of Hingham made a bid to have World's End selected as the site of the United Nations headquarters. Obviously, United Nations planners opted for New York. Then, in 1965, the peninsula experienced another close call by nearly becoming the foundation for a nuclear power plant. This last threat proved fortuitous, as it prompted The Trustees of Reservations to ensure its preservation by buying it two years later.

## NEARBY ATTRACTIONS

Camping, mountain biking, and more hiking trails are available at Wompatuck State Park, in Hingham. To get there from World's End, take MA 128 west toward US 3, and turn left onto Free Street.

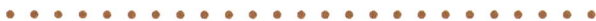

• • • • • • • • • • • • • • • • • • • • • • • • • • •

**GPS TRAILHEAD COORDINATES** N42° 15.550'  W70° 52.300'

**DIRECTIONS** From Boston, take I-93 south to MA 3 (to Cape Cod). Take Exit 14 and take MA 228 north 6.5 miles toward Hingham. Turn left onto MA 3A and follow it 0.4 mile. Go through the rotary, turn right onto Summer Street and continue straight to the intersection with Rockland Street. Turn left onto Martin's Lane and drive 0.7 mile to its end.

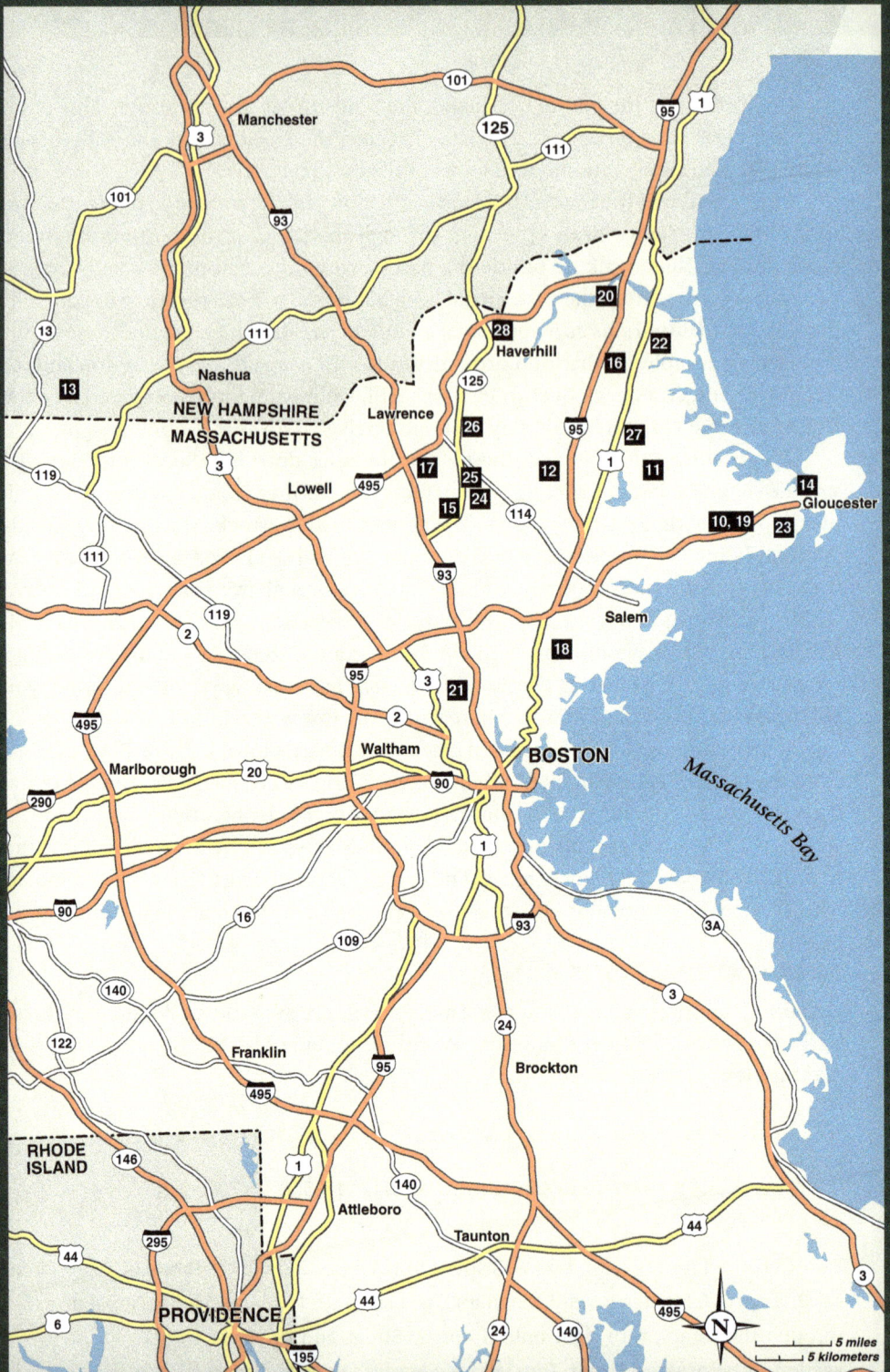

# NORTH OF BOSTON

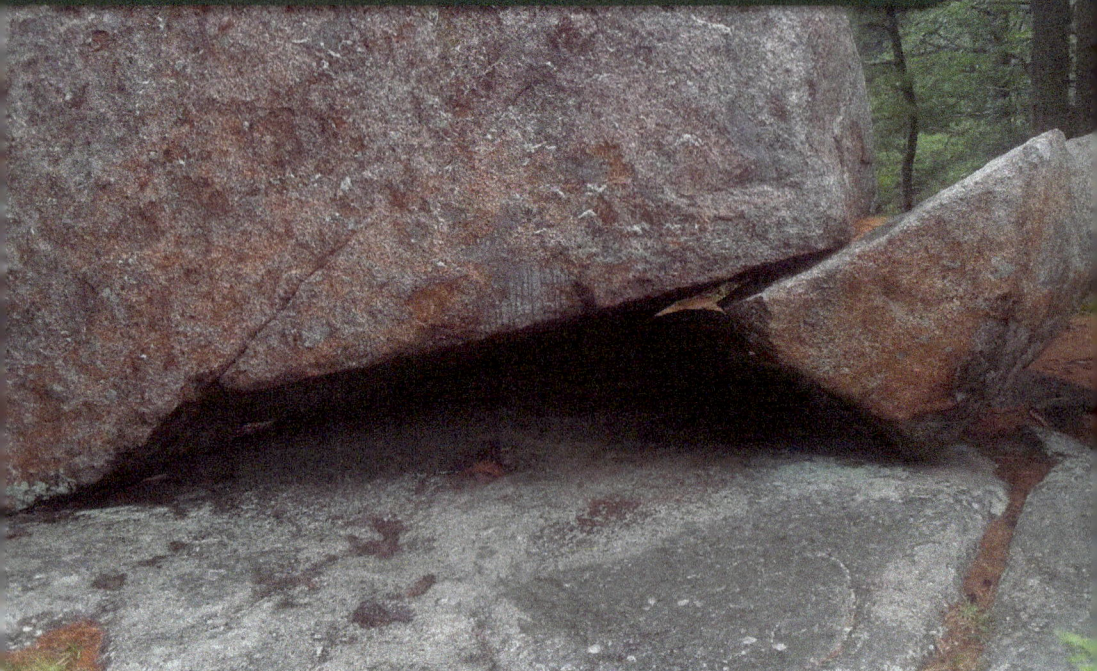

# 10 AGASSIZ ROCK RESERVATION

Kids of all ages (and their parents) will enjoy exploring the rock formations at Agassiz Rock Reservation.

**THIS SHORT, RUGGED HIKE** tours a hillside made spectacular by the handiwork of the Wisconsin Glacier. Two granite monoliths are the stars of the show, but plan to spend some time on the open granite cap at the top of the hill.

## DESCRIPTION

From the gate at the trailhead, follow the broad, rocky path as it climbs abruptly into the woods. Sweeping southeast, the path meets a stream running from a source high on the hill. You'll traverse a wooden-plank bridge and pass a vernal pool sided with granite rubble and adorned with ferns and luxuriant moss. The trail is firmly packed, well defined, and well marked. Nestled in a cleft between hills, the trail runs on level ground briefly before beginning its climb. Switching east and northeast over protruding rocks and roots, the path eases downhill and soon arrives at a short causeway with a small pool to the right.

Immediately ahead, a sign directs you left to Big Agassiz and right to Little Agassiz. Take the left path to complete a clockwise loop. Heading north under overhanging branches, the trail passes another pool. Continuing on flat ground, step around a grand orb of granite on the right, brushing past bayberry bushes on the way.

Curving north, the slender trail runs downhill through a thick growth of bushes on either side. Tumbling through tangled brush, the trail suddenly emerges at a bog.

**DISTANCE & CONFIGURATION:** 0.75-mile out-and-back with small loop

**DIFFICULTY:** Easy–moderate

**SCENERY:** Astonishing glacial erratics, hilltop view of Gloucester

**EXPOSURE:** Mostly shaded, but exposed at the top

**TRAFFIC:** Light

**TRAIL SURFACE:** Packed dirt with exposed roots and stones

**HIKING TIME:** 40 minutes

**DRIVING DISTANCE FROM BOSTON COMMON:** 30 miles

**ELEVATION:** 45' at trailhead, 171' at highest point

**SEASON:** Year-round

**ACCESS:** Sunrise–sunset; free

**MAPS:** Posted at the entrance

**WHEELCHAIR ACCESS:** No

**FACILITIES:** None

**CONTACT:** The Trustees of Reservations, thetrustees.org/places-to-visit, 617-542-7696

**LOCATION:** School Street, Manchester-by-the-Sea, MA

**COMMENTS:** Swiss glaciologist and Harvard professor Louis Agassiz was the first to reason that enormous boulders often caught in precarious positions like those found on this hike were moved and arranged on the landscape by sheets of glacial ice.

Look left and you will see Big Agassiz emerging from the brush like a massive ship. Resting in this spot for thousands of years, the rock is said to be far more massive than it appears. Like the iceberg that sank the *Titanic,* most of Big Agassiz lies hidden.

Take a moment to walk off the trail toward Big Agassiz, as it is somewhat set back from the hiking trail. Only by hiking up to its sweeping gray granite walls can you truly appreciate the enormity of this geologic oddity. You can only imagine the size of the glacier that was moving around a boulder of this magnitude.

During the 19th century, Swiss geologist Joseph Agassiz convinced his peers and the general population that glacial forces led to the curious placement of Big Agassiz and other such boulders. By his explanation, this boulder and the others of all shapes and sizes that litter New England are called "glacial erratics," the stranded victims of ice long melted away.

After gazing at the massive Big Agassiz rock for a while, return to the trail, taking it east (left) as it continues upward from the edge of the wetland. Along this part, the trail is surfaced with coarse grit. It's not yet sand but finer than gravel that may once have been a part of the famous boulder.

You'll pass a grove of beeches to the left and hemlocks to the right. Then the trail steepens as it bends south. Along here, you will see one or two lichen-bedecked boulders on the right. Although they are also glacial erratics, you have not yet reached Little Agassiz. Even the smaller of the two Agassiz erratics is larger than these boulders. Continue until you reach a flat expanse of granite to the left at the top of the hill. Walk out onto this for a look southeast over the treeline to Cape Anne. The garden of glacial erratics and the views from the hillside of the surrounding towns and coastline are well worth exploring for hours on end.

Once you reach this dramatic hilltop, walk to the right and you will find Little Agassiz behind another unnamed but nevertheless impressive boulder. Propped

## Agassiz Rock Reservation

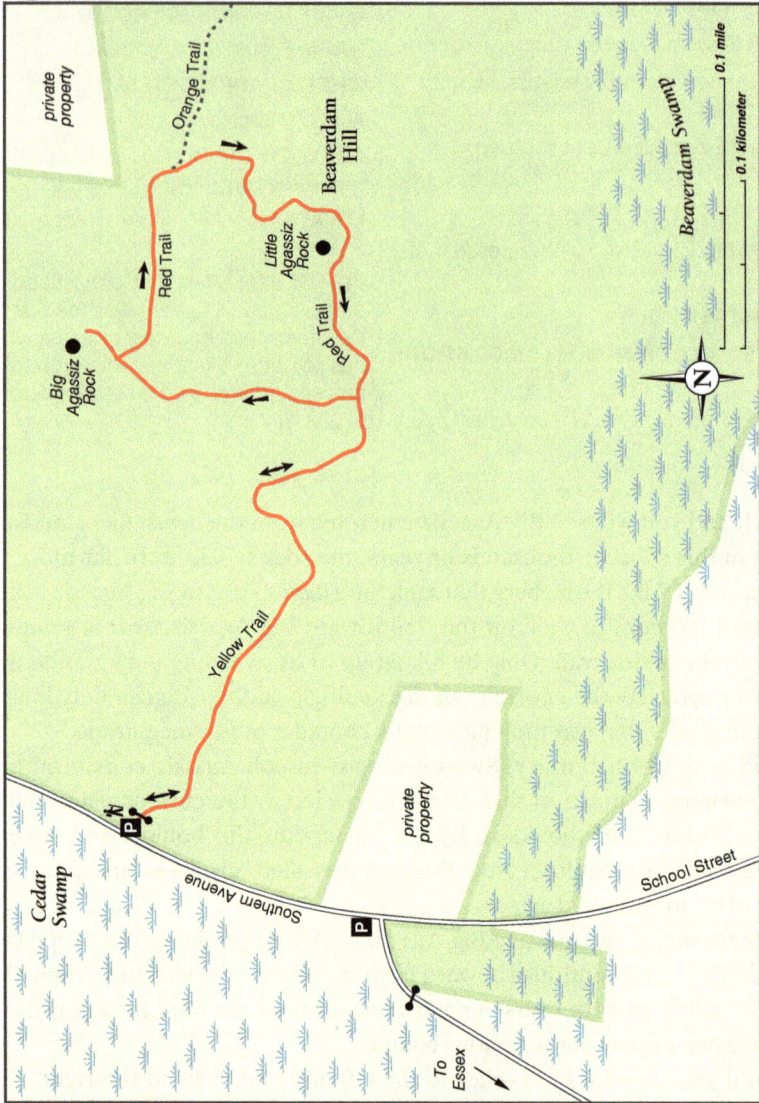

precariously on a tilted triangular stone, Little Agassiz seems to pulse with potential energy. The rock garden these glacial erratics form atop the hill begs much exploring, especially on a sunny day.

After spending some time surveying the view, pick up the path just below Little Agassiz to the left. Checking the ground, you might spot the tiny columbine that grows from the gritty soil. Blooming in June, its minute flowers are pink with yellow pistils.

After a steep pitch, the trail eases as it returns to the shaded woods. Wintergreen grows profusely along the mossy path's edge. Soon the steeper incline grows more gentle and the walking gets easier as you arrive back at the junction. Here the path bears right to Big Agassiz. Keep left to return to the trailhead at Southern Avenue and complete your Big Agassiz/Little Agassiz loop.

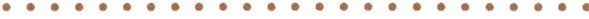

• • • • • • • • • • • • • • • • • • • • • • • •

**GPS TRAILHEAD COORDINATES** N42° 35.900'  W70° 46.017'

**DIRECTIONS** From Boston, take US 1 N for 13 miles. Merge onto I-95/MA 128 north. Drive 14 miles on MA 128 N. Take Exit 15 and travel 0.5 mile north. The entrance is off Southern Avenue on the right. A roadside pulloff will accommodate 10 cars.

Be ready for a rocky hike up and around Agassiz Rock.

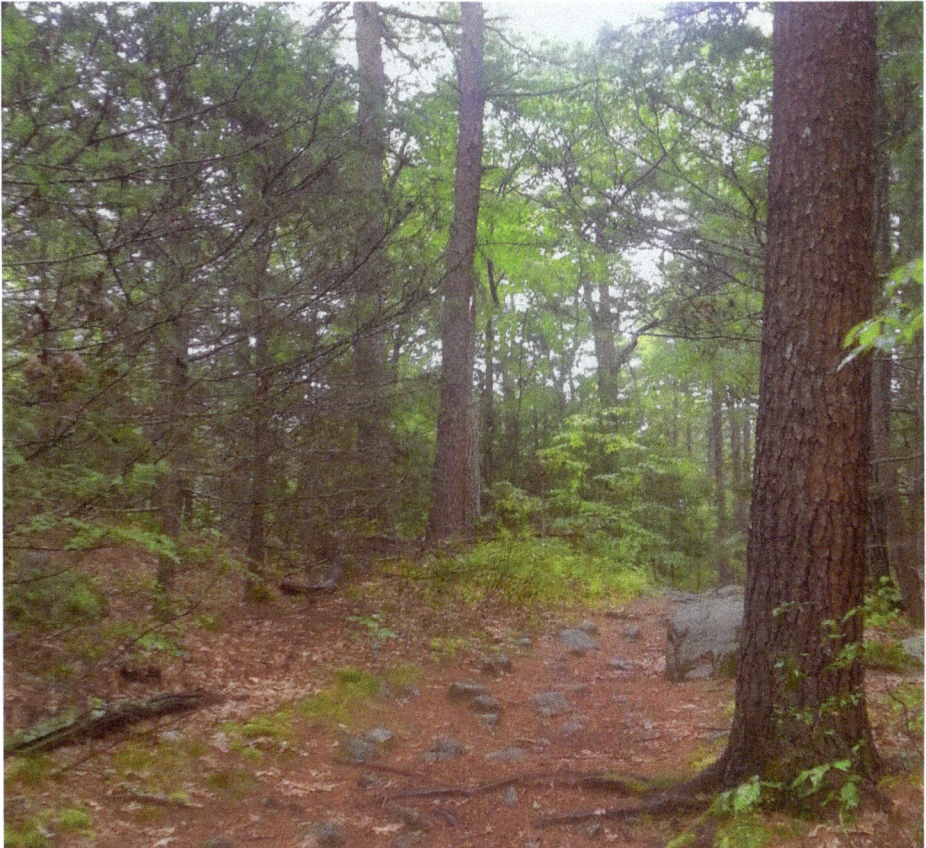

# 11 APPLETON FARMS: Grass Rides

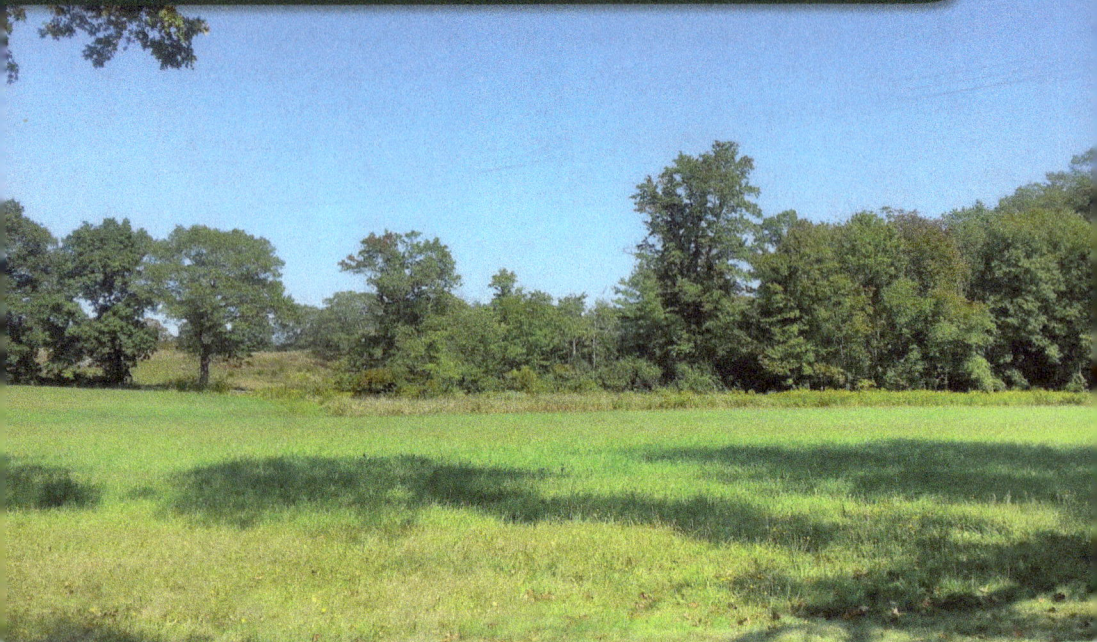

The pastoral beauty of Appleton Farms is truly spectacular.

**EXPLORE THE NORTHWESTERN ACRES** of Appleton Farms, following an old steeplechase course and trails through forested wetlands.

## DESCRIPTION

In 1638, the King of England granted Samuel Appleton a 460-acre parcel of land spreading between the towns of Ipswich and Hamilton. Over the centuries, nine generations expanded and maintained what grew to be a magnificent 1,000-acre farm. Today Appleton would be delighted to know the property has passed into the protective care of The Trustees of Reservations and continues as a productive farm.

Starting at the parking area, cross the field, following the avenue of maples over a wide, firm, and flat carriage road to an entrance to the Grass Rides located beyond the bog at the edge of the woods. Enter through a break in a stone wall to access trails cleared generations ago for the purpose of equestrian sport. Head immediately left, and follow the path along the edge of the woods to where it meets another gap in the wall. Turn left again and continue uphill just beyond the shadows of the hemlocks and oaks to your right.

Over your left shoulder you will see the soft contours of the wide-open field known as the Great Pasture. Where the path levels off, there's a well-placed bench that invites you to stop and marvel at this vast field. At 133 acres, it is the largest grassland in northeastern Massachusetts.

**DISTANCE & CONFIGURATION:** 2.6-mile loop

**DIFFICULTY:** Easy

**SCENERY:** Forested wetlands and views across massive pastures granted to the original owner by the King of England

**EXPOSURE:** Mostly shaded

**TRAFFIC:** Light

**TRAIL SURFACE:** Packed dirt, grass

**HIKING TIME:** 2 hours

**DRIVING DISTANCE FROM BOSTON COMMON:** 30 miles

**ELEVATION:** 43' at trailhead, no significant gain

**SEASON:** Year-round

**ACCESS:** Sunrise–sunset; free

**MAPS:** Posted at the entrance and available at tinyurl.com/appletonfarmsgrassrides

**WHEELCHAIR ACCESS:** No

**FACILITIES:** None

**CONTACT:** The Trustees of Reservations, thetrustees.org/places-to-visit, 617-542-7696

**LOCATION:** Highland Street, Hamilton, MA

**COMMENTS:** Managed by The Trustees of Reservations, Appleton Farms is still a working farm, producing high-quality hay, milk, meat, and produce.

Leave the bench and continue along the pasture. Follow the path as it winds through the loose forest, descends for a bit, and then climbs to the peak of Pigeon Hill—the highest point in Appleton Farms. Break from the path here and walk out into the Great Pasture. In the center of the hill, you will see a large granite pinnacle. Salvaged from Gore Hall of Harvard University, the pinnacle was placed on the hill to commemorate Colonel Francis Randall Appleton Jr. (1885–1974). Looking southeast from Pigeon Hill, you can see as far as Hog Island and Crane Beach.

Continue along the edge of the Great Pasture to where the trail eases southwest downhill and turns northwest. Spilling off the hill, the trail widens as it meets another route joining in from the right. This broad, even track once served as a steeplechase course. You can imagine riders atop thoroughbred horses tearing through this turn.

Before long the trail arrives at a four-way intersection. Take a sharp left to go west. The trail is raised through here, forming a causeway between wetland on either side. Soon the trail bends left as it passes a small meadow surrounded by woods. Resuming a straight course, the path takes you to a second pinnacle positioned at the center of a clearing shaped like the hub of a wheel with trails radiating in all directions.

Stay your course, walking south beyond the pinnacle to the next trail on the right, and proceed northwest. Unlike the avenues radiating from the pinnacle, this new trail has curves. Look for the occasional swamp oak among more plentiful beech and shagbark hickory trees. Shortly you will reach a stand of exotic evergreens planted in clean rows on the left and right. Directly ahead, look for a stone wall and, beyond it, a lightly traveled road. Turn right to parallel the wall on your left.

Following alongside wetland once more, you will pass a trail on the right, but continue straight. Soon you will notice a brown house on the left across the dirt road beside the Grass Rides Trail. Follow the trail as it arrives at a three-pronged fork, and continue up a short rise. Just beyond the rise, the trail arrives at another elegant avenue of cultivated evergreens.

## Appleton Farms: Grass Rides

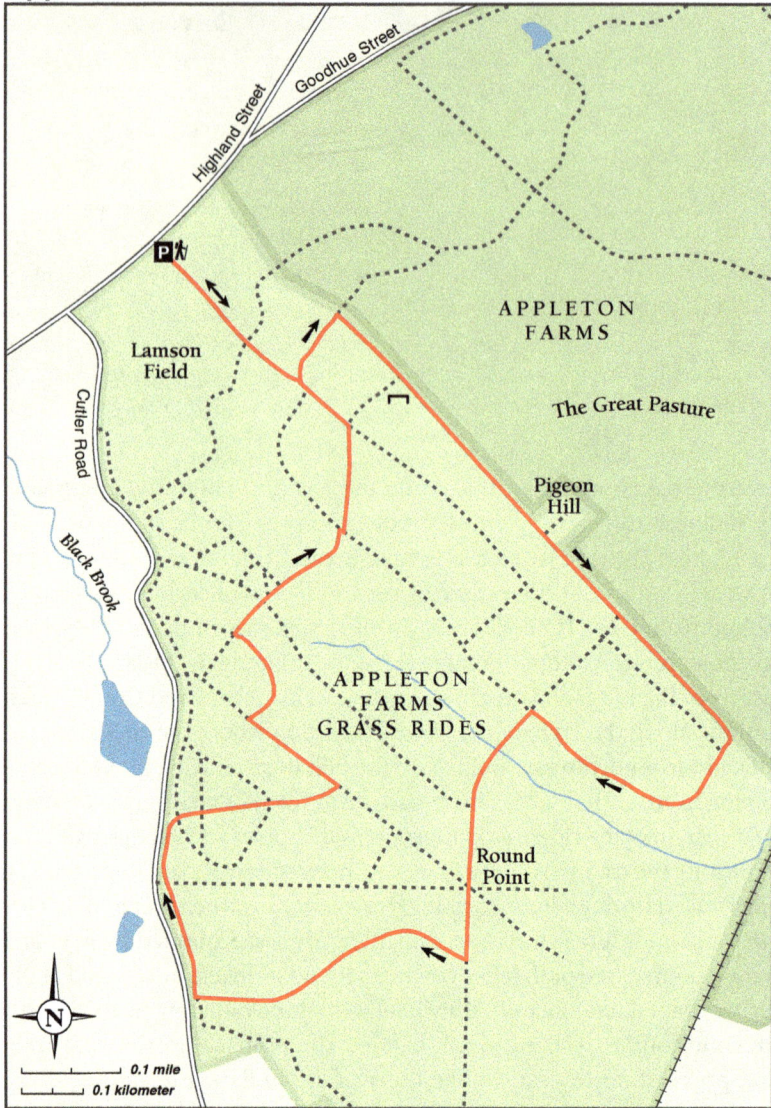

Heading east now, the trail takes you downhill briefly over soft footing. Passing through another intersection, continue straight and cross wetland via a short causeway. Just beyond this the trail joins one of the avenues that leads to the second pinnacle off to your right. Across the avenue lies a small meadow.

Turn left to head northeast. Evergreens stand on either side of the trail, with wetlands behind them. Upon reaching another grove of conifers, turn right to travel northwest. At the next intersection, bear right to cross a narrow causeway. Continue straight, heading northeast. Following a dip, the trail rises again and forms a T with another path. Cross here, bearing slightly left to follow the trail as it heads upward beneath a canopy of hemlocks. When you reach the next junction, turn left to head back past the column of maples that welcomed you as you began the hike.

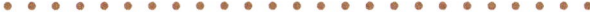

• • • • • • • • • • • • • • • • • • • • • • • • • •

**GPS TRAILHEAD COORDINATES**  N42° 38.967'  W70° 52.167'

**DIRECTIONS**  From Boston, take US 1 N to MA 128 N. Drive 6.5 miles on MA 128 N, and take Exit 20A to MA 1A N. In 4.5 miles, turn left onto Cutler Road and go 2.2 miles. At the intersection with Highland Street, turn right. There is a parking area immediately on the right.

This stately column of trees welcomes you to the farms.

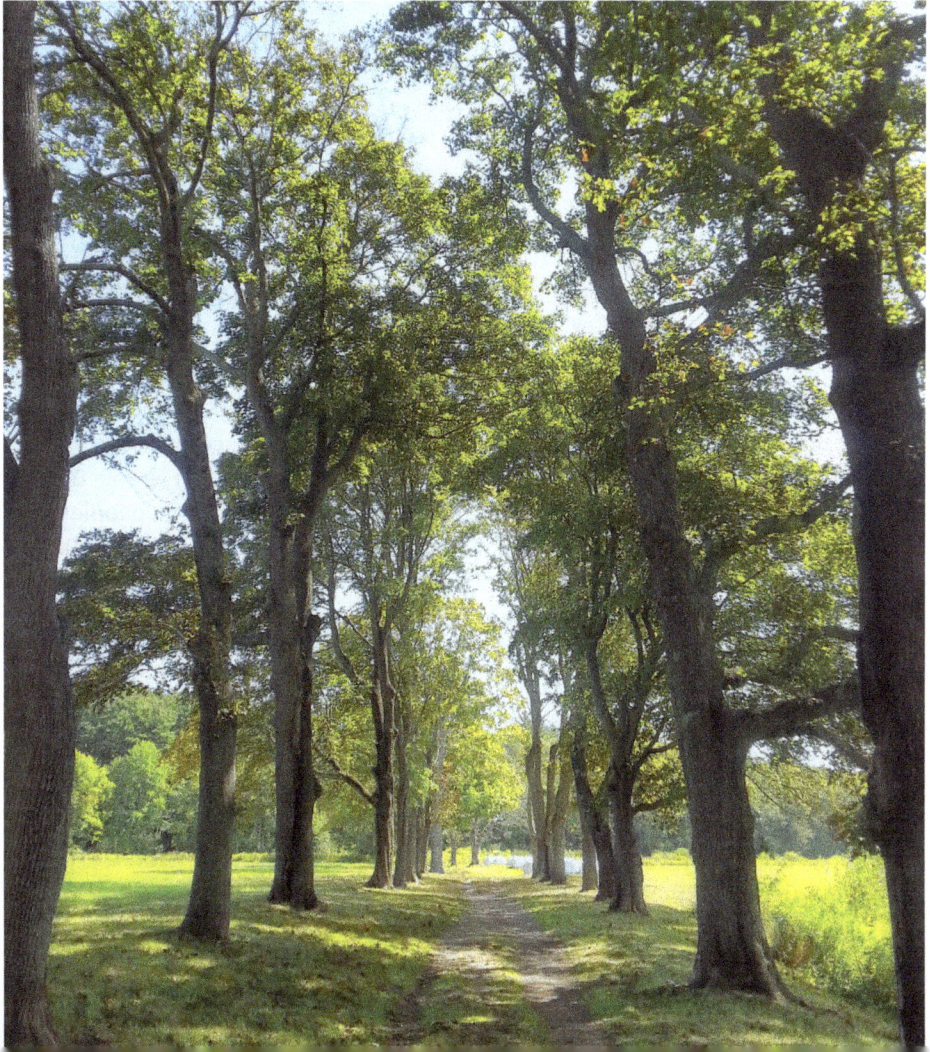

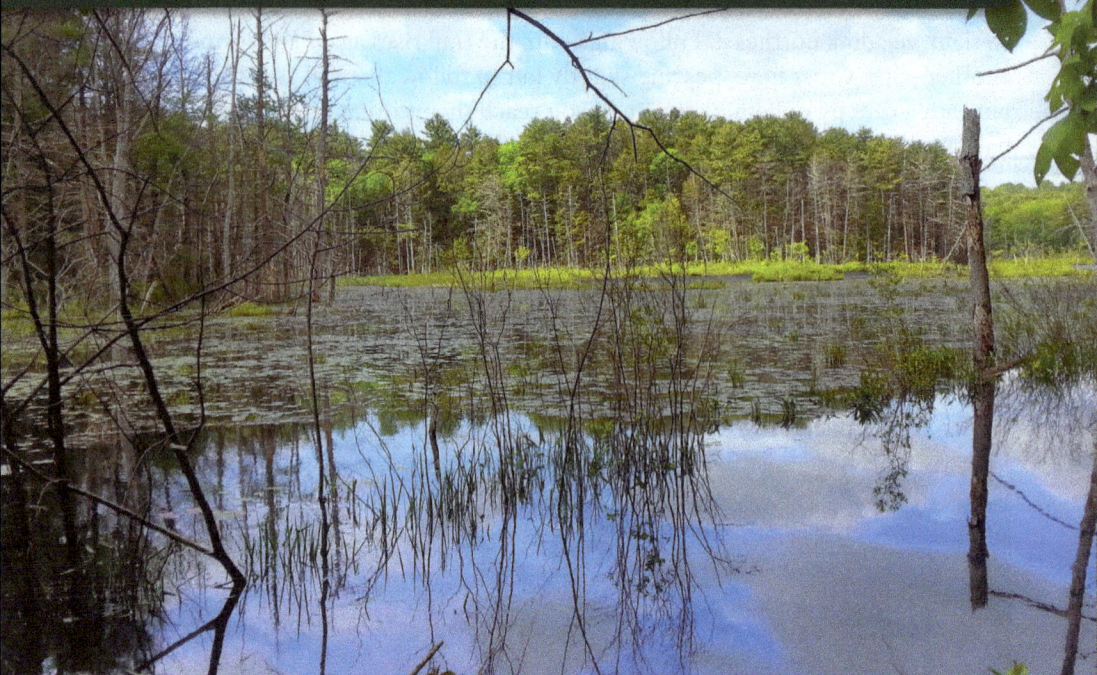

You'll need to pay attention to landmarks such as ponds to stay on the right trail.

**THIS HIKE CIRCLES** a great outwash plain of the Wisconsin Glacier and, while scaling Bald Hill, passes through an 18th-century farmstead once owned by a veteran of the American Revolution.

## DESCRIPTION

There is more to these quiet woods than first meets the eye. Sometime before or after the Wisconsin Glacier bulldozed through, volcanic forces convulsed at Crooked Pond. Drawn by abundant game, sheltering hills, and ponds rippling with fish, people of the Agawam tribe settled here. Colonial farmers came and went, and in the early 1900s the Diamond Match Company literally reduced much of the forest to matchsticks.

Start the hike directly behind the parking area on the wide cart road running west into a wooded landscape reminiscent of an unmade bed. At the first junction, marked number 19, bear right to continue southwest. Ascending a fold in the earth, the trail passes two kettle ponds, one on either side, as it bridges wetland. After winding over and between hillocks in the company of red squirrels and chipmunks, the trail meets up with an old stone wall. At an unmarked junction beyond the wall, bear left to descend a rocky but gentle slope.

As you get deeper into the woods, the clarity of the trail markers and sometimes even the definition of the trail itself are not always obvious. It even says at the bottom

**DISTANCE & CONFIGURATION:** 6.53-mile loop

**DIFFICULTY:** Moderate

**SCENERY:** Farmland reverted back to dense woodland, kettle ponds, vernal pools, massive beaver dam, remains of an 18th-century farmstead

**EXPOSURE:** Mostly shade

**TRAFFIC:** Light

**TRAIL SURFACE:** Firmly packed dirt, loose gravel, mud, flooded areas

**HIKING TIME:** 3 hours

**DRIVING DISTANCE FROM BOSTON COMMON:** 26 miles

**ELEVATION:** 88' at trailhead, 223' at highest point

**SEASON:** Year-round

**ACCESS:** Sunrise–sunset; free

**MAPS:** Available from the Boxford Trail Association/Boxford Open Land Trust (978-887-7031) or the Boxford town hall (978-887-6000), or at tinyurl.com/baldhillmap

**WHEELCHAIR ACCESS:** No

**FACILITIES:** None

**CONTACT:** Essex County Greenbelt Association, ecga.org/property/bald-hill-conservation-area, 978-768-7241

**LOCATION:** Middleton Road, Boxford, MA

**COMMENTS:** Sturdy water-resistant boots are recommended.

of the trail map, "Bald Hill trail loops are not marked in the field. Due to numerous small foot paths throughout Bald Hill, there are more trails on this property than shown on this map." Just pay attention and keep an eye on your orientation relative to significant landmarks, such as the ponds.

Upon reaching a clearing, stay with the cart road as it undulates northwest. Though not identified by trail markers, the rutted cart road is easy to follow. Passing by more vernal pools and kettle ponds, the trail meets another stone wall and then narrows as it arrives at junction 18. Bear left here and left again at the next split to continue south.

Proceeding along the edge of an enormous expanse of wetland, the cart road is now bordered by stone walls on either side as it rolls over waves of earth and stone. Ferns thrive in the understory beneath spindly oaks and vigorous pine saplings. Velveteen moss blankets the rocks underfoot. Coasting down a long slope to intersection 8, the cart road meets the Bay Circuit Trail. Bear left. Where the trail overlaps part of the Bay Circuit Trail, you'll find the Bay Circuit Trail more clearly identified.

Curving southwest along a floodplain that is perpetually flooded thanks to industrious beavers, the trail clings to eroding land. Here roots pop from the banking like veins on the back of an old man's hand. Barely a foot away, there's a small pool of swampy water darkened by shadows and oak tannins. The trail then climbs away from the wetlands and travels along a slope of rocky silt, known in glacial terms as a kame terrace. As the trail continues beside a stone wall on a level stretch and the woods thin, it feels as though there's more room to breathe.

Gaining momentum as it passes a hemlock grove beside a vernal pool, the trail descends and quickly devolves into muddy chaos. Immediately to the left, you'll

## Bald Hill Conservation Area

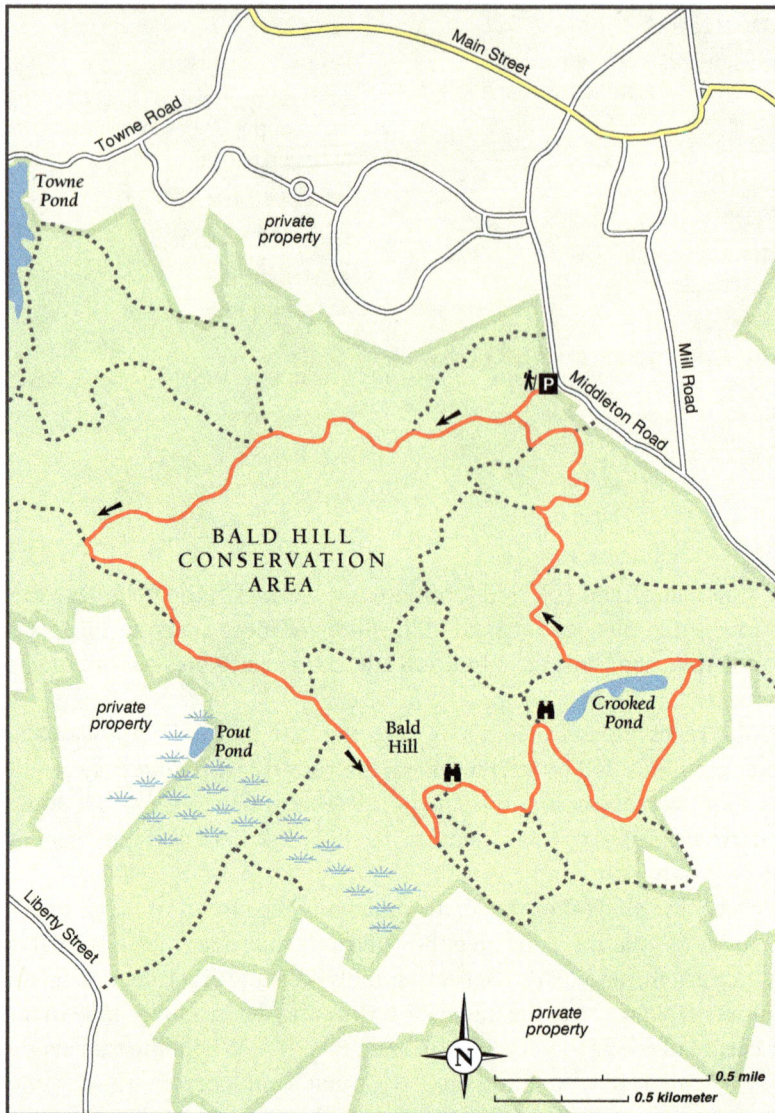

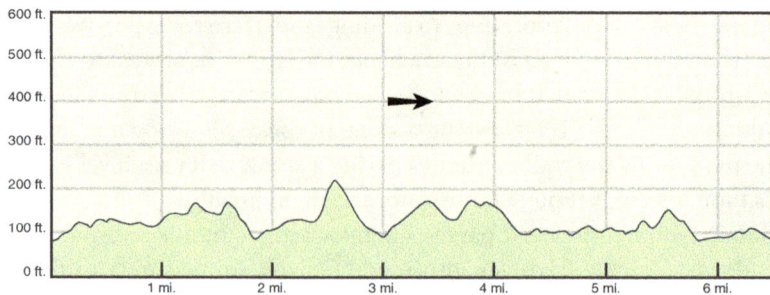

Main Street

Towne Road

Towne Pond

*private property*

Mill Road

Middleton Road

P

BALD HILL
CONSERVATION
AREA

*private property*

Pout Pond

Bald Hill

Crooked Pond

Liberty Street

*private property*

N

0.5 mile

0.5 kilometer

600 ft.
500 ft.
400 ft.
300 ft.
200 ft.
100 ft.
0 ft.

1 mi.  2 mi.  3 mi.  4 mi.  5 mi.  6 mi.

likely still see a beaver dam constructed of maple, oak, birch, and any other fellable tree stacked on a 20- to 30-foot diagonal and packed with mud.

Characteristic of construction sites, the dam has obstructed traffic and altered the trail. On a bank opposite the mire, the trail climbs back onto upland beneath the boughs of hemlock trees. Continuing uphill in this quieting evergreen wood, the trail comes to a tree marked with two white dashes, an indication that the Bay Circuit Trail is about to change course. Shortly after that, you'll come to junction 8A. At this three-way split, hike straight through, staying on what appears to be one of two branches of the Bay Circuit Trail.

The western slope of Bald Hill lies ahead. Composed of rock, silt, and topsoil squeezed together as two sheets of glacial ice collided, the drumlin amounts to a farmer's dream because the deep loam supported by layers of rock and gravel is fertile ground with excellent drainage.

Tracing the hillside between parallel stone walls, the old cart road leads up a gravel slope to a turn indicated by marker number 10. This junction is just beyond a pasture. Swing left at the turn to climb northwest to the site of the Hooper family farmhouse. Though the house is long gone, the foundation and remnants of the garden remain. Vines still climb the garden steps behind the house, and rhododendrons continue to flower each spring. Two or three hundred yards farther up the rugged slope, the trail reaches a mowed field atop Bald Hill.

From the 247-foot peak, follow the track as it bends southeast and descends back into oak woods. At junction 12, bear left and continue northeast. As the trail descends farther, water seems to percolate from all sides. And as conditions get wetter, more species of ferns appear, along with birches. Sweet pepperbush (*Clethra alnifolia*) and spicebush (*Lindera benzoin*) give the air a spicy scent. Late-summer blossoms of white alder or pepperbush attract hummingbirds and honeybees.

Ahead, where a vast pond becomes visible through brush, the trail arrives at junction 13A. Leave the cart road here, and bear right onto a lightly etched path heading southeast along the edge of Crooked Pond. Aim for higher ground as the trail ducks under hemlock cover on the pond's eastern side, veering wide of the wetland. In the dark woods bereft of underbrush, it can be difficult to be sure of the way. Ignore the arrow pointing uphill to the right, and instead continue straight (northeast).

Easing downhill, then up again, the trail meets with several stone walls. On the north side of Crooked Pond, the trail rushes downhill over a streambed. Markers disappear for a spell, but the north-pointing route is easy to follow. By now the pond is starkly visible on the left, constrained by upland immediately to the right. From this point on, the true route is tough to follow, as it is neither well marked nor well defined. Use the water as a guide until a marker for Bay Circuit Trail materializes near a stone wall close to the pond. A few feet farther on, there is a blue marker and then a sign posted by the Boxford Wildlife Sanctuary asserting the rights of the beaver. At this junction, bear left to follow Bay Circuit Trail markers as they lead northwest.

Still following the border of the expanding pond, the trail aims west then arcs northward to higher ground. At the fork ahead, stay to the right with Bay Circuit Trail to climb away from the pond. After scaling the rocky side of another basin, the trail slips back down to wetland, then, negotiating sloping deposits of sand and gravel, arrives at junction 23. At this split, bear left, staying on Bay Circuit Trail. Junction 22 is just beyond a wet patch crossed by wooden planks; turn right to continue northeast. Where it approaches a stone wall, the trail bends resolutely east. Ignore an arrow pointing north, and stay with the trail until it reaches junction 20A, soon after. Bear left and continue to the fork marked number 20. At this split, turn right, and follow the trail north to junction 19. At this final fork, bear right once more to return to the parking lot.

## NEARBY ACTIVITIES

The Topsfield Fair is held every year from the last week in September through the first week in October and is open daily 10 a.m.–10 p.m. To reach the fairgrounds from Boxford, take I-95 S to Exit 53 (MA 97). Follow MA 97 S to US 1, then follow US 1 S to the sign on the left. In addition to the fair, the fairgrounds host other events year-round. Visit topsfieldfair.org to view the schedule.

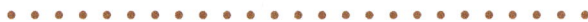

• • • • • • • • • • • • • • • • • • • • • • • • •

**GPS TRAILHEAD COORDINATES** N42° 39.067' W71° 00.200'

**DIRECTIONS** From Boston, take US 1 N toward Tobin Bridge/Revere. At 15.2 miles, merge onto I-95 N, and continue 6.3 miles to Exit 51. Take Endicott Road toward Topsfield/Middleton; head west from the exit ramp 0.2 mile. Turn north onto Middleton Road and travel 2.4 miles to the pullout on the left just beyond a small, white house.

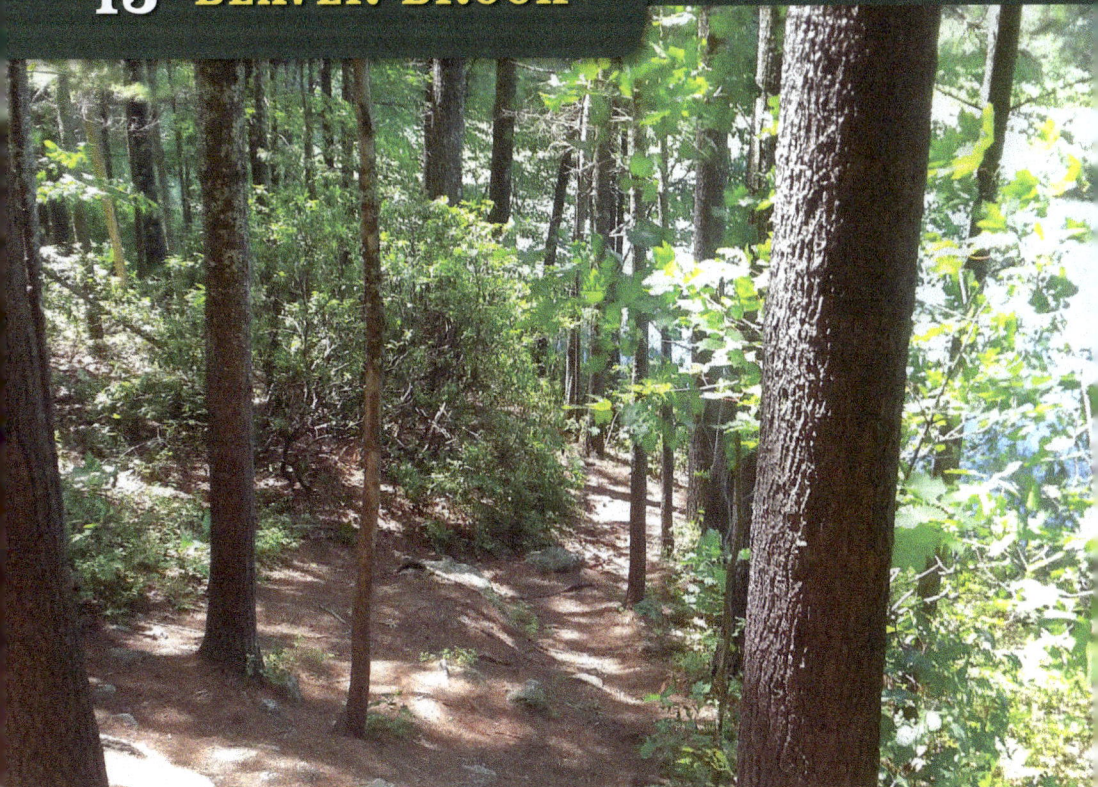

Beaver Brook is a large reservation with ponds, swamplands, and deep woods.

**LOCATED JUST OVER** the Massachusetts–New Hampshire border, Beaver Brook presents a landscape where beavers abound and loons or even a wandering moose wouldn't come as a big surprise.

## DESCRIPTION

Like many conservation projects, the 2,000-acre Beaver Brook exists because a small group of individuals with a passion for the environment got an idea and acted on it. It all began in the early 1960s when two cousins, Hollis Nichols, a Boston mutual fund manager with a love of nature and the outdoors, and Jeff Smith, a farmer, forester, horticulturalist, and already active conservationist, put their heads together and founded the Beaver Brook Association.

Today Beaver Brook consists of 90 separate parcels located in the Merrimack River watershed, most of which lie in the town of Hollis. An additional 200 acres lie in neighboring Milford. Invested in more than conserving land and protecting wildlife, the Beaver Brook Association runs a sustainable farm, educational programs for children, public festivals, and horticultural classes. All told, the overarching goal is to demonstrate how forestry, recreation, and wildlife can thrive side by side.

**DISTANCE & CONFIGURATION:** 5.69-mile loop

**DIFFICULTY:** Moderate

**SCENERY:** Forested wetlands, beaver ponds

**EXPOSURE:** Mostly shaded

**TRAFFIC:** Light

**TRAIL SURFACE:** Packed dirt, wooden footbridges, some rugged rocky areas

**HIKING TIME:** 2.5–3 hours

**DRIVING DISTANCE FROM BOSTON COMMON:** 50 miles

**ELEVATION:** 357' at trailhead, 504' at highest point

**SEASON:** Year-round

**ACCESS:** Sunrise–sunset; free

**MAPS:** Available at beaverbrook.org/bbtmaps .htm and the Beaver Brook Association office (open Monday–Friday, 9 a.m.–5 p.m., and Sunday, 10:30 a.m.–3:30 p.m.; closed Saturday)

**WHEELCHAIR ACCESS:** No

**FACILITIES:** None

**CONTACT:** Beaver Brook Association, beaverbrook.org, 603-465-7787

**LOCATION:** MA 130, Hollis, NH

**COMMENTS:** The Beaver Brook Association manages a cabin facility that accommodates up to 22 people, with two bunkhouses, a cookhouse, a well house, a campfire circle, and a primitive latrine.

From the notice board located in the right corner of the parking lot, hike north on Wildlife Pond Loop Trail, passing through woods along a stone wall. Starting out wide and level, the path soon reaches a junction, where it splits in two. Take the path on the right to continue on Wildlife Pond Loop Trail, marked with yellow diamonds.

Becoming narrower, the trail dips and bends over soft ground riddled with roots to reach the southwestern end of Wildlife Pond. Turning east and briefly leaving the bank, the trail returns to the water's edge, and what first appears to be a modest pond is revealed to be something more. Greatly elongated, this magnificent pond stretches on and on.

Five hundred feet ahead, Wildlife Pond Loop Trail is bisected by Old City Trail, which runs northwest. Crossing NH 130, this trail links the northern and southern halves of Beaver Brook.

Rising from the water just past this junction is a Taj Mahal of beaver lodges. Beyond this impressive structure, the trail leads to a bench arranged on a mossy nub of turf. Stop here to scan the watery landscape for a moose, a flashy wood duck, or a heron standing in shallows like a frozen shaft of lightning.

Winding onward, Wildlife Pond Loop Trail encounters a path to the right and a small footbridge. Mountain laurel adds elegance, and the plump fruit of well-irrigated highbush blueberries entices as the pond reaches north. Close by, too, is another beaver lodge similar in size to the first. Finally, rounding the slender tip of the pond, the trail turns and traces the opposite bank to its western end. Yellow-flowered lily pads grow densely on this murkier side, and flycatchers swoop from drowned trees to chase damselflies.

Short of completing the loop around the pond, the trail veers away from the wetland into a hemlock wood. A few yards farther, after a stone wall interrupts the trail, the path rejoins Old City Trail. Turn right toward upland here to hike along a

# Beaver Brook

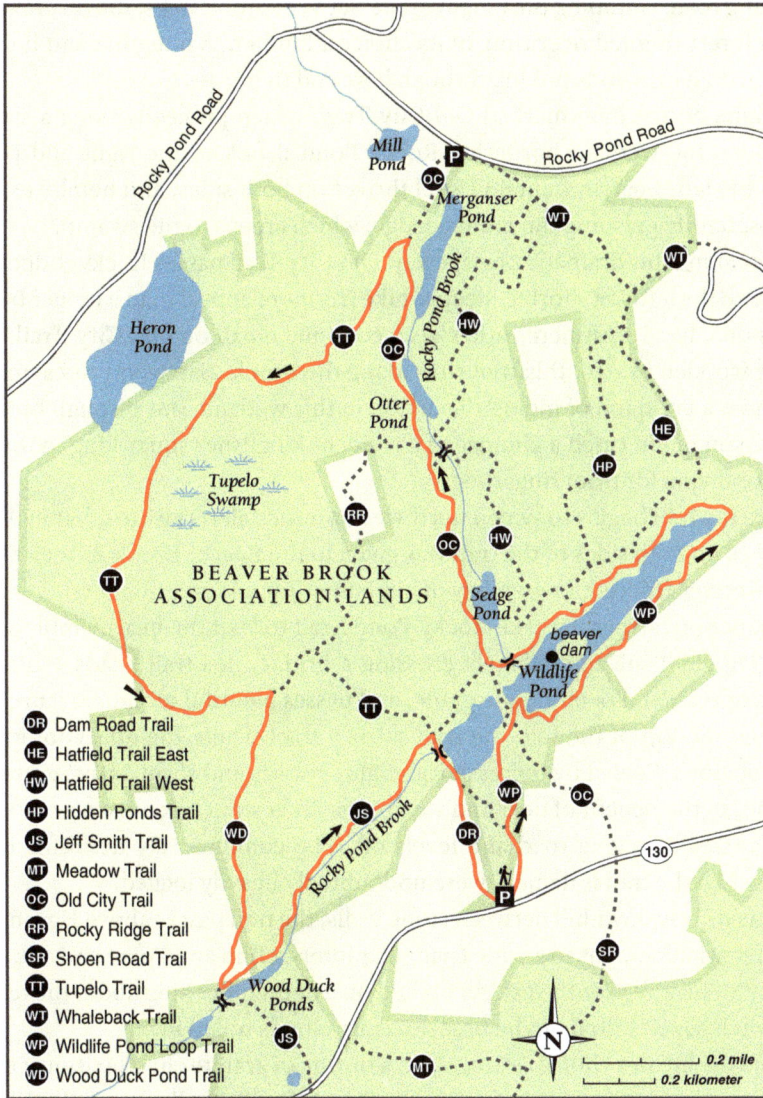

**DR** Dam Road Trail
**HE** Hatfield Trail East
**HW** Hatfield Trail West
**HP** Hidden Ponds Trail
**JS** Jeff Smith Trail
**MT** Meadow Trail
**OC** Old City Trail
**RR** Rocky Ridge Trail
**SR** Shoen Road Trail
**TT** Tupelo Trail
**WT** Whaleback Trail
**WP** Wildlife Pond Loop Trail
**WD** Wood Duck Pond Trail

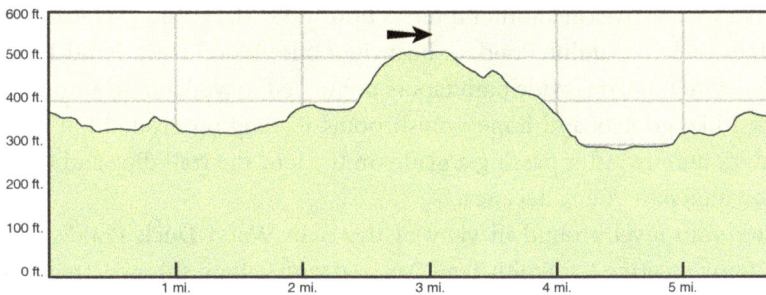

wide logging road. Climbing on a slight grade between stone walls, the dirt road cuts through a forest thinned over time of its choicest lumber. White pine and hemlock dominate with hardwoods poking through here and there.

Continue on the blue-marked Old City Trail, which proceeds along a sliver of land between the wetland bordering Rocky Pond Brook to the right and rugged upland to the left. Leafy mountain laurel thrives on both sides, and hemlocks tilt at odd angles, tightly grasping the granite ledge, which creeps to the swamp.

Not far along this dramatic passageway, Old City Trail passes Rocky Ridge Trail, which cuts to the left. If a shorter, steeper hike has more appeal than a longer but less strenuous one, head west here; otherwise, continue north on Old City Trail. Soon crossing a wooden bridge, this trail runs along the brook. Basswood trees, maples, and aspen do a good job of hiding the action in this wetland, but through breaks in the foliage you might catch a glimpse of a resident kingfisher squawking in the high branches or diving for trout fingerlings.

Where the trail begins to sweep northwest, a notice alerts visitors that in August 2005 acreage on both sides of the trail was given to the Beaver Brook Association by Debra Worcester Hildreth in memory of her father, John Worcester.

At a junction farther on, take Rocky Pond Trail to visit the nearby mill, or turn left onto Tupelo Trail. Immediately crossing a bridge, this trail heads southwest, narrowing as it ascends a moderate grade, and passes plentiful mountain laurel.

Nearing the top of the hill, the trail skirts a tract where the effects of logging are more obvious. Fueled by increased sunlight, grasses and shrubs have gotten the upper hand, to the benefit of deer and songbirds. A chestnut oak or two grow where the trail crosses a logging road and levels off. The commercially desirable tupelo trees, for which the trail is named, were undoubtedly heavily logged.

Making its way downhill between stone walls, the trail passes above Heron Pond and, moments later, opens to a wide triangular intersection amid pine and oak. Continue straight, heading southwest. As I hiked on a September afternoon, the lemony smell of witch hazel drifted on the breeze as rain clouds rolled in.

Behind the hill in a choice resting spot, a throng of granite chunks sits just off the trail like weary bystanders. Hereafter, the incline shifts decidedly downhill. Winding east, the trail soon arrives at another intersection. Take Mary Farley Trail on the left for a shortcut back to Wildlife Pond, or bear right onto Wood Duck Pond Trail.

Marked with blue, this wide path tapers unhurried to wetland. In autumn, amanitas shaped like goblets and honey mushrooms feeding on eroded life poke out from the dark humus. After passing a glade on the left, the trail dips and then rolls steadily downhill past young beeches.

Settling onto level ground in view of the twin Wood Duck Ponds, the trail makes a T upon meeting Jeff Smith Trail. Marked with yellow, this new trail emerges from between the ponds to the right and heads abruptly east. Whatever the season, I highly recommend the pond detour on Jeff Smith Trail.

Having been coaxed back to life by Beaver Brook Association volunteers, the Wood Duck Ponds are always beautiful—even in the smudgy gray light of an impending storm. In dim light, the red blossoms of cardinal flowers (*Lobelia cardinalis*) spark like flares. Like Old City Trail, Jeff Smith Trail connects the north and south sides of Beaver Brook. A half-mile or so past the Wood Duck Ponds, this trail crosses NH 130. But to complete the loop back to the parking lot, return to the intersection at the end of Wood Duck Trail and follow Jeff Smith Trail northeast.

Weaving between rocks, roots, and trees in a valley at the foot of the hill, the trail follows a brook connecting Wood Duck Pond to Wildlife Pond. Coarse granite rubble makes for uneven footing, while moist conditions bring orbs of pure quartz to a mysterious glow. After passing through a stone wall and over a footbridge, the trail breaks from the woods and arrives at a junction at the head of Wildlife Pond. Turn right to cross a constructed causeway and, once on the southern side, follow Dam Road back to the parking lot.

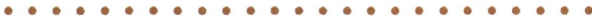

• • • • • • • • • • • • • • • • • • • • • • • • • •

**GPS TRAILHEAD COORDINATES** N42° 44.017' W71° 37.283'

**DIRECTIONS** From Boston take Storrow Drive E to I-93 N. After 5.4 miles, merge onto I-95 S/MA 128 S via Exit 37B toward Waltham. After 2.4 miles, take the US 3 N/Middlesex Turnpike (Exit 32B-A). Merge onto US 3 N via Exit 32A toward Lowell/Nashua, and continue 27.1 miles. Take Exit 6 (Broad Street) toward Hollis. Turn left (west) onto NH 130 W/Broad Street. Pass through one roundabout and continue 5.4 miles. Turn right onto Ash Street to stay on NH 130. Continue to follow NH 130 to the sign for the Beaver Brook parking lot on the right (note that you will first pass another Beaver Brook parking lot on the left).

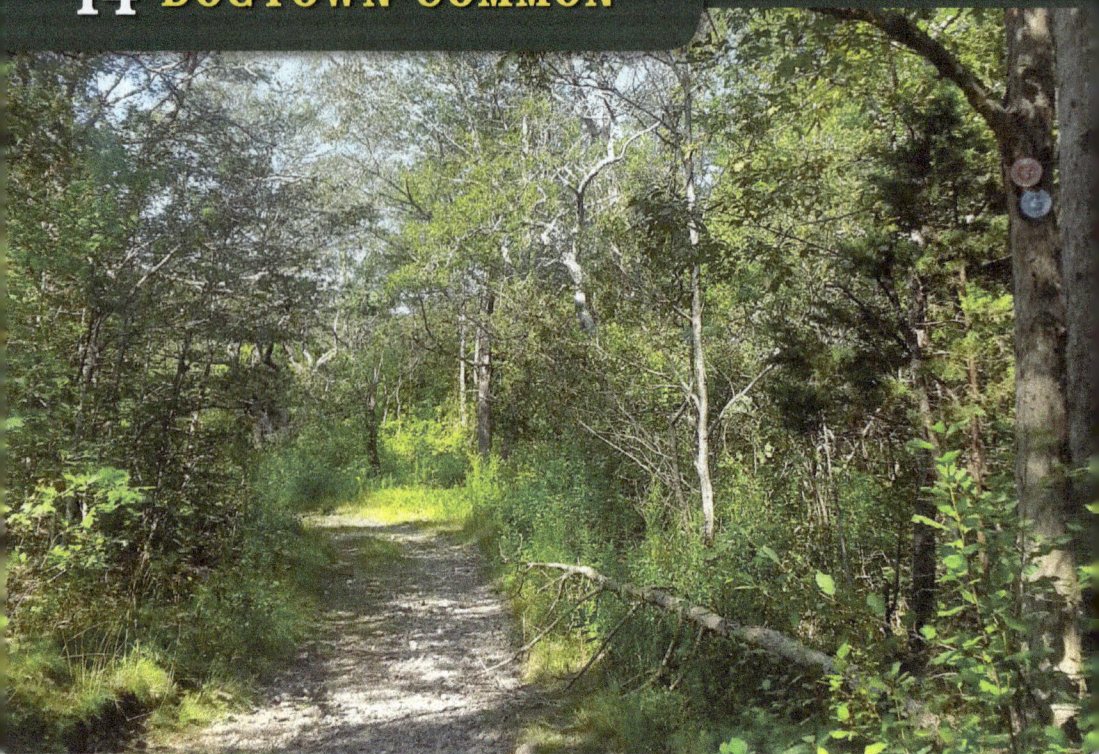

Bring a map and be ready for an afternoon of exploring.

**MEANDERING FOOTPATHS WEAVE** through beech woods piled high with granite rubble, skirt swamplands, and pass overgrown cellar holes and boulders engraved with words of inspiration.

## DESCRIPTION

Named for the many dogs that watched over the women and children of the village while the men were at sea, Cape Ann's Dogtown is seemingly as mysterious as its name. In the 1600s, farmers built modest homes here and spent their days striving to eke out a living from the unforgiving land, eventually turning to the sea as fishermen.

From the parking area, walk along Dogtown Road, heading southeast a short way to where it curves left and the pavement cedes to gravel. You'll come to a gate limiting access to pedestrians and mountain bikes.

Look right to find the trailhead. The trail winds gently through woods, first uphill then down. Boulders of all sizes and weatherworn shapes lie amid spindly oaks and cedars stunted and stooped due to scant nutrients and the granite ledge at their roots. After passing a stand of birch, you will see the Babson Reservoir at the bottom of the slope in front of you. Glacial erosion has stripped away topsoil, leaving massive chunks of rock.

**DISTANCE & CONFIGURATION:** 5.25-mile loop

**DIFFICULTY:** Moderate

**SCENERY:** Oak, pine, and beech forest; ancient cellar holes; granite boulders inscribed with inspiring words

**EXPOSURE:** Mostly shaded

**TRAFFIC:** Light

**TRAIL SURFACE:** Varies from packed earth to rough, rocky spots

**HIKING TIME:** 3 hours

**DRIVING DISTANCE FROM BOSTON COMMON:** 30 miles

**ELEVATION:** 109' at trailhead, 183' at highest point

**SEASON:** Year-round

**ACCESS:** Sunrise–sunset; free

**MAPS:** Available at parking lot

**WHEELCHAIR ACCESS:** No

**FACILITIES:** None

**CONTACT:** Essex National Heritage Area, tinyurl.com/dogtowncommon, 978-740-0444

**LOCATION:** 0.5 mile from MA 127, Gloucester, MA

**COMMENTS:** Because of Dogtown Common's rugged terrain and interweaving trails, both named and unnamed, it is a good idea to bring a map, a compass, and plenty of water.

Make your way down the embankment 100 feet or so to the water, following the trail as best you can. It appears the course of the trail has been interpreted in many ways over the years, and as a result no one way is the right way. Once at the water's edge, bear left. A passing train on the Boston–Gloucester line may draw your attention to the train tracks running along the opposite shore. Don't feel bad if you get a bit mixed up here at Dogtown. Bring a map if you can, and leave yourself time to explore. Not all the trails are well marked or defined, so don't feel obliged to follow a specific route. It still is a great place to hike though.

Continue northeast, through a split in a stone wall, and straight ahead you will see a large stone inscribed TRUTH. This startling find confirms that you have reached the Babson Boulder Trail. During the Great Depression, millionaire Roger Babson hired stonecutters to carve words of inspiration into 23 boulders scattered along this route.

Stay to the left of "Truth," and follow a rocky stretch along an esker. Soon after, you'll see a sign marked 22. Another trail forks left here, but stay on the esker as the Babson Boulder Trail heads right.

Peering between beech limbs, you will notice a neat network of stone walls laid out in a tumbling grid. A little farther along, you will find another of Babson's boulders, this one inscribed WORK. Continuing east you will begin to notice mountain laurel adding softness to the hardwood forest. A bit farther along, you will encounter a boulder inscribed COURAGE.

Note that several colors seem to denote the same trail; follow the blazes without concerning yourself with a particular color. After cutting through a gap in a stone wall, bear left. The other route leads across the railroad track to the Babson Museum.

Hiking north takes you to the "Loyalty" boulder. The trail then narrows and winds like the cow path it may once have been. Farther along, heading northwest while stepping among stones, keep an eye out for a boulder on the left with the inscription KINDNESS.

## Dogtown Common

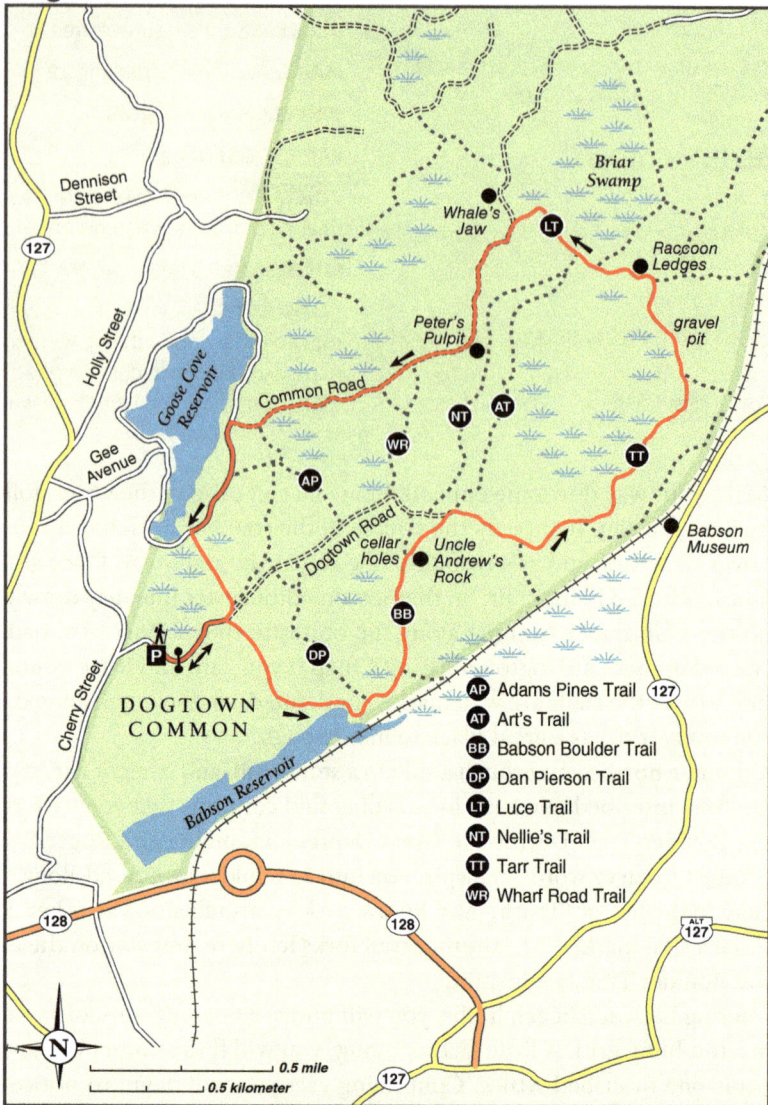

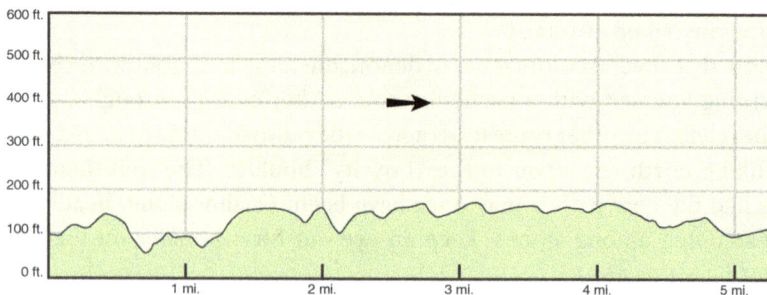

Dennison Street

127

Holly Street

Goose Cove Reservoir

Gee Avenue

Cherry Street

Briar Swamp

Whale's Jaw

LT

Raccoon Ledges

Peter's Pulpit

gravel pit

Common Road

NT    AT

WR

TT

AP

Babson Museum

Dogtown Road

cellar holes

Uncle Andrew's Rock

BB

DP

DOGTOWN COMMON

Babson Reservoir

127

AP  Adams Pines Trail
AT  Art's Trail
BB  Babson Boulder Trail
DP  Dan Pierson Trail
LT  Luce Trail
NT  Nellie's Trail
TT  Tarr Trail
WR  Wharf Road Trail

128    128    ALT 127

N

0.5 mile
0.5 kilometer

127

At this point, the trail levels and begins to smooth. The beeches thin, making way for blueberries. Up ahead you will find two more Babson stones, the first marked IDEAS, and the second, INDUSTRY. Just beyond these, the trail forks right to take you to the enormous Uncle Andrew's Rock, bearing the words SPIRITUAL POWER.

Make a semicircle around Uncle Andrew's rock, and rejoin the Babson Boulder Trail. From here, the footing becomes grassy and flat, and the tangled thickets give way to pretty stands of birches. A short distance ahead, the path leads into a circular clearing with a large tree at the center.

As trails radiate seemingly from all points, walk across the circle to a path slightly left of a large cedar tree. When this trail forks, bear right. A little farther along, look for a sign marked 10, denoting Art's Trail. Instead of taking this route, pick up the Tarr Trail, which heads right to another gathering of dwarfing boulders. Tarr Trail immediately turns squirrelly, becoming narrow and winding as it heads southeast.

At the end of a tricky downhill, the trail arrives at a wide intersection. A tree standing directly ahead is marked with red, white, and blue. Turn left here and ascend the facing slope. Here again you will see blazes of all colors marking the way. Try to follow the lime-green ones. The trail then weaves erratically north as ragged rocks heaved together by glacial force make forging a straight route impossible.

As you twist through crevices to make your way along this goat path, listen for a stream to the west. The volume of both sound and water increases as you reach a wetland at the foot of the Tarr Trail esker. Red pine replaces beech as the dominant tree in these parts. Several large pines disgorged by lightning stand near the trail.

Reaching another clearing, you will notice a sign marked 13, denoting an old gravel pit. Continue left (northwest). Young beeches crowd out pines, and barbed-wire fencing subdued by rust lines the path.

Arriving at a rise called Raccoon Ledges, the trail splits to the left and right. Choose the left route, and continue northeast. Following the groove of the trail—not the colored blazes—you'll soon come to a small vernal pool on the left.

After turning northwest, the trail runs downhill to the boardwalk at Briar Swamp. Be careful not to be lured to the right by another trail running southeast. Look north to see a stone dam or causeway. The boardwalk is to the right, hidden in reeds. If you like, split off here for a short walk through the briar; otherwise, hike across the causeway. Up ahead, you come to a broad intersection where the boardwalk ends and Luce Trail starts. Continue northwest, passing trails heading sharply left.

Leaving the wetland, the trail becomes wider and much easier to follow. Passing another trail heading right, continue as the trail bends distinctly west. After running southeast for a stretch, the trail passes to the right of Peter's Pulpit, another extraordinary boulder. Beyond, the gravel route veers west along woods of cedar.

Pass another trail heading left, and continue on what is now called Common Road. Looking into the woods, you might spot a stone carved with the number 34. This and others like it mark where Dogtown homes once stood.

On arriving at junction 2, turn left onto Adams Pine Trail. When you come to a split, continue left to head southeast. The trail makes a loop then bisects another path. Cross this intersection and continue straight to travel west. Before long, the trail ends at the service road for the Goose Cove Reservoir. Follow this paved road downhill to the right, keeping an eye out for a trail heading left back into the woods.

Follow this trail as it turns southwest, climbs past a pond, and continues over a narrow concrete dam. Winding on farther, the trail converges with a stone wall, crosses a boardwalk, then comes to an end directly across from where the hike began. Again, if you get a bit mixed up in here and don't end up following this precise hike, don't beat yourself up. Just enjoy the trail you're on when you're on it, and enjoy the sights and sounds of Dogtown Common.

## NEARBY ATTRACTIONS

If sightseeing interests you after your hike, consider Rockport's Bearskin Neck. This small peninsula located at one of Cape Ann's easternmost points has been the center of activity since settlers arrived in the 1600s. Once a busy docking area for fishing boats and the ships that ferried Cape Ann's granite to Boston and ports as far away as South America, Bearskin Neck is now a bustling artist colony with galleries, bookstores, boutiques, and eateries. From Cherry Street drive south 0.5 mile, and turn right onto Poplar Street. At 0.2 mile turn left onto Washington Street/MA 127 S, and take the third exit from the rotary onto MA 128 N. Turn left onto MA 127 and continue 2.8 miles. Turn right onto High Street then left onto MA 127A N to Bearskin Neck.

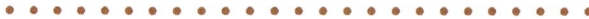

• • • • • • • • • • • • • • • • • • • • • • • • • •

**GPS TRAILHEAD COORDINATES**  N42° 38.033'  W70° 39.983'

**DIRECTIONS**  From Boston, take US 1 N to MA 128 N and continue to Gloucester. At the large traffic circle in Gloucester, exit left onto MA 127 toward Annisquam and follow it 0.5 mile, crossing a small bridge. Turn right onto Reynard Street. Follow Reynard Street to the end and turn left onto Cherry Street; soon after, turn up a steep road to the right, marked with a sign for Dogtown Common.

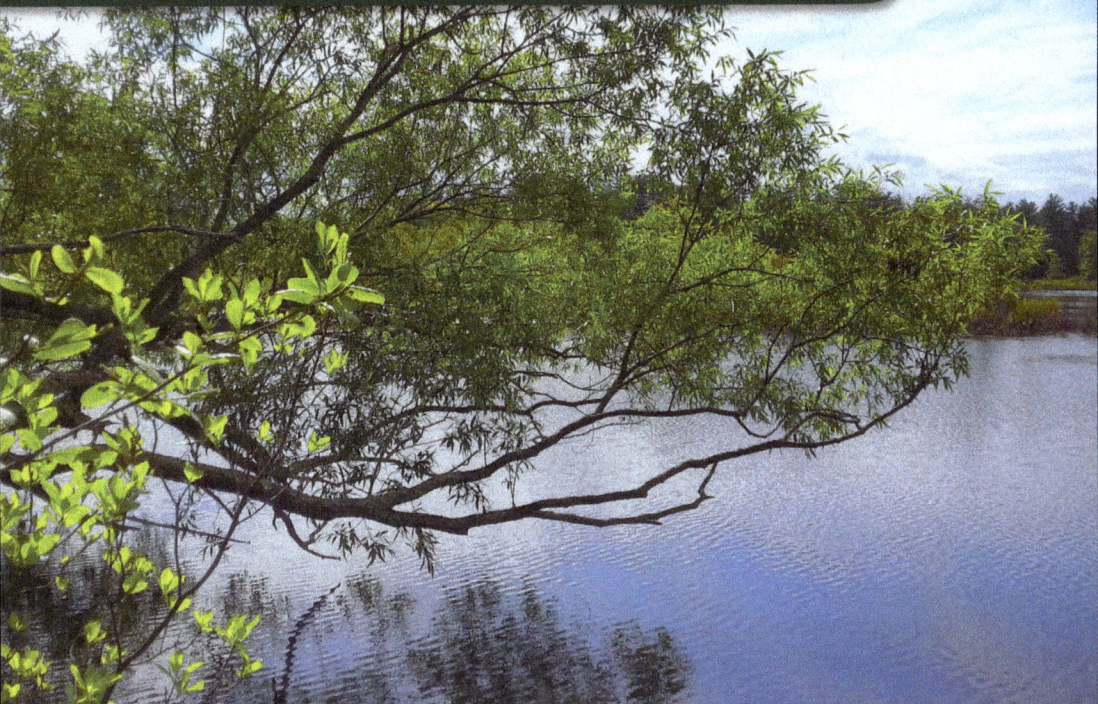

The pondside trees at Goldsmith Reservation evoke the feeling of a Japanese Zen garden.

**THIS HIKE EXPLORES** the fabulously glaciated woodland landscape around a large pond named for one of Andover's first settlers.

## DESCRIPTION

From the trailhead at the far end of the parking area, start your hike heading west on Zack's Way, a smooth, firm, level path about the width of a farm cart. Easing downhill alongside a brook past a kiosk and AVIS signs, this old-time service road nests on the bank beneath rock, sand, and gravel shoved high by glacial ice 10,000–12,000 years ago. A bit farther ahead, Zack's Way swings left. Bear right on the High Trail to ascend a great ridge rimming wetland to the north. Dark, tall, straight pines mixed with a few birches fill in the view of the gurgling waters of Frye's Brook down below.

Edged for a while by a weathered stone wall, the trail traces the ridge west, passing an unmarked path to the left before leaving the wall and descending to a clearing on the shore of an old millpond. Steer left, taking up the Pine Trail, which joins in off the hillside and travels south, keeping within sight of Foster's Pond and its swampy border. Rolling over gentle dips and swells through mixed woods accented with young aspens, the trail soon rises to a broad junction cut into a stand of black pines. Noting Zack's Way entering from the left and a new trail, make a beeline for

**DISTANCE & CONFIGURATION:** 3.67-mile loop

**DIFFICULTY:** Easy–moderate

**SCENERY:** Woods, wetlands, large pond

**EXPOSURE:** Mostly shaded

**TRAFFIC:** Light

**TRAIL SURFACE:** Packed dirt, gravel, a few boardwalks

**HIKING TIME:** 1–1.5 hours

**DRIVING DISTANCE FROM BOSTON COMMON:** 22 miles

**ELEVATION:** 95' at trailhead, no significant gain

**SEASON:** Year-round

**ACCESS:** Sunrise–sunset; free

**MAPS:** Find maps to Goldsmith Reservation at avisandover.org/assets/maps/goldsmith.pdf

**WHEELCHAIR ACCESS:** Zack's Way, which leads from the parking area to Foster's Pond, is fairly rough but passable.

**FACILITIES:** None

**CONTACT:** The Andover Village Improvement Society, avisandover.org/goldsmith.html

**LOCATION:** MA 28, Andover, MA

**COMMENTS:** Though short in miles, Goldsmith Woodlands Loop is long in interest. Be sure to allow enough time for birding, admiring the plants, relaxing at Bessie's Point, and blueberry picking at the right time of year.

the pond by heeding the sign for Bessie's Point. The trails here are quite well defined and well marked.

Sloping downhill on a gentle grade, the path quickly dovetails with another then carries on through an avenue of black pines up to an elevated enclave that is rich with rhododendrons and laurels planted nearly a century ago. Landowner Bessie Goldsmith kept house on this peaceful hummock in a rough-hewn cabin from World War II through the Nixon years. She is said to have been more than a little possessive of her blueberries in picking season. Any trespasser she caught harvesting was met with a shotgun pointed at the bucket. Though indeed strong in her convictions, Bessie was not ungenerous—in 1974 she entrusted her entire property, blueberry bushes and all, to the Fund for Preservation of Wildlife and Natural Areas.

From the crest of the hill where Bessie's cabin once stood, follow the trail as it tapers to a slender spit of moss-covered rocks sleeved in highbush blueberries and honeysuckle. There is water all around, rippling with all sorts of life, from polliwogs and water striders to wood ducks and painted turtles.

To continue the hike, reverse direction and ascend the steps to a bench beside Bessie's homesite. When you're ready, head back and bear right at the junction encountered earlier, staying with the cart road as it leaves the pines behind and enters a wood of oak and maple to soon arrive at a crossroad. Here a sign alerts you to the former location of Zack's cottage on the right and his hop pit (where he apparently grew hops for brewing beer) nearby. Zack likely never met with the butt of Bessie's shotgun, as Bessie employed him as a caretaker for the woods and as a seasonal handyman in the summer months when she rented out cottages to vacationers.

After surveying the cellar hole of Zack's cottage, follow Pond Road west back toward Foster's Pond. After meeting with a path to the left, this rutted cart road bears north and rolls downhill, rounding a shrub-hidden bend or two to meet the

## Goldsmith Reservation

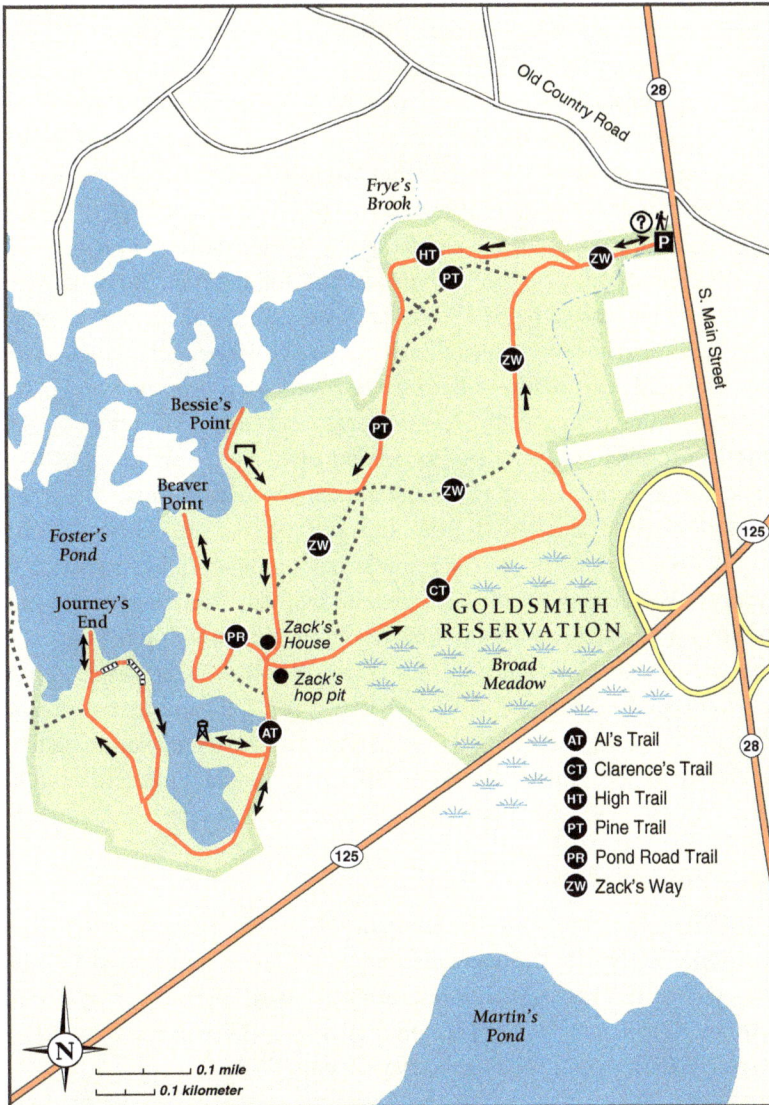

Map legend:
- **AT** Al's Trail
- **CT** Clarence's Trail
- **HT** High Trail
- **PT** Pine Trail
- **PR** Pond Road Trail
- **ZW** Zack's Way

water's edge at Wind Landing. To vary the route on the return trip, split to the right when the trail forks and hike along the pond's steep banking to loop back to Pond Road, heading east again.

Returning to the site of Zack's house, turn right and follow Al's Trail south, first downhill then across a causeway between wetland and Foster's Pond. Don't be turned away by the chain—its purpose is to bar vehicles, not hikers. Opposite a path that ventures up a steep rise pondside, the trail travels past meadowland fringed by woods to the east. Once around a weedy cove, the trail ascends into a hemlock grove arcing high and wide of the water to follow an earthen finger to Journey's End.

From the peninsula's narrow point, backtrack to a path branching left, and follow its lead across a boardwalk to the tiny island of Point Judith. Follow the path as it crosses to another oblong island via boardwalk and loops back to the hemlock wood. Aiming southeast now, retrace your steps over Al's Trail past Birch Cove back to the junction at Zack's house—detouring to the left along the way for one more gander across the pond. Turning from the pond, pass Zack's hop pit, and follow Pond Road as it dives east. Continuing over and through great swells and swales, the trail swerves west at a brook then converges with the level plane of Zack's Way. At this triangular junction, bear right and follow the sandy cart road east back to the reservation's entrance and parking lot.

This area is rich in history. In 1634 the Great and General Court of Massachusetts set in motion the establishment of an inland plantation northwest of the already burgeoning settlement of Boston. To encourage colonists to leave the comfort and security of the coast for the wild frontier, the court offered the first settlers three years of immunity from taxes, levies, and services, except military obligations. Thus encouraged, Andrew Foster and another 21 game individuals from Newbury and Ipswich ventured forth and, together by pooling resources that amounted to £6 of currency and a coat, transacted a land deal with Chief Cutshamache of the Pennacook.

According to the evidence, Andrew Foster won the gamble, for after amassing a sizable parcel of land, including the pond that now bears his name, he lived to the remarkable age of 106. His widow, Ann "Goody" Foster, did not fare as well. During the Witch Trials of 1692, she was condemned and died during her 21st week in jail.

## NEARBY ATTRACTIONS

Extend your stay in Andover by camping at the nearby Harold Parker State Forest (1951 Turnpike St., North Andover, 978-686-3391). The campground has 91 spacious and wooded sites, hot showers, and restrooms. The campground is open mid-April–mid-October. Trails in the 3,000-acre park also connect with the Skug River Reservation (see Hike 24, page 130) and the Bay Circuit Trail.

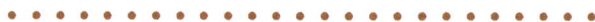

• • • • • • • • • • • • • • • • • • • • • • • • • •

**GPS TRAILHEAD COORDINATES** N42° 36.633' W71° 07.433'

**DIRECTIONS** From Boston, take Storrow Drive E and merge onto I-93 N via the ramp on the left toward Concord. At 16.5 miles, take Exit 41 to MA 125 toward Andover. Drive 2.3 miles on MA 125 and take the MA 28 N ramp. Merge onto MA 28/S. Main Street and drive 0.3 mile. An AVIS sign marks the entrance to the parking area on the left.

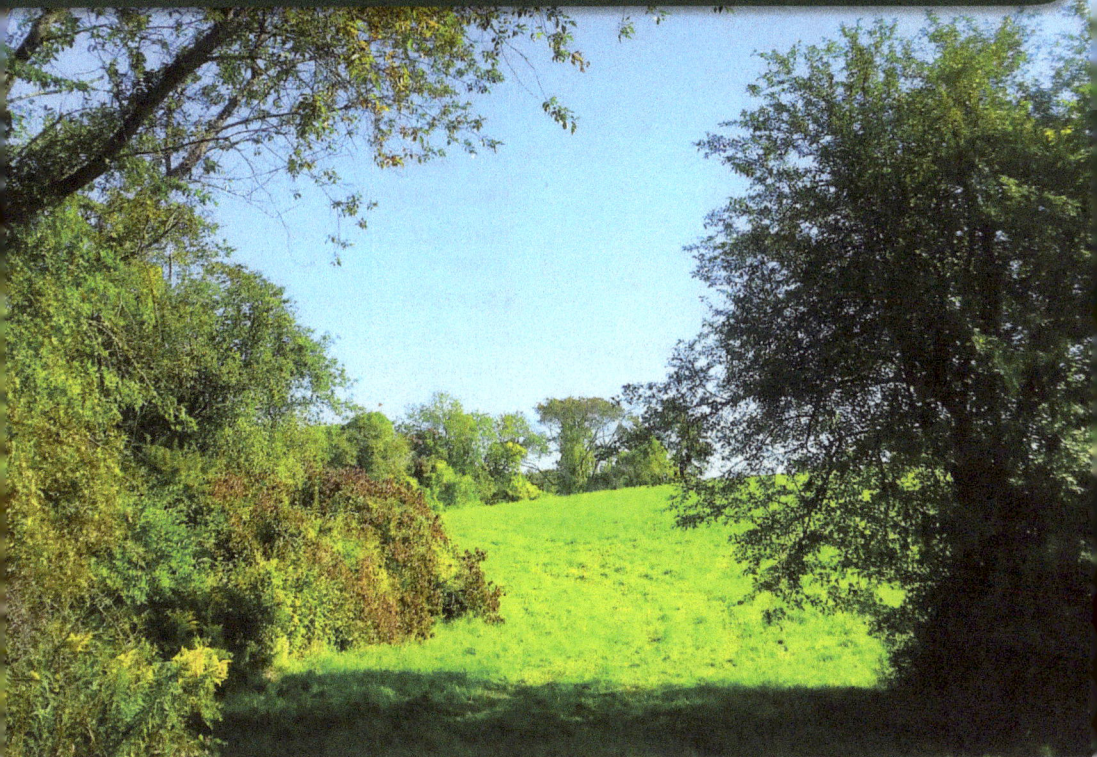

Great Meadow is a short but spectacularly scenic hike.

**IF MEASURED IN FOOTSTEPS** or time, this hike across the meadows of a 17th-century farm to salt marshes cleaved by a tidal river could be described as short. But if measured in beauty or ecological and historical relevance, it is boundless.

## DESCRIPTION

Great Marsh is a tract of 20,000 acres that includes salt marsh, barrier beach, tidal rivers, estuaries, mudflats, and upland islands across northeastern Massachusetts and into New Hampshire. An ecological gem, the Great Marsh has rightfully received a healthy amount of attention from environmentalists and land preservation groups. Because it is both a breeding ground and refuge for migratory birds, the Great Marsh—including the Parker River—enjoys international renown as an important birding area.

In the late 1970s, a small group of people and a fledgling organization called the Essex County Greenbelt thankfully saved a portion of the Great Marsh from development—the 100 or so acres that today make up Great Meadow. Today, the property is public parkland maintained and managed by the Town of Newbury.

**DISTANCE & CONFIGURATION:** 0.8-mile out-and-back

**DIFFICULTY:** Easy

**SCENERY:** Meadows bordered by woods overlooking the Parker River

**EXPOSURE:** Mostly sun, some shade

**TRAFFIC:** Light

**TRAIL SURFACE:** Grass, earth

**HIKING TIME:** 30 minutes

**DRIVING DISTANCE FROM BOSTON COMMON:** 33 miles

**ELEVATION:** 18' at trailhead, no significant gain

**SEASON:** Year-round

**ACCESS:** Sunrise–sunset; free

**MAPS:** Not needed, as this hike is truly straight out and back

**WHEELCHAIR ACCESS:** No

**FACILITIES:** None

**CONTACT:** Great Marsh Coalition, greatmarsh.org

**LOCATION:** 1.5 miles east of I-95, Newbury, MA

**COMMENTS:** As part of the Great Marsh, the largest salt marsh in New England, Great Meadow is internationally recognized as a significant birding area.

This is a supershort hike across a vast grassland to the salt marshes of the Parker River. And while it may be a short hike, it is long in its value for being peaceful, scenic, and restorative.

The sign that identifies Great Meadow may sneak up on you as you come around the corner on Orchard Street. If you happen to pass it, simply turn around at your next opportunity and backtrack to the road leading into the reserve. After parking in the small parking area at the end of a short dirt road bordered on either side by private homes and private property, walk east on the dirt drive to the trailhead at a metal gate. Immediately ahead, past a fringe of woods, lie two sprawling fields separated by landlocked wetland. It can be a little tough to spot the path initially, especially if the grass is grown in a bit higher, but you'll see it soon enough. Follow the narrow footpath worn into the ground over the grassland, heading southeast. After the tractor path bears left, the path climbs steeply up the side of a softly contoured hill. There is little to see here but acres of hay fields rolling beneath the sky like great ocean swells. Towering groves of various deciduous trees border the fields, containing them like rocky cliffs encircling an ocean inlet.

As you crest the hill, the peaceful grassland falls away, and the Parker River becomes the focus. You'll catch your first glimpses of the salt marshes through a buffer of trees. The slender waterway snakes east to west through rich salt marsh, looking much as it did in 1635 when Henry Sewall first established one of Newbury's first plantations on this location.

From this first lookout point, the path curves east along the topmost edge of the field then leaves the grassland through a split in a stone wall hidden by bushes. Continuing several hundred yards farther along a narrow peninsula, the path comes to an end at Gerrish's Rock. This narrow point faces a channel of the Parker River. Sheltered by salt marsh, the bowl-shaped creek just off Gerrish's Rock has been a favorite swimming spot for generations of hearty locals. This part of Great Meadow

## Great Meadow–Gerrish's Rock

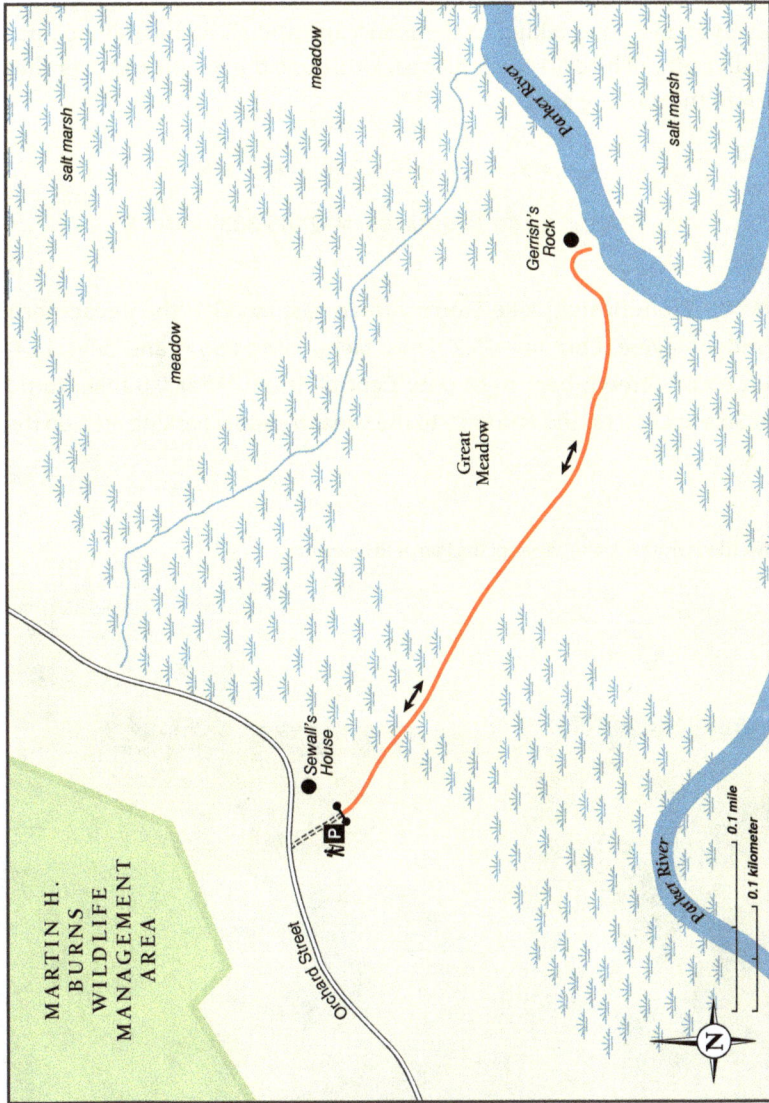

is also a perfect spot for a picnic lunch, birding, or photography. You could spend the better part of the day before feeling inclined to turn around and head back.

Fall is a good time for a hike anywhere around Boston, but this one is particularly spectacular, as the meadow has been tamped down somewhat and the massive stands of trees that define the border of the meadow on the far left and far right and along the banks of the salt marsh are ablaze in colors.

Once you are done taking in the landscape and all its inhabitants, particularly the rich diversity of bird life, meander back through the woods and over the meadow to return to the parking area.

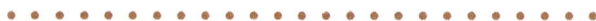

• • • • • • • • • • • • • • • • • • • • • • • • • • •

**GPS TRAILHEAD COORDINATES** N42° 45.333' W70° 55.250'

**DIRECTIONS** From Boston, take Storrow Drive east to US 1, then head north toward Tobin Bridge/Revere. Continue 15.2 miles. Merge onto I-95 N and drive 15.4 miles to Exit 55 (Central Street); bear right onto Central Street. After 0.6 mile, turn left onto Orchard Street. Look for the entrance to the Great Meadow parking area on the right.

You're rewarded with sweeping views of the Parker River estuary.

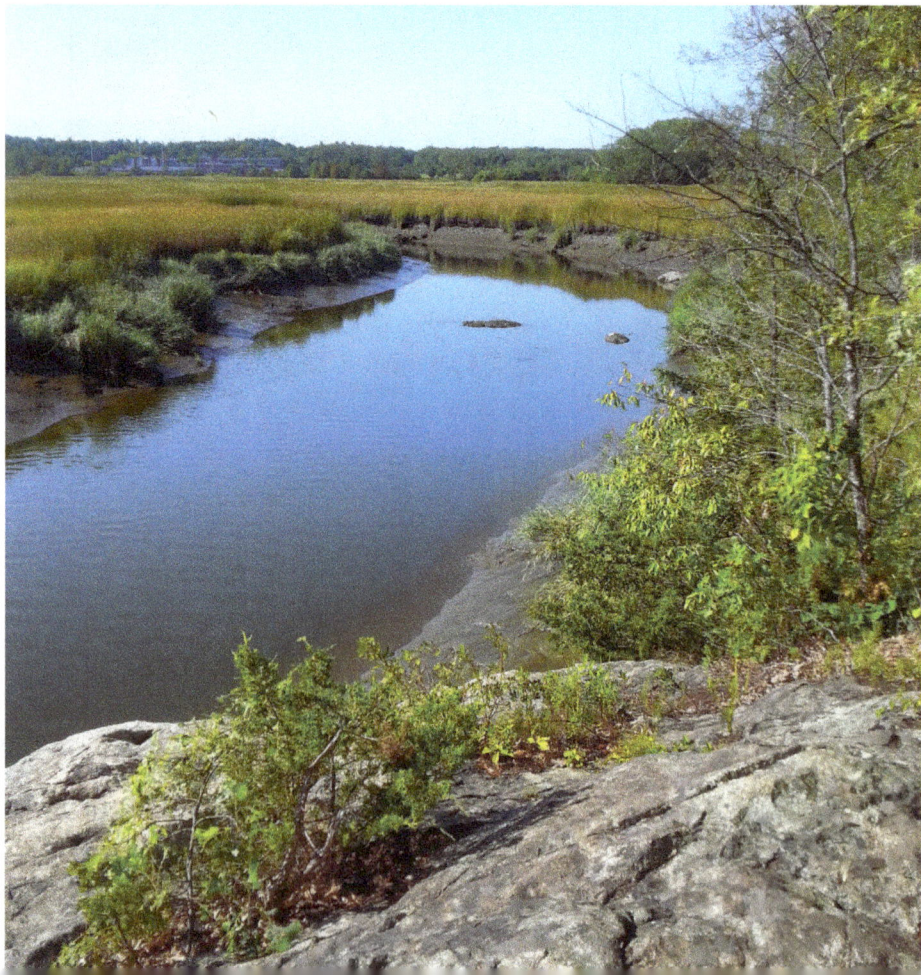

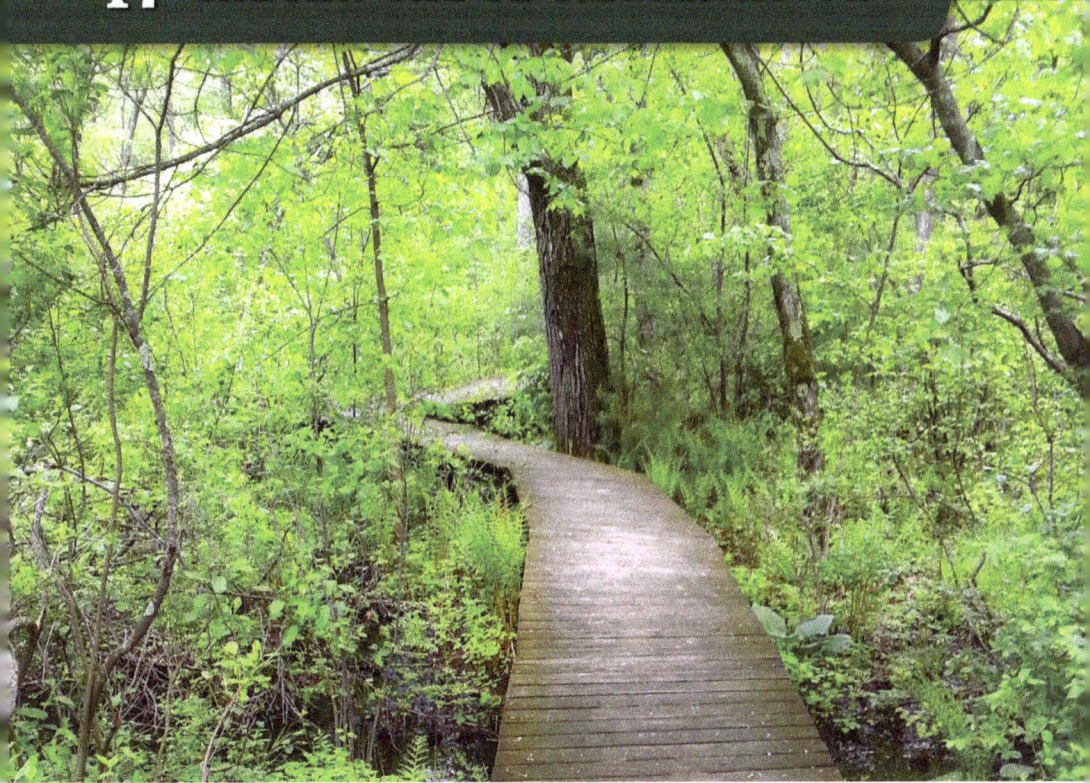

The Indian Ridge Reservation is a varied hike with woodlands, grassy fields, and swamp marshes.

**STARTING IN WOODS** not far from Andover's historic West Parish Church, this hike crosses a meadow, negotiates a 50-foot-tall esker, dips to wetland, continues over a second esker, and then loops around a large beaver pond.

## DESCRIPTION

This hike links three properties conserved and managed by The Andover Village Improvement Society (AVIS): Baker's Meadow Reservation, Sakowich Reservation, and West Parish Meadow Reservation. Starting at Oriole Drive, find the AVIS trail marker, and hike downhill toward the marsh. Continue hiking to the left several hundred yards around the Baker's Meadow marshland (with the marsh on your right). The pond eventually retreats from view as the trail enters the heavy shadows of woods and eases along the side of a sharply sloped hill. In spots where water percolates through underfoot, a boardwalk ensures dry crossing. Joining up close to a stone wall on its left, the trail soon makes a final climb to Reservation Road. You'll see the AVIS sign indicating the trailhead on the left of Reservation Road, then continue northeast across a wooden footbridge several yards into woods brightened in summer by blossoming waist-high jewelweed and other ground cover.

**DISTANCE & CONFIGURATION:** 2.95-mile loop

**DIFFICULTY:** Easy–moderate

**SCENERY:** Woods, meadows, pond, views from 2 tall eskers

**EXPOSURE:** Mostly shaded

**TRAFFIC:** Light–moderate

**TRAIL SURFACE:** Gravel, grass, firmly packed dirt, long boardwalks over muddy areas

**HIKING TIME:** 1.5–2 hours

**DRIVING DISTANCE FROM BOSTON COMMON:** 24 miles

**ELEVATION:** 117' at trailhead, no significant gain

**SEASON:** Year-round

**ACCESS:** Sunrise–sunset; free

**MAPS:** Online at tinyurl.com/indianridgemap

**WHEELCHAIR ACCESS:** No

**FACILITIES:** None

**CONTACT:** The Andover Village Improvement Society, avisandover.org/indianridge.html

**LOCATION:** 1.5 miles east of I-93, Andover, MA

**COMMENTS:** Andover offers hikers numerous trails through hundreds of acres of conservation land. By accessing the 200-mile-long Bay Circuit Trail, you can easily expand short jaunts into lengthy expeditions.

After traveling along the level banking of a stream, the trail departs the damp shade of the woods to cross a beautiful open meadow. In the near distance, the white spire of the West Parish Church stretches to the sky. Curving east over the domed field once grazed close by cows and now mowed by AVIS on a schedule that coordinates with bobolink nesting, the narrow trail parts clusters of milkweed and clover before returning to woods.

Wetland formed 10,000–12,000 years ago by the Wisconsin Glacier lies at the base of the field. Here the trail continues across a lengthy span of boardwalk over the marsh. A harbor for species such as highbush blueberry, ferns, and skunk cabbage, this primordial morass sets the stage for the equally striking glacier work that lies ahead.

At the gravelly crossroads on the far side of the boardwalk, the trail continues to the right, heeding Bay Circuit Trail markers as they lead up the side of an esker's slope of cascading glacial grit. Climbing higher, the trail eventually reaches the height of the rooftops of neighboring houses.

As suburbs spread and tracts of land are leveled and filled by graders and bulldozers, it is easy to lose sight of the terrific geologic activity that shaped the New England landscape. However powerful and transformative the human impact on the land may be, this enormous mound demonstrates the superior strength of nature. Formed of silt carried by meltwater beneath hundreds of feet of ice, this esker is a subtle but vivid reminder of the significance of climate conditions.

Passing well over the heads of the students and faculty of the school nestled on the esker's northwestern flank, the trail continues south, rising and dipping along the rocky ridge. Sheathed in the foliage of oaks, hickories, maples, and birches, the esker provides a well-camouflaged vantage point—a fact that wasn't lost on the generations of Algonquians and Pennacook who hunted here until Chief Cutshamache of the Pennacook sold the territory to white settlers for £6 and a coat in the early 17th century. That is likely the source of the reservation's name.

## Indian Ridge Reservation

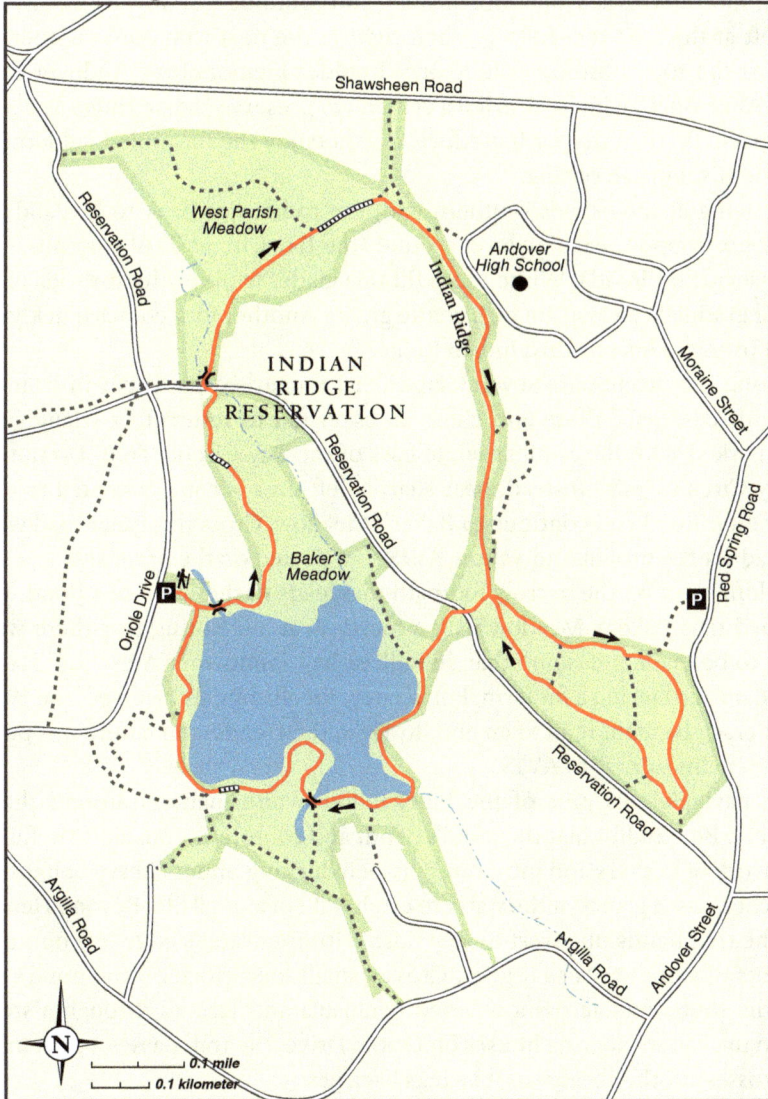

The esker eventually subsides and lists southwest. Another, smaller esker joins in to the right, forming a deep valley between them. Continue straight, following Bay Circuit Trail markers, ignoring the paths entering and departing from either side. Beyond a stand of young pines, a vale, and a rise, the trail arrives at an AVIS bench placed on one of Indian Ridge's highest points.

At the split on this downhill run, bear left onto a trail that leads to an oak-filled dell lying between wetland and the esker now tapering east. Crossing this floodplain, the trail soon arrives at a junction. Bear left and continue east on the Bay Circuit Trail. Bear left at the split that follows, then right at the next to mount another, smaller esker. At the top, a bronze plaque on a boulder memorializes Andover conservationist Alice Buck, who in 1896 led a crusade to preserve Indian Ridge as permanent open space. Be thankful for her efforts as you enjoy the unspoiled wilderness in its convenient suburban setting.

Arriving at the esker's southern end, the route dips back to lowland, turning sharply north upon reaching level ground (the Bay Circuit Trail continues south to join Reservation Road). White pines fill this glade, with few hardwoods in sight as the trail gradually rises again on a gentle grade. Another fork comes quickly; choose the left prong to hike toward Indian Ridge.

Along this stretch are several superficial unmarked paths cut in from the left and right. Disregard these and climb an esker tail to return to a triangular crossroads marked with the familiar white bars of the Bay Circuit Trail. Do not pick up the Bay Circuit Trail—instead, bear sharply left on a second esker tail to exit onto Reservation Road and continue to Baker's Meadow. Cross this quiet road with care, and head for the brown-and-yellow AVIS sign posted on the other side.

Hiking west on the narrow footpath that leads to the shore of a pond, you'll be reminded that Baker's Meadow isn't a meadow at all. Noting that there was more money to be made in fashion than in milk or hay, landowner Alexander Henderson built a dam and started a fur farm. Fortunately for all animals involved, the 1929 stock market crash brought it all to an end. In 1958, the Henderson family was persuaded to sell their "meadow" to AVIS.

To navigate this part of the hike, follow white markers around the pond's periphery. Be mindful that the pond's depth and contour is constantly in flux thanks to the work of beavers and muskrat. Between ducking under cherry boughs and lilting birches, cast a glance at the water to catch sight of animal life. Beyond Henderson's dam, the trail bends due west to stay flush with the water's edge, encountering the remnants of stone walls as it goes. Cross a small footbridge on the pond's far side. Then the route cuts across a wooded peninsula and weaves through a stone wall close to the water. Nearing houses on Oriole Drive, the trail passes a path on the left then crosses another bridge as it swings back east.

Upland banking closes in to the left as the trail eventually winds north, passing wetland extending from the pond. To finish the hike, take a trail back up to parking on Oriole Drive.

The name Indian Ridge recalls the rich history in this area between the English settlers and the native tribes. Before King Philip's War (1675–76), the Algonquians, the Pennacook, and the settlers of the Massachusetts Bay Colony kept a tenuous peace. Practical knowledge the Pennacook passed on to the settlers of Andover certainly helped keep many alive through the plantation's early years before farms were well established. The Pennacook and Algonquians, who had long been subjected to

Mohawk aggression, gained a crucial ally in the English. Change was set in motion, however, in 1662, when the Wampanoag chief Massasoit's eldest son, Alexander (Philip's brother), was summoned at gunpoint to a meeting by the Plymouth Court and died soon after of what was suspected to be poisoning. The incident enraged the Wampanoag, who read the hostile actions of Plymouth's leaders as part of a power play intended to control and subdue them. This precipitated the ultimate collapse of King Philip's well-tested tolerance of the white settlers.

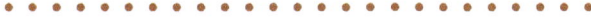

• • • • • • • • • • • • • • • • • • • • • • • • • •

**GPS TRAILHEAD COORDINATES** N42° 39.317'  W71° 09.867'

**DIRECTIONS** From Boston, take I-93 N to Exit 43. Go right on MA 133 E toward Andover and continue 0.8 mile. Turn right onto Cutler Road and follow it approximately 0.4 mile to the intersection at Reservation Road. Turn right on Oriole Drive and park at either of a couple of on-street parking areas on the left.

Be sure to bring bug repellent when you're hiking Indian Ridge.

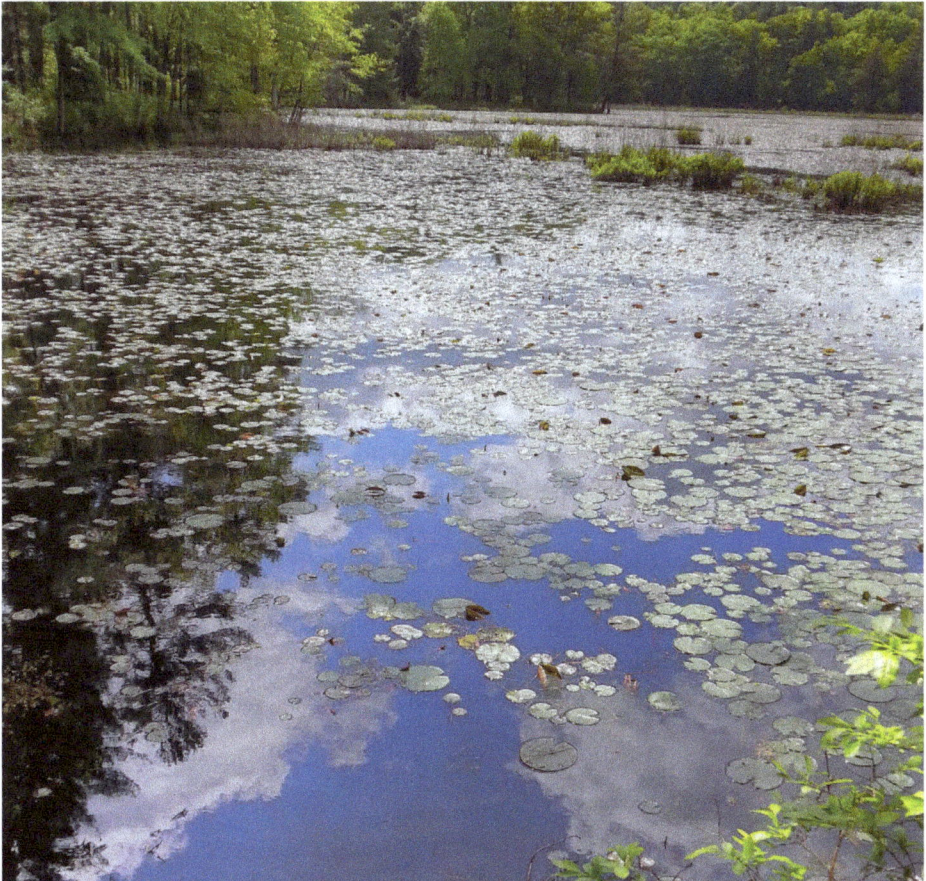

# 18 LYNN WOODS

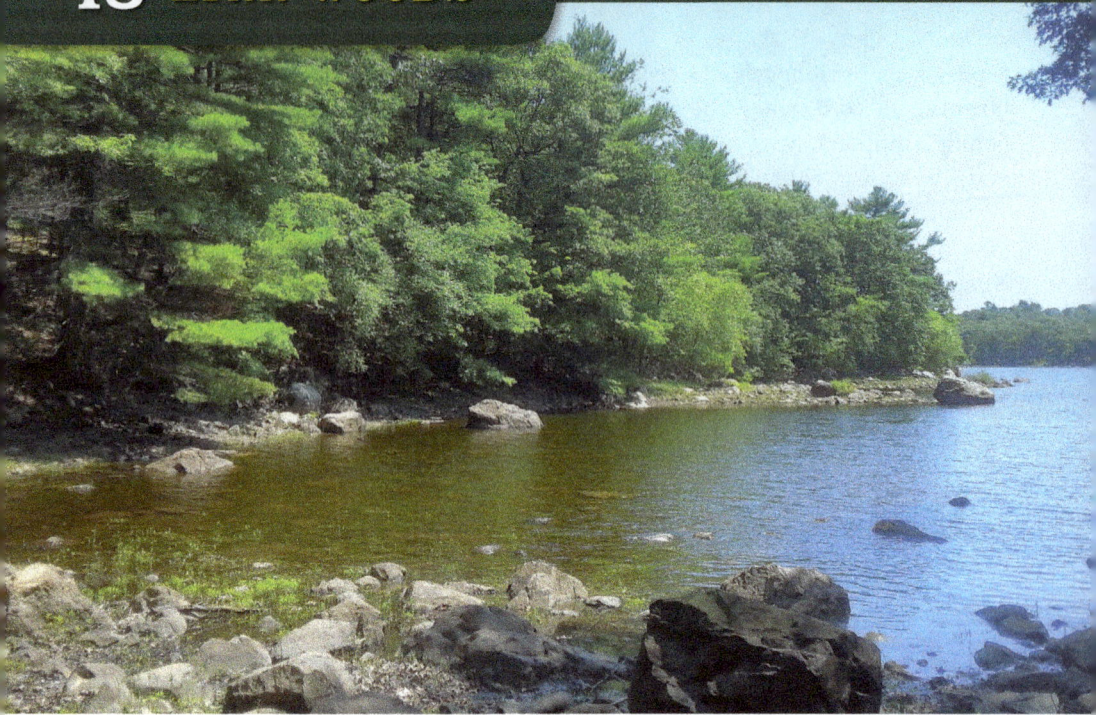

Well-traveled carriage roads and twisting narrow trails lead to peaceful pondside views at Lynn Woods.

**TRAVEL OVER THE** rugged hiking trails and old carriage roads of Lynn Woods Reservation to the top of Mount Moriah and along the shores of Walden Pond.

## DESCRIPTION

Lynn Woods is a remarkable 2,200-acre oasis within the busy city of Lynn. It's similar in its scope and proximity to the Middlesex Fells and Boston. This parcel of woods was first declared common land by English settlers in 1629. Turned over to private ownership in 1702, when the townspeople voted to divide the land among the town's landowners, the woods were gradually made public again after 1881, when a group of activists intent on creating a park organized to purchase lots.

From the parking lot, hike up the driveway to the special-needs camp. A blue arrow painted on a rock points to the trailhead to the right of the cul-de-sac located behind the buildings. At the immediate fork in the woods, take the green trail left, and continue west up a rocky slope. You are instantly out of the city and wandering through a twisting, narrow hiking trail, over roots and rocks.

Widening as it rounds Cedar Hill, the trail passes a granite outcropping just before a short path to the hilltop. Have a look, or better yet, bypass this detour, because the view from Cedar Hill is of nothing but trees. To reach a superior view, proceed northwest from intersection B7-5.

**DISTANCE & CONFIGURATION:** 5-mile loop

**DIFFICULTY:** Easy–moderate

**SCENERY:** Majestic forest, Walden Pond, scores of vernal pools, view of Boston from a rocky peak

**EXPOSURE:** Mostly shaded except on peaks, where the trail is in full sun

**TRAFFIC:** Light–moderate

**TRAIL SURFACE:** Packed dirt, some rocky slopes

**HIKING TIME:** 2.5–3 hours

**DRIVING DISTANCE FROM BOSTON COMMON:** 15 miles

**ELEVATION:** 101' at trailhead, 276' at highest point

**SEASON:** Year-round

**ACCESS:** Sunrise–sunset; free

**MAPS:** Available on a first-come, first-serve basis at the reservation; Friends of Lynn Woods also provides maps at lynnwoods.org.

**WHEELCHAIR ACCESS:** Pennybrook Road and the many other gravel cart roads are traversable by scooters and other motorized wheelchairs. However, the other trails included in this hike are not.

**FACILITIES:** Picnic tables and an amphitheater where open-air concerts are held in the summer

**CONTACT:** City of Lynn, ci.lynn.ma.us, 781-598-4000; Friends of Lynn Woods, lynnwoods.org, 781-593-7773

**LOCATION:** 2 miles east of US 1, Lynn, MA

**COMMENTS:** Many seasonal events are hosted at the reservation; additional information can be found at lynnwoods.org.

Where Cedar Hill meets Mount Moriah, stay left to continue on the green trail heading north. After crossing a ridge strewn with rock cut, carried, and spewed by glacial action, the trail bears left at a two-way split.

Beyond a basin piled high with blocks of granite, the trail ascends up a gravel-laced incline. Surfacing on flat ground once again, the trail then runs relatively free of stone cover to another two-pronged fork marked B6-3. Together these paths form a ring around Mount Moriah. To reach the hilltop by the more circuitous of the routes, opt for the path to the left. Making its way around the peak, the trail dips to wetland then levels at a sort of causeway. You'll see granite cliffs off to one side and blueberry bushes concealing bog and vernal pools to the other.

Descending past oaks interspersed with white pine and tender birch saplings, the trail swings east at junction B5-4, bending around a tree charred by lightning. Mount Moriah stands off to the right. Arcing around the peak, the trail, now marked with blue, crosses a sheet of granite then rises to a plateau where in autumn oak trees the color of flames all but singe the soft green of pine and moss.

Beyond another vernal pool, the trail splits yet again. At this junction, B5-2, the dark-blue trail veers left, and the (reappearing) green trail curves right. Follow the green trail through a grove of spindly beech to junction B5-3, which lies just beyond. This section of trail, which winds south along the side of Mount Moriah, is edged with carefully laid stone and, being well above treetops, provides an excellent vantage point. During fall migration, from late August to early December, raptors coast by, taking advantage of powerful wind currents.

For a 360-degree view of the surroundings, turn right on a short path ahead, and scale the last few yards to the top of Mount Moriah. Boston's skyline on the northwest horizon is hard to miss.

## Lynn Woods

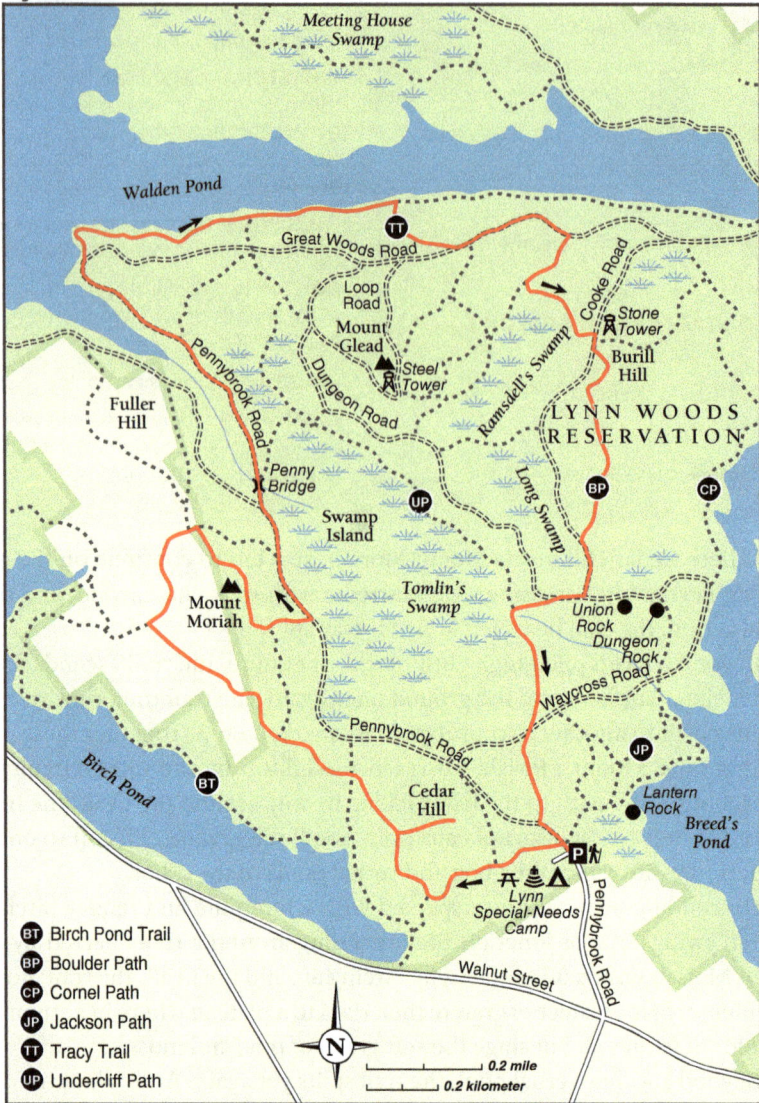

**Legend:**

- **BT** Birch Pond Trail
- **BP** Boulder Path
- **CP** Cornel Path
- **JP** Jackson Path
- **TT** Tracy Trail
- **UP** Undercliff Path

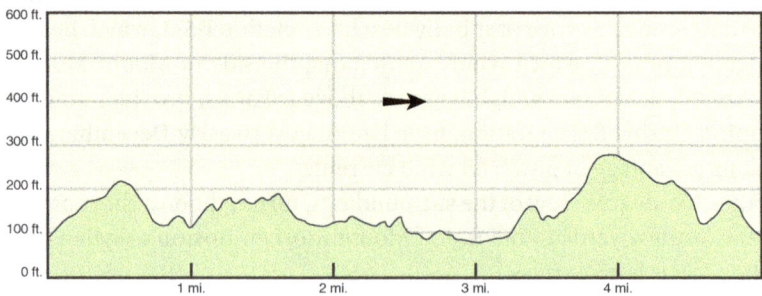

To continue the hike, double back to the green trail, bearing right to descend south. Upon reaching an intersection, turn left and follow this short linking trail to its end on Pennybrook Road. Leaving rocky elevations for a spell, turn left to pick up this centuries-old cart road.

Built for draft animals to haul out timber, this wide road tips gently toward the bridge for which it was named. After about 0.25 mile, at a broad intersection, Walden Pond Road departs to the left. Continue straight, following Pennybrook Road to where it meets a stream that is spanned by a fieldstone bridge. The trail rises slightly here.

Stay on the cart road as it travels along Pennybrook Road's tall banking beneath the overarching branches of maples, hickories, and hemlocks. Farther along the brook, the road's grade steepens. Soon hemlocks gripped tight to a precipitous slope hide the water below. Shortly, however, the magnificent Walden Pond comes into view.

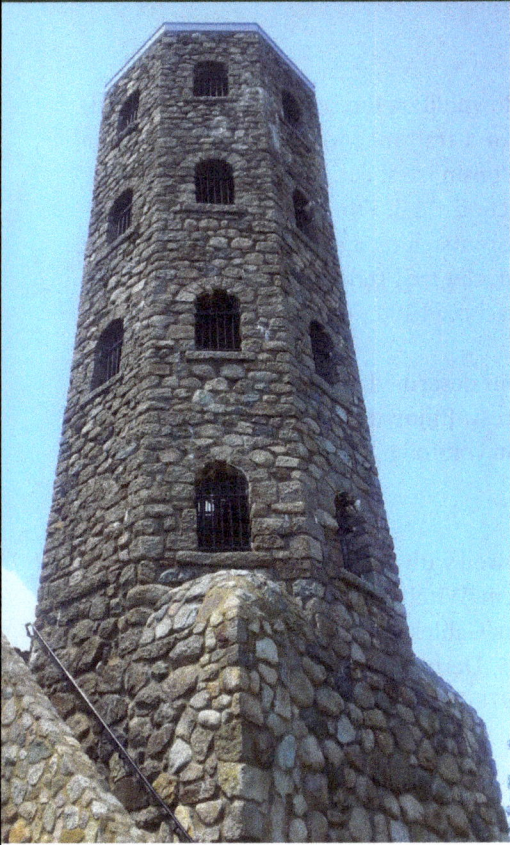

The stone tower presides over Lynn Woods.

Before meeting the water, Pennybrook Road bends east. Where it commits to the new direction, a sign alerts visitors to dos and don'ts, and arrows point left and right. Here take the Pennybrook Trail (B4-3), marked with blue, which dips immediately to the pond. Clear across, far enough off to look like a toy, a railroad line makes a silhouette against the sky and water.

The slender Pennybrook Trail traces a sketchy route beside the pond. Blue markers can be hard to find, but with the water's edge to guide, there's no losing the trail. At a little over 0.5 mile, diagonally across from a water tower protruding from trees on the opposite bank, Tracy Trail diverts to upland. Leave the shores of Walden Pond here, and follow this new route south to where it soon joins Great Woods Road. Turning left onto this cart road, hike onto the second path to the right, D5-6.

Zigzagging west to east, navigating Burrill Hill's granite ghosts of the last ice age, the trail emerges after 0.25 mile at the foot of a 48-foot tower. Although it looks medieval, this fieldstone fire lookout was built in 1936 under the auspices of the Works Progress Administration (WPA). At 285 feet, Burrill Hill is Lynn's highest point.

With the tower to the left, hike 0.1 mile downhill on the cart road (Cooke Road) to Boulder Trail. For 0.36 mile, this sliver of a trail meanders through a garden of granite vagrants dropped here by the Wisconsin ice sheet. At the trail's end, bear left back onto Cooke Road, then right at junction C6-3. From here hike left, traveling downhill to pass the Undercliff Path before reaching a stream trickling toward Tomlin's Swamp. Climbing from the wetland, the trail traverses Waycross Road to connect with Pennybrook Road. Follow the cart road 100 yards or so south to return to the parking lot.

As with many of the parks and reservations described in this book, Lynn Woods has myriad trails winding throughout the forest. Enjoy the hike described here, or equip yourself with a map and go exploring on your own.

## NEARBY ATTRACTIONS

A hike at Lynn Woods combines wonderfully well with a visit to Salem. Three attractions especially worth visiting are The Salem Witch Museum (19½ Washington Square, 978-744-1692); the House of Seven Gables, made famous by Nathaniel Hawthorne's book by the same name (115 Derby St., 978-744-0991); and the Peabody Essex Museum (East India Square, 978-745-9500).

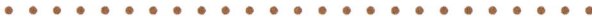

• • • • • • • • • • • • • • • • • • • • • • • • • • • •

**GPS TRAILHEAD COORDINATES** N42° 28.617'  W70° 59.200'

**DIRECTIONS** From Boston, take US 1 N to the Walnut Street exit in Saugus, then head east on Walnut Street into Lynn. After 2 miles turn left at a blinking light onto Pennybrook Road. Follow Pennybrook Road to its end to reach the parking area.

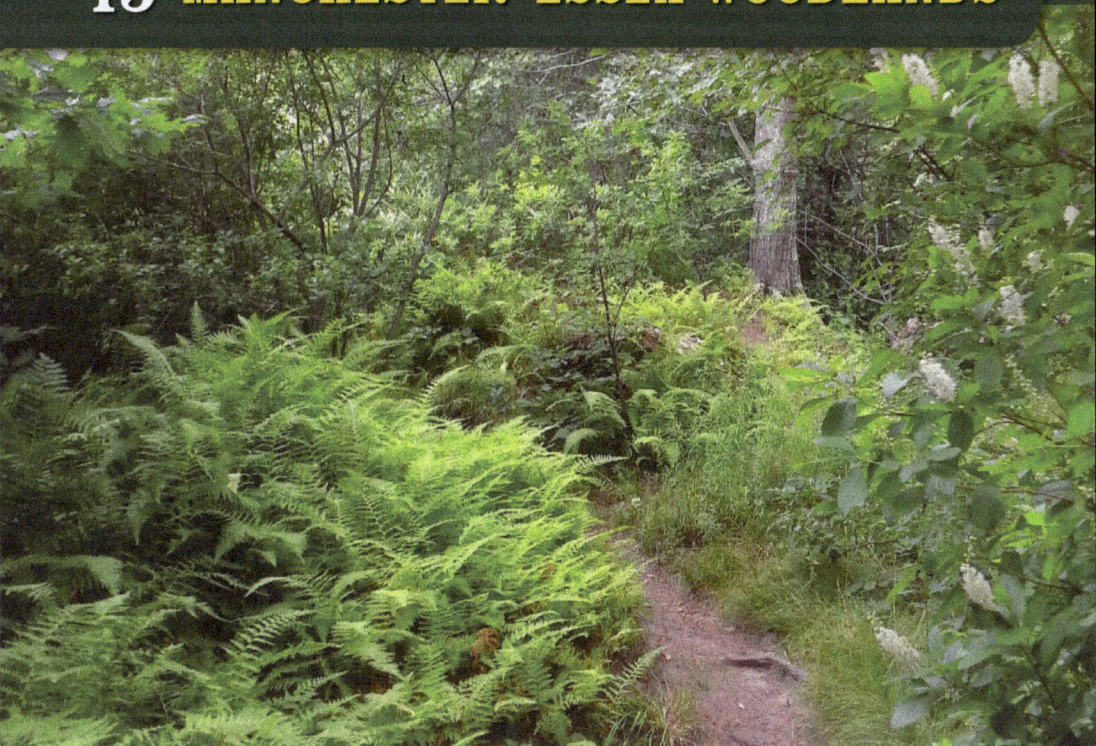

Lush vegetation at Manchester–Essex Woodlands

**AFTER TAKING A** 0.15-mile boardwalk across a cedar swamp teeming with life, this hike explores granite hills, an old cart road, and bogs dense with bayberry, maples, and blueberries.

## DESCRIPTION

Set out on the crushed-gravel road (Old School Road) heading southwest beyond a metal gate barring vehicle access. Running along the edge of wetland past dense marsh undergrowth, the road reaches the trailhead of the Cedar Swamp Trail after 0.1 mile.

Crossing this spectacular long footbridge, you'll see a rich array of birds, insects, and wildflowers. Close to the opposite bank, the boardwalk widens to include a lookout platform. Below that are steps to a dock at water level. After enjoying the view, and perhaps stopping to apply some bug spray, continue west to the boardwalk's end. Along the trail, you'll see gnawed stumps chiseled to points and nibbled trunks swaddled in chicken wire—evidence of the ongoing battle of man versus beaver. Hard to tell who will win this one.

After stepping off the boardwalk at a well-marked junction, continue left to hike south flush with Cedar Swamp below a heavy brow of granite and lashes of hemlock. A short distance ahead, the trail reaches a sign that appears to identify two trails as

**DISTANCE & CONFIGURATION:** 4.75 miles, 2 linked loops

**DIFFICULTY:** Easy–moderate

**SCENERY:** Cedar and maple swamps, vernal pools, hemlock woods

**EXPOSURE:** Mostly shaded

**TRAFFIC:** Moderate

**TRAIL SURFACE:** Packed dirt with rugged areas of loose gravel and exposed rock

**HIKING TIME:** 2.5–3 hours

**DRIVING DISTANCE FROM BOSTON COMMON:** 30 miles

**ELEVATION:** 41' at trailhead, no significant gain

**SEASON:** Year-round

**ACCESS:** Sunrise–sunset; free

**MAPS:** A map is posted at a kiosk at the parking area. You can also get one from the Manchester–Essex Conservation Trust, mect.org.

**WHEELCHAIR ACCESS:** No

**FACILITIES:** None

**CONTACT:** Manchester–Essex Conservation Trust, mect.org, 978-890-7153

**LOCATION:** School Street, Essex, MA

**COMMENTS:** Beware of biting insects from spring until the first frost. Saxifrage, spicebush, marsh marigold, goldthread, bluets, and hepatica all begin blooming in early spring.

the Millstone Hill Trail. Both are marked with orange blazes. Follow the trail to the left, following the border of the swamp.

Mosses and ferns pulsing green contrast with the black-brown mud underfoot and the gray feldspar-blended granite that punctuates the hillside to the right.

Continuing southwest toward the sound of cars on MA 128, the trail follows the course of an old stone wall. Bearing left to pass through, the trail then reaches a sign on the right that states PRIVATE PROPERTY—NO TRESPASSING. Stay with the trail as it climbs a rise and soon meets Old School Road. Leaving the woods and swamp behind, you'll be on the dirt road once more, traveling west. After paralleling MA 128 approximately 0.3 mile, the trail curves north to the base of Millstone Hill. Follow as it ascends a rocky slope. When you reach a split, bear left onto a wide gravel trail.

Passing an adjoining path on the right, the trail retreats gently downhill next to a stone wall. A hundred yards or so farther, another path splinters to the right, reconnecting with the Millstone Hill Trail. Continue straight to promptly intersect Ancient Line Trail, marked with both a red blaze and a wooden sign posted high on a tree. Bear left, traveling northwest into a stand of hemlock growing in a cleft between two small hills.

You are well away from MA 128 and any other road now, so the silence of the woods returns. It feels wonderfully remote and silent as the sound of traffic is replaced with the sound of woodland critters. Beech and linden trees blend in with the ubiquitous hemlocks. The bog emerges once again, with its great density of water, mosses, and ferns. Grit and chunks of granite bespeak the glaciers that left behind a vast array of debris.

The trail rises and falls through the woods, zigzagging in all directions. Here it is also quite narrow and fairly rugged with roots and rocks. Despite your relative proximity to civilization, the trail feels quite remote. Heading southeast then west, you

## Manchester–Essex Woodlands

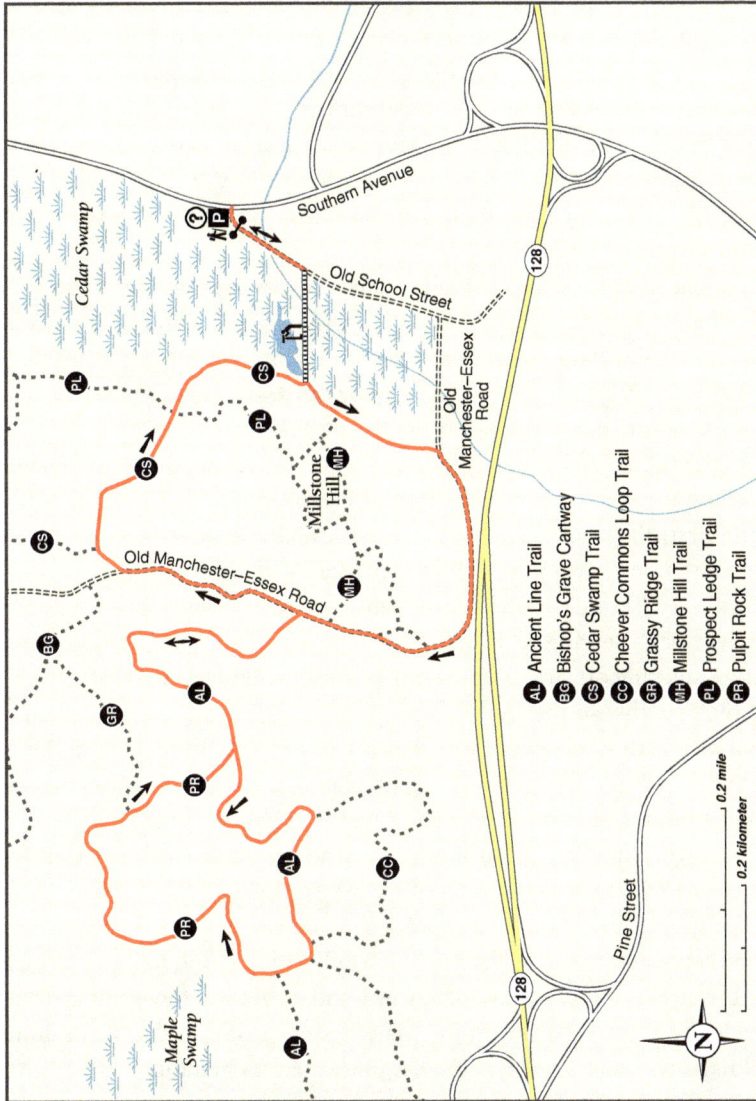

swing upland, passing a good many birches, though the ground is fairly blanketed with pine needles. Randomly strewn boulders, pools of water, and woven tree roots will keep you stepping carefully.

At the next junction, a sign for the Ancient Line Trail Detour points east. From here, follow red blazes west several hundred yards to a three-way intersection. Stay right to pick up Pulpit Rock Trail. Blue blazes lead the way north along the edge of a hill. Ahead, a spring marks a junction where Grassy Ridge Trail bears right and Pulpit Rock Trail keeps left on its northwest trajectory.

This wetland is fittingly called Maple Swamp. Being perpetually damp, the area fosters an abundance of mushrooms. In June especially, delicious oyster mushrooms spread out like fans from the sides of dead and dying hardwoods.

Climbing uphill over a mostly gravel surface, the trail parts the forest. Because of scant topsoil and unyielding ledge, trees remain small in diameter. This lends the immediate forest an intimate feel. Gaining elevation, the trail reaches open areas with stretches of exposed bedrock. As you reach the pulpit, the woods clear to a panoramic view.

Rounding southeast, the trail follows blue blazes back downhill toward wetland in a valley below, passing over logs tossed together to bridge mud then climbing west to the relatively dry flank of another hill. After some twisting and turning, the trail bends decidedly south on upland, passing a pool and stream. On arriving at a junction, continue left, bearing away from Pulpit Trail and another route that climbs steeply to the right. Ahead, partly hidden by hemlock boughs, a sign for the Ancient Line Trail points southeast. Two junctions lie ahead, one following the other. Bear left at the first, then left again at the second, hiking northeast and away from the Cheever Commons Loop Trail, which is marked with light-blue blazes.

A stone wall beside the trail confirms that these were once fields filled with grazing livestock. Bearing east, the trail climbs steadily uphill, keeping flush to the wall before splitting off. You'll see a scruffy meadowland to the right.

Turning southeast, the trail meets up again with the Cheever Commons Loop Trail, but stay with Ancient Line Trail as it cuts tightly left, tucking under the steep upland banking. Running northwest again, making an elongated loop, the trail passes through a grouping of vernal pools and cavernous spaces made by lichen-encrusted boulders heaved together. Continuing on nearly level ground, the trail weaves its way northeast to return to the start of Pulpit Trail. Stay with Ancient Line Trail to double back to where it began.

Upon returning to the Millstone Hill Trail, turn left and follow what used to be the north–south track of Old Manchester Road. A granite town-line marker carved with the letter *M* stands erect on the Manchester–Essex border. Continuing north, the trail narrows and looks less and less like a road as hemlocks and birches crowd in. At 0.26 mile Old Manchester Road reaches a fork where the Cedar Swamp Trail diverts east. A moment later, you encounter a two-way split. Both routes lead to rock formations, one called Baby Rock and the other Ship Rock. If you're curious to see these glacial erratics and how they might have earned their monikers, hike left. Otherwise, bear right to follow blue blazes east.

Proceeding down a gentle grade, the trail passes through a dramatic rockscape fringed with hemlocks. Gradually oaks and beeches fill in, and before long the trail arrives at Prospect Ledge Trail. At this and the next junction, Ship Rock Trail winds through the woods. Keep an eye out for blue blazes to once again reach Cedar

Swamp. Hiking over the firm ground on the swamp's perimeter, the trail winds back to the boardwalk, which leads you back to the trailhead.

## NEARBY ATTRACTIONS

If you have a taste for seafood, plan your hike around lunch or dinner at J. T. Farnham's (88 Eastern Ave., 978-768-6643, jtfarnhams.com), located 4 miles from the trailhead in Essex. From the parking area at the Manchester–Essex Woods, drive 2.5 miles north on Southern Avenue, and turn right onto Eastern Avenue (MA 133). Farnham's is 0.6 mile ahead on the left.

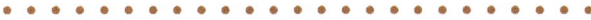

• • • • • • • • • • • • • • • • • • • • • • • • • • •

**GPS TRAILHEAD COORDINATES**  N42° 35.811'  W70° 46.054'

**DIRECTIONS**  From Boston, take US 1 N. After 13.6 miles, merge onto I-95/MA 128 north toward Peabody/Gloucester and continue 1.3 miles to Exit 45 toward Gloucester. At 13.2 miles, take Exit 15, School Street, toward Manchester/Essex. At the end of the ramp, turn left onto Southern Avenue. Parking for the Manchester–Essex Woodlands is about 0.5 mile ahead on the left.

A long boardwalk brings you across the swamp at the beginning and end of your hike.

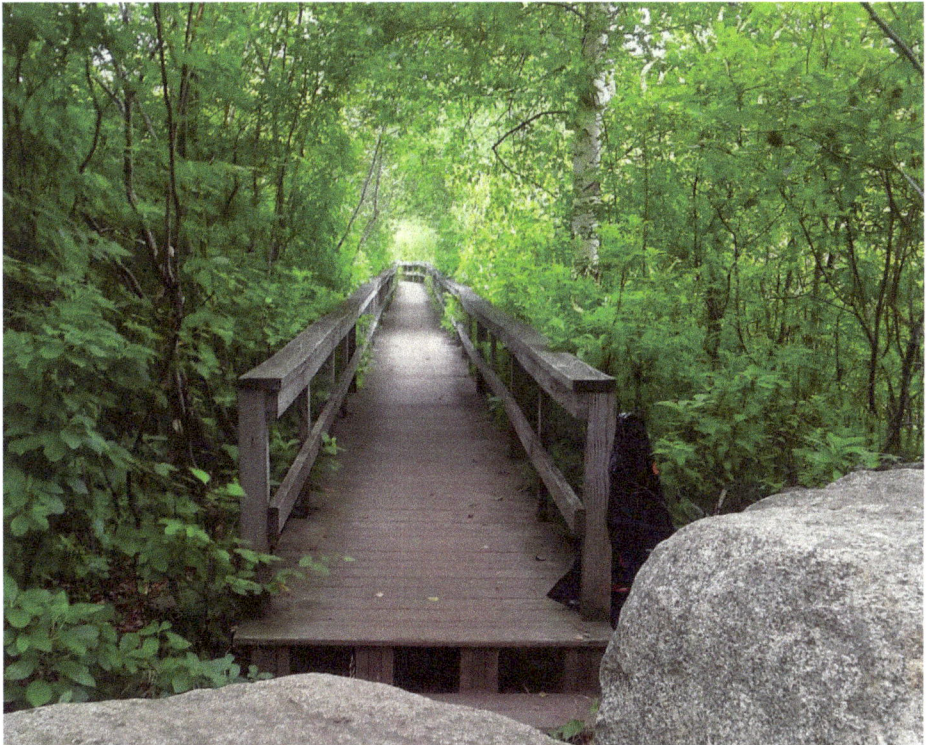

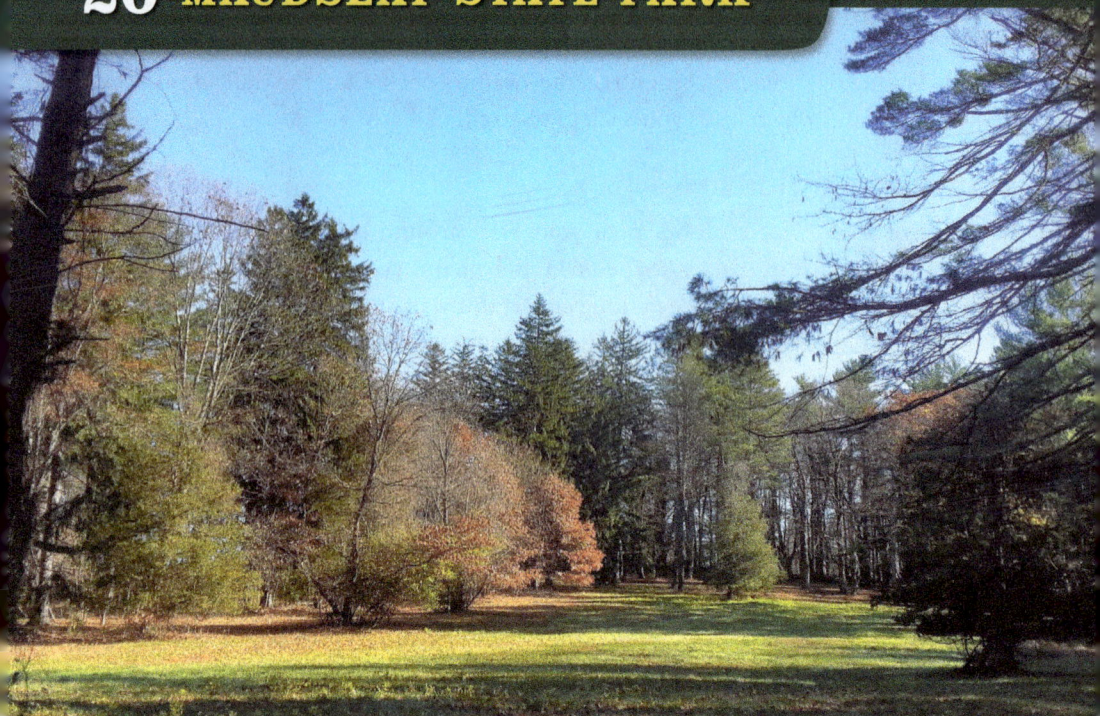

The grounds of Maudslay State Park are an inspiring blend of woods and open fields.

**FOLLOWING TRAILS AND** carriage roads, the hike takes you through meadows, woodlands, and formal gardens. From the site of the Moseley mansion, the hike follows Merrimack River north through hemlock woods where bald eagles roost in winter.

## DESCRIPTION

When you first start out at Maudslay State Park, you're faced with a massive open field, punctuated by impressively large columns of shade trees. Start your hike by crossing Pine Hill Road from the parking lot to the start of Pasture Trail. Hike over the arc of the open field, keeping left when the slender path splits. On meeting a gravel carriage path, follow as it descends left. In summer, goldfinches dart among lilting blossoms of black-eyed Susans and Queen Anne's lace growing in the meadow beneath open sky.

Where the trail turns northwest, the sun-drenched pasture meets shady woods. On the right is a stand of white pine planted by Frederick Moseley. To the left is a deciduous wood of shagbark hickory, beech, and various species of oak. Where the trail levels, another, less-pronounced path breaks off to the right. Bear left to enter the woods. The trail here is firm, level, moderately wide, and quite well marked and defined.

Before long, this broad trail reaches a three-way intersection. Detour onto a narrow path sweeping left. At the next fork, bear left again and follow the path downhill,

**DISTANCE & CONFIGURATION:** 3.9-mile loop

**DIFFICULTY:** Moderate

**SCENERY:** The grounds of a 450-acre estate designed by landscape architects Charles Sprague Sargent and Martha Brookes Hutcheson, with views of the Merrimack River

**EXPOSURE:** Mostly forests with some open fields

**TRAFFIC:** Moderate

**TRAIL SURFACE:** Mostly firmly packed dirt

**HIKING TIME:** 3 hours

**DRIVING DISTANCE FROM BOSTON COMMON:** 38 miles

**ELEVATION:** 96' at trailhead, no significant gain

**SEASON:** Year-round

**ACCESS:** Sunrise–sunset. Parking is $5 for MA residents, $6 for nonresidents

**MAPS:** Available at parking lot or at tinyurl.com/maudslaymap

**WHEELCHAIR ACCESS:** The trail called the Main Road is mostly wheelchair accessible; the other trails in this hike are not.

**FACILITIES:** Restrooms and picnic tables

**CONTACT:** Massachusetts Dept. of Conservation and Resources, mass.gov/locations/maudslay-state-park, 617-626-1250

**LOCATION:** Just west of I-95, Newburyport, MA

**COMMENTS:** The park hosts a full schedule of cultural events in the summer months, and permits are available for special events.

brushing by bushes and sassafras saplings. Ahead you come to a small footbridge, one of three that Moseley had constructed in 1915. Rhododendrons surround you here. Bear left, climbing to ascend stone steps to emerge at the eastern end of the Garden Walk. At the end of this path, you come to a gravel drive and an entryway through an imposing hedge. Slip into the peaceful garden through this passage to reach the spot where Maudslay Hedges, the home of Moseley's daughter Helen, once stood. Built in 1939, the house mysteriously burned to the ground in 1978, four years after her death.

Exit through the hedge and turn right on the gravel drive and right again onto a path heading southeast through an orchard. Past a spruce hedge, you come to a small granite building that is now shuttered. Ahead, the path leads to the shattered shells of the greenhouses and cold frames that Moseley had constructed in 1900.

Continue on the gravel road as it curves sharply right to reach a formal garden currently being rehabilitated with help from the Garden Conservancy. After taking in the neatly geometric perennial beds and imported marble ornaments, depart through the gate at the far end of the garden. A meadow lies off to the left, as does the well for which the path is named. At the next junction, the path to the left leads to the site of the coachman's house and barn. To reach the site of the Moseley mansion, continue straight through to a yard of several barns in disrepair and, beyond these, to a sprawling lawn overlooking the Merrimack River.

Head toward the river, keeping the water to your left, and pick up Merrimack River Trail. Here the hike begins to feel more like a hike. The trail narrows slightly, and the woods become a bit denser. Staying with Merrimack River Trail, walk beneath the pines and hemlocks growing along the steep riverbank. This part of the trail overlaps the Bay Circuit Trail, which begins at Plum Island and runs out around the Boston area to Duxbury and Kingston on the south shore.

## Maudslay State Park

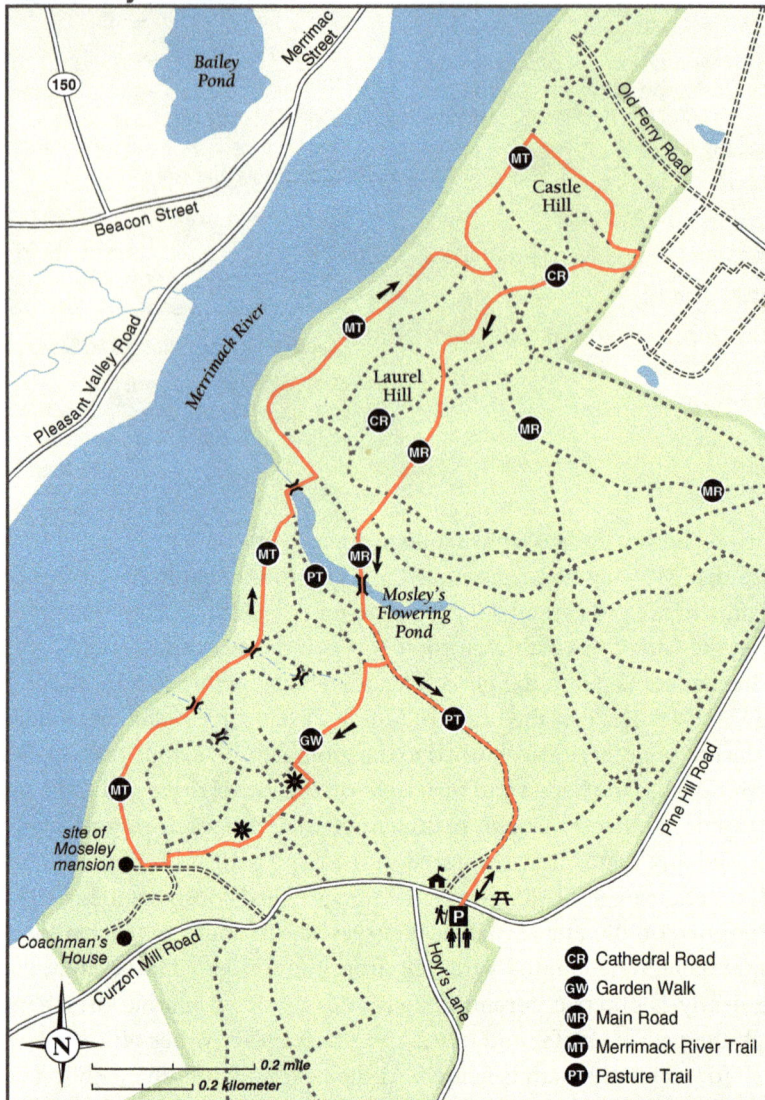

Map legend:

CR Cathedral Road
GW Garden Walk
MR Main Road
MT Merrimack River Trail
PT Pasture Trail

Continuing downhill, you soon come to a wooden bridge. Ahead, a swath cut in the mountain laurels affords a view of the river below. On the other side of the clearing, the trail resumes its course under heavy branches of oak, hickory, and white pine. After encountering two sections of chain-link fence and a concrete dam, the path merges with another hard-packed trail. Climbing the banking, the route leads to a memorial bench.

Merrimack River Trail continues uninterrupted until it reaches Moseley's Flowering Pond, where it detours to a gravel road. From the road, descend left to a stone bridge and dam at the foot of the pond.

Midway through the estate, the Merrimack River Trail climbs Laurel Hill. Watch for the great horned owls and pileated woodpeckers that nest here, and if winter is setting in, keep an eye out for bald eagles. In fact, this trail is closed November 1–March 31 to provide peace and protection for a number of these spectacular raptors that retreat from Canada to this spot every year. If the trail is closed when you are there, please respect the closures.

From the eagles' roosting grounds, stay with Merrimack River Trail until it reaches a broad fork. At this juncture, proceed left up a rocky slope to arrive at a large intersection. Stay beside the river until the trail arrives at an avenue of sugar maples ascending in a regal line to the top of Castle Hill. From this high point, follow the gravel road as it corkscrews around the other side of the hill. Arriving at the bottom, make a hairpin turn to take up a westward trail on the right.

The trail forks twice in quick succession; hike right at the first split and left at the second to travel downhill on a gravel carriage route. Pass through the next junction to continue straight on this path, which is aptly named Cathedral Road. Stay on Cathedral Road through each four-way intersection, and upon arriving at a fork, hike downhill to the left. Soon after this junction, the trail reaches yet another split; continue straight, and at the next fork bear left. Proceed straight on the wide carriage path. Before long you will see a sign that reads PARKING with an arrow pointing to a trail to the left. Resist this direct route to the parking lot and bear right. In a moment, the road passes a narrow footpath running off into underbrush to the left. This also takes you back to the start, but stay on the gravel carriage road to pass over a magnificent stone bridge. This is called the Main Road, and it promptly reaches a T intersection. Travel straight to rejoin Pasture Trail and retrace your steps back to the parking lot.

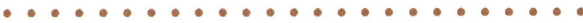

• • • • • • • • • • • • • • • • • • • • • • • • • •

**GPS TRAILHEAD COORDINATES** N42° 49.317' W70° 55.567'

**DIRECTIONS** From Boston take US 1 N 13.9 miles to I-95 N. Get off I-95 at Exit 57 to MA 113 E. Follow MA 113 east 0.5 mile and turn left on Noble Street. At the stop sign, turn left onto Ferry Road, bear left at the fork, and follow the signs.

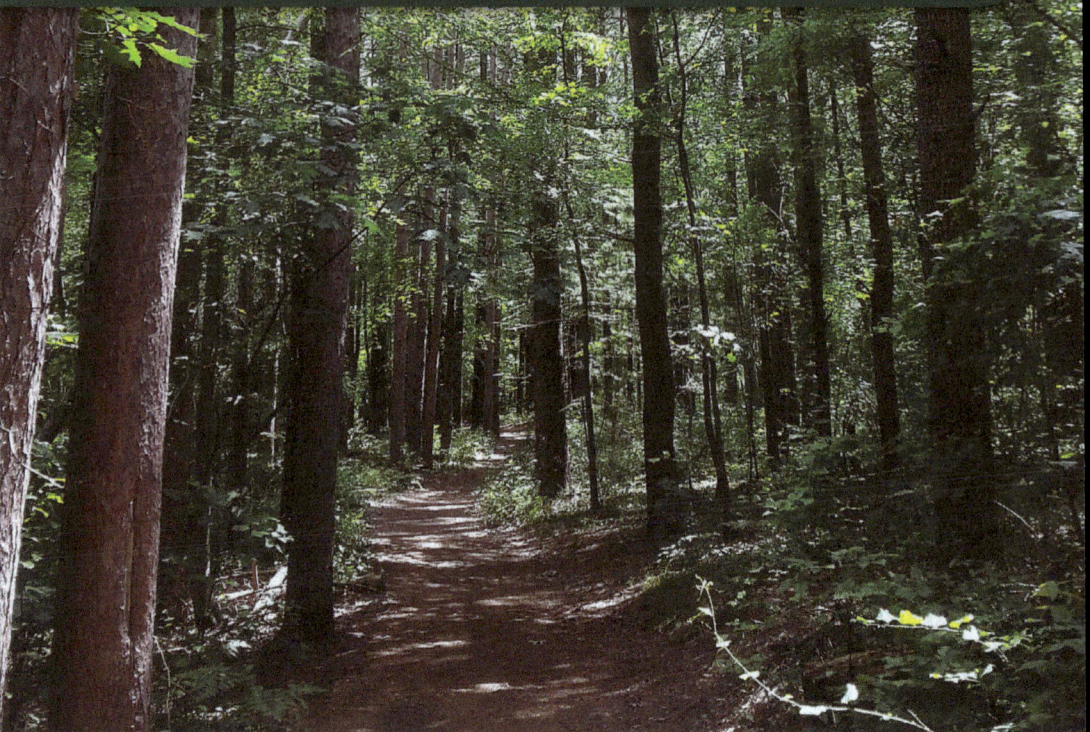

Hiking the full Skyline Trail at the Middlesex Fells will certainly test your endurance.

**SETTING A COURSE** over jagged upland surrounding wetland and three enormous reservoirs, Skyline Trail circles the entire 2,060-acre Middlesex Fells Reservation.

## DESCRIPTION

The 2,575-acre Middlesex Fells Reservation is fairly unique in its proximity to Boston and its massive size. It is fortunate indeed that such a large wooded area so close to the center of Boston would be set aside as a reservation. The term *fells,* which is what the local hikers and mountain bikers call the reservation, actually comes from an old Saxon word for "hilly terrain." The Fells certainly qualifies. Hike the full Skyline Trail, and you will know you've done something by the end of the day.

From the parking area off South Border Road, begin by setting out on the gravel fire road heading northwest. Several hundred yards in, you'll find a tree decorated with several colorful trail blazes, including white for the Skyline Trail. That is somehow appropriate, as the Skyline Trail is like the Fells' miniature version of the Appalachian Trail.

**DISTANCE & CONFIGURATION:** 7.5-mile loop

**DIFFICULTY:** Strenuous

**SCENERY:** A landscape composed of granite out-croppings, hemlock forest, and hardwood stands surrounding a chain of ponds; the two peaks you'll traverse reward you with views of Boston.

**EXPOSURE:** Mostly shaded

**TRAFFIC:** Moderate

**TRAIL SURFACE:** Packed dirt, roots, rugged boulders, granite outcroppings

**HIKING TIME:** 4–5 hours

**DRIVING DISTANCE FROM BOSTON COMMON:** 10 miles

**ELEVATION:** 129' at trailhead, 276' at highest point, with a considerable amount of rise and fall along the trail

**SEASON:** Year-round

**ACCESS:** Sunrise–sunset; free

**MAPS:** Available from the Friends of the Middlesex Fells (fells.org) or at tinyurl.com /middlesexfellsmap

**WHEELCHAIR ACCESS:** Reservoir Trail (orange) is recommended for wheelchair users.

**FACILITIES:** None

**CONTACT:** Massachusetts Dept. of Conservation and Resources, mass.gov/locations /middlesex-fells-reservation, 617-626-1250

**LOCATION:** South Border Road, Medford, MA

**COMMENTS:** Prepare for a hike in the Middlesex Fells as you would for a hike in remote moun-tains. Wear sturdy shoes, and bring plenty of water, food, and a flashlight. The full loop is a fairly long, strenuous hike.

This spot where you leave the gravel fire road and enter the woods marks where several trails run concurrently up a hill to the left. It's also amusing when the white-blazed Skyline Trail overlays the orange- and green-blazed trail. At one point, there's a tree marked with green, white, and orange blazes—three trails at once or the Irish flag? It is the Boston area, so either is plausible. Following Skyline's white blazes, leave the fire road here to hike north.

Set back in the woods away from South Border Road, the trail sets a rugged course from the outset due to the Fells' glacier-hewn topography. This is what you think of when you think of a hiking trail. It's narrow; the trail surface is root- and rock-bound; and it twists, winds, and undulates throughout the forest. It's some-times surreal while hiking on a trail like this, feeling like you're a million miles from anywhere, yet you can occasionally hear a truck on I-93 or a plane coming into Logan.

Following many and varied undulations, the trail soon arrives at a small pond at the tip of a tree-hidden reservoir contained deep within the reservation. Cross the gravel access road on a diagonal to the left, and resume Skyline Trail.

Climbing an easy uphill grade, the trail of compounded routes briefly passes close to the reservoir then tunnels back under tree cover. Long-established hemlocks, oaks, and maples stand their ground, though the occasional growth of pine indicates periodic clear-cutting—some of which was done under General Washington to pro-vide timber to fortify Dorchester Heights.

The trail frequently intersects some of the wider, doubletrack trails that wind throughout the park. These are quite popular with mountain bikers, so keep an eye out left and right when crossing them. It can sometimes be like crossing a paved road in the Boston area. You can't be too careful.

## Middlesex Fells Reservation: Skyline Trail

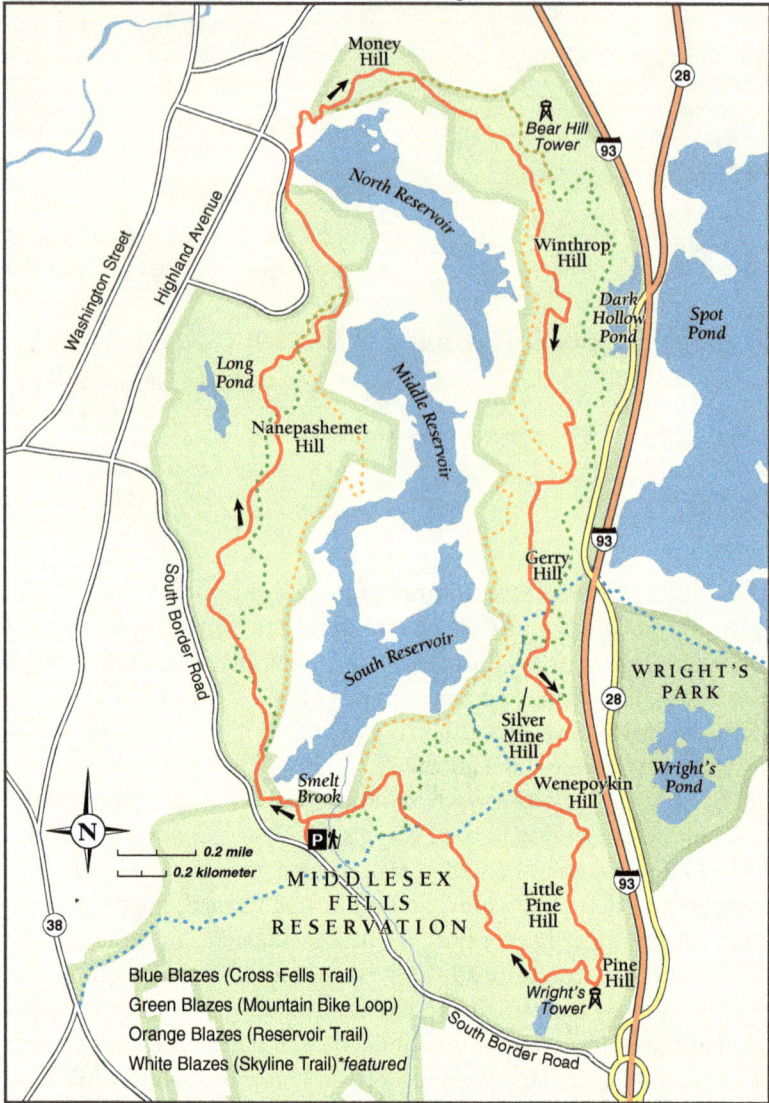

Money Hill

Bear Hill Tower

North Reservoir

Winthrop Hill

Dark Hollow Pond

Spot Pond

Long Pond

Middle Reservoir

Nanepashemet Hill

Gerry Hill

WRIGHT'S PARK

South Reservoir

Silver Mine Hill

Wright's Pond

Smelt Brook

Wenepoykin Hill

N

0.2 mile
0.2 kilometer

MIDDLESEX FELLS RESERVATION

Little Pine Hill

Pine Hill

Wright's Tower

Blue Blazes (Cross Fells Trail)
Green Blazes (Mountain Bike Loop)
Orange Blazes (Reservoir Trail)
White Blazes (Skyline Trail)*featured

South Border Road

Washington Street

Highland Avenue

South Border Road

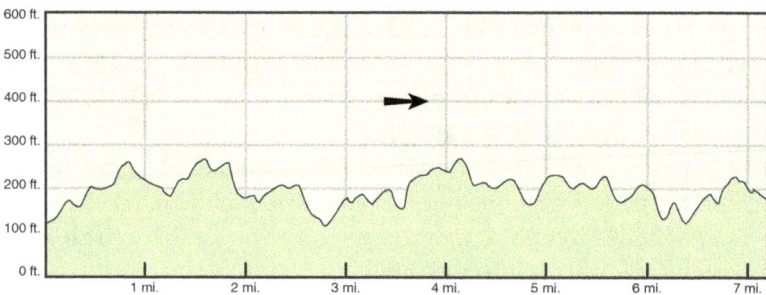

600 ft.
500 ft.
400 ft.
300 ft.
200 ft.
100 ft.
0 ft.

1 mi.  2 mi.  3 mi.  4 mi.  5 mi.  6 mi.  7 mi.

Making its way north, now and again joining a cart road named for Nanepash-emet, the Skyline Trail passes over Nanepashemet Hill then dips within sight of the second in a chain of three reservoirs that lie at the center of the Fells. After crossing Willow Spring Path, Skyline Trail clings to the westernmost edge of the fells, squeezing between North Reservoir and the houses of a Winchester neighborhood. It then bears east and climbs up and over Money Hill before heading back into woods a hair short of the reservation's northern boundary.

Sloping into wetland on the outskirts of the reservoir, the trail navigates a series of small bridges then climbs sharply as it meets the base of Bear Hill. Beyond Bear Hill Trail, joining in to the left and marked with blue, Skyline Trail drops straight south, narrowing to something like a goat path as it edges up the grizzled face of Winthrop Hill.

Proceeding from Winthrop Hill—named for John Winthrop, who in his journal described an exploratory expedition to the Fells by the governor, the Reverend John Eliot, and others in 1632—the trail leads to a large meadow called the Sheepfold. In the park's early years, a herd of sheep grazed here, adding a pastoral touch to the dense forest and granite-laden hills. The paved road beside the sheepfold is a soapbox-derby track built by the Metropolitan District Commission after World War II.

Arriving at a parking area, follow the white and orange trail markers right, onto Chandler Road. Skyline Trail soon diverts sharply left; take this turn onto a rocky slope, and resume hiking south to ascend Gerry Hill. At the foot of the hill's western slope, after being bisected by Brooks Road, Skyline Trail takes on another hill. This one is named Silver Mine Hill for the efforts of F. W. Morandi, who tried to mine the area for precious metals between 1881 and 1883.

The next, more rock-strewn peak is Wenepoykin Hill, which offers an exhilarating vantage point. Bearing west and descending back into woods, the trail arrives at a junction in a clearing. Here Skyline Trail meets Cross Fells Trail, marked with blue. If daylight is starting to fade on you, forgo the rest of the Skyline Trail and continue straight on Cross Fells Trail—the parking lot on South Border Road is less than a mile away.

The next leg of Skyline Trail is marked, as always, with white blazes. Starting with a lengthy downhill over loose granite rubble into dense woods of pine and hemlock, the trail twists its way to the top of twin peaks—Little Pine Hill and the stone knuckle of Pine Hill, where it arrives at Wright's Tower.

From this stone tower, Skyline Trail meanders generally west, clambering up sheets of granite grooved from the wear of glacial action and easing along placid stretches of cool, packed earth, passing the cave of a long-gone panther to rejoin Cross Fells Trail.

To stay with Skyline Trail to the end, bear right for one more climb and descent before rejoining the orange and green trails and concluding the hike with an easy amble back to the fire trail that leads to the South Border Road parking area.

## NEARBY ATTRACTIONS

The Stoneham Zoo, founded in 1905, is located close by at Spot Pond on the Fells' eastern side (149 Pond St., Stoneham; 781-438-5100; zoonewengland.org/stone-zoo). Those interested in learning more about the American Indians of the Middlesex Fells should visit the Peabody Museum of Archaeology and Ethnology (11 Divinity Ave., Cambridge; 617-496-1027; peabody.harvard.edu) at Harvard University.

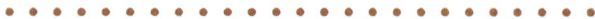

• • • • • • • • • • • • • • • • • • • • • • • •

**GPS TRAILHEAD COORDINATES** N42° 26.300'  W71° 07.167'

**DIRECTIONS** From Boston, take Storrow Drive east to the ramp for I-93 N toward Concord. Take I-93 N 5.2 miles to Exit 33 toward Winchester. Stay straight to access MA 28 N. Enter the next roundabout and take the second exit, onto South Border Road. Continue approximately 1.3 miles to the parking area on the right.

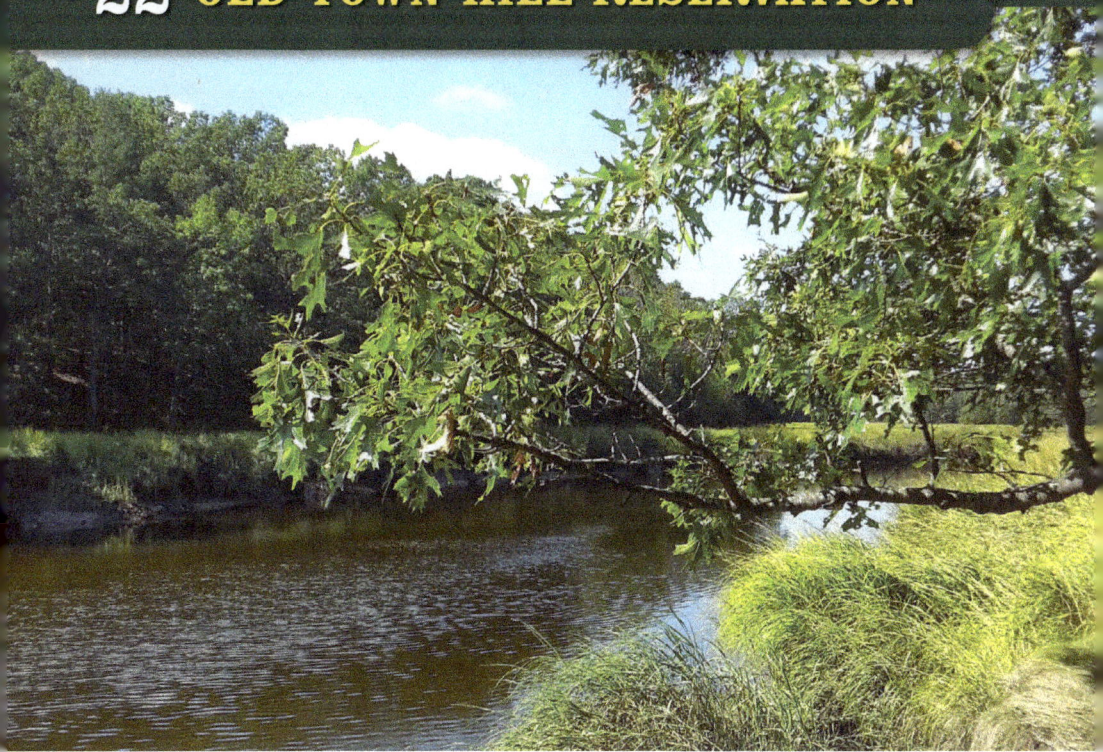

Old Town Hill is like two hikes combined into one.

**SURVEYING SALT MARSHES** and Newbury's tallest hill, this hike explores a landscape that remains much as it was in the 1600s when a small group of colonists first settled the area.

## DESCRIPTION

Old Town Hill was farmed for generations, and the landscape remains largely unchanged from the days when horse and buggy traversed the land. From the parking area on Newman Road, hike southwest on the wide packed-earth trail. Several hundred feet along, you will pass a trail heading uphill to the left. Continue descending the hill to arrive at a causeway leading between tracts of marshland. Looking west, you will see the Little River, a tributary of the Parker River. To the northeast, you can see acres and acres of fragrant wetland dominated by a hardy, salt-tolerant grass called spartina.

On the far side of the causeway, a path splits off to the right, but continue straight up a slight rise to reach a cedar and oak grove on an island surrounded by tidal-zone marshland. The narrow path winds as it leads to a lovely, small "beach." If the day is hot and the tide high, pull off your shoes and jump in, for the water is clean and the current gentle.

**DISTANCE & CONFIGURATION:** 2.6-mile loop

**DIFFICULTY:** Moderate

**SCENERY:** Salt marshes, woods, hayfields, view of Plum Island from the hilltop

**EXPOSURE:** Mostly shaded

**TRAFFIC:** Light

**TRAIL SURFACE:** Mostly packed dirt with grass sections and some gravel roads

**HIKING TIME:** 1.5 hours

**DRIVING DISTANCE FROM BOSTON COMMON:** 38 miles

**ELEVATION:** 19' at trailhead, 168' at highest point

**SEASON:** Year-round

**ACCESS:** Sunrise–sunset; free

**MAPS:** Posted at entrance

**WHEELCHAIR ACCESS:** No

**FACILITIES:** None

**CONTACT:** The Trustees of Reservations, thetrustees.org/places-to-visit, 617-542-7696

**LOCATION:** Newman Road, Newbury, MA

**COMMENTS:** If you're planning a hike here in the summertime, bring a bathing suit. If the tide is high enough on a hot day, a swim in the nearby creek is a pleasure you won't want to miss.

From this spot, the trail continues northwest along the edge of the woods, switching east to cross a hayfield thick with timothy, vetch, and patches of milkweed. At the end of the field, the trail descends to the causeway crossed earlier.

Double back a short distance to the path running up a steep hill to the right. A climb up this banking leads to a wooden bench where you can relax and look out over a gorgeous view of the river below. From this spot, continue hiking east, following the course of a stone wall on the left. Ducking into the shade of hickory branches, bristly cedars, and scrappy black cherry boughs, continue until you come to a break in the wall marked with daylilies and an arrow pointing left. Heed the arrow and hike north alongside the hayfield. It is still a working field, so you may well see huge shrink-wrapped bundles of hay waiting to be hauled off to feed the county's horses and remaining cattle. At the corner of the field, the path continues through a parting in the weeds, reenters the woods, then quickly links back to the trail on which you originally entered.

To expand your hike to Old Town Hill, cross Newman Road, heading north to find the trailhead marked by a white sign bearing a hiker symbol. Another sign posted nearby identifies this path as part of the Bay Circuit Trail. Traveling east through woods bordering Newman Road, the trail leads to an intersection near a pine grove planted in rows. Bear left to pick up a wide, packed-gravel trail.

Swinging southwest as it gains elevation, this old wagon route leads to a pasture atop Old Town Hill. Now the meadow is a butterfly haven choked with milkweed and Queen Anne's lace. Turning southeast to cross the hilltop, the mowed-grass path passes several old fruit trees holding out among the vigorous Norway maples. The path reenters woods briefly before spilling out to a second field. From here, the township's highest point, you can see for miles on a clear day. Thick clouds or summer haze may hide Plum Island and the sea from view, but you'll know they are there by the fresh scent on the breeze.

## Old Town Hill Reservation

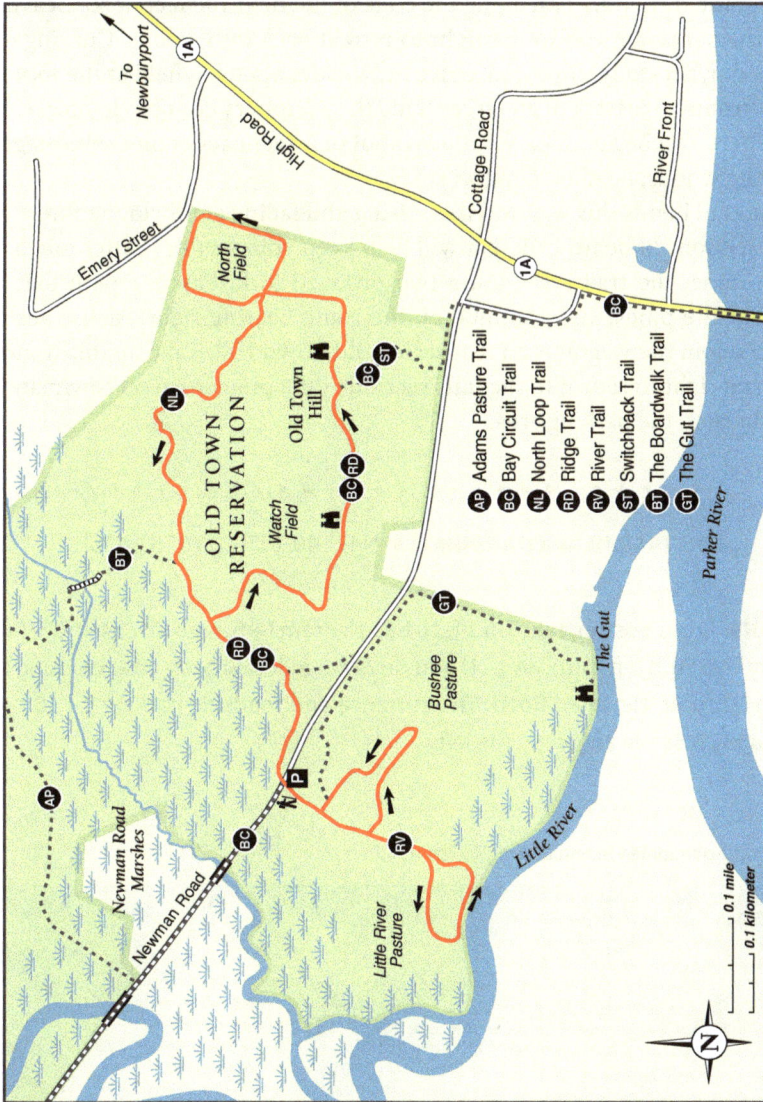

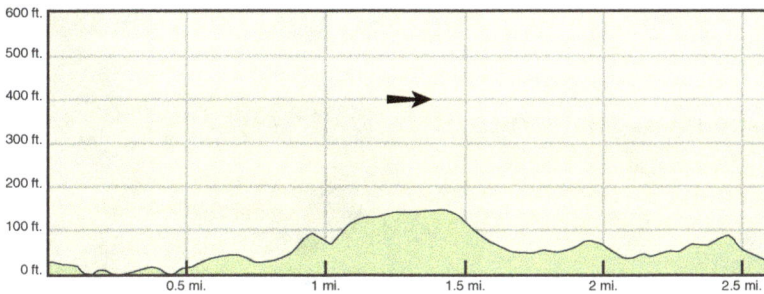

To Newburyport

1A

High Road

Emery Street

Cottage Road

River Front

North Field

NL

OLD TOWN RESERVATION

Old Town Hill

BC ST

BC RD

Watch Field

BT

AP

Newman Road Marshes

RD
BC

P
NL

BC

Newman Road

Little River Pasture

RV

GT

Bushee Pasture

The Gut

Little River

Parker River

N

- AP  Adams Pasture Trail
- BC  Bay Circuit Trail
- NL  North Loop Trail
- RD  Ridge Trail
- RV  River Trail
- ST  Switchback Trail
- BT  The Boardwalk Trail
- GT  The Gut Trail

0.1 mile
0.1 kilometer

600 ft.
500 ft.
400 ft.
300 ft.
200 ft.
100 ft.
0 ft.

0.5 mi.    1 mi.    1.5 mi.    2 mi.    2.5 mi.

To find the trail, walk east along the edge of the field 100 feet or so. Leaving the clearing, the path slants off to the right to retreat back into woods. Curving east, it then spills down a stony slope and arrives at a wide, open hayfield at the foot of the hill. Loop around this tract of green, walking the periphery counterclockwise. When nearing where you began, look for the symbol of a backpacker on a white sign, and return to the woods, heading northwest.

As the trail bends this way and that, rising and falling gently in the forest, you'll pass over sections of boardwalk that will help keep your feet dry. After much twisting and turning, the trail arrives at a two-pronged fork. Pass the path that heads uphill under the pines, and continue on the route bearing right. At the next split, stay left to rejoin the wagon road that scales Old Town Hill. Take up this route once more, hiking right to return to the intersection at the pine grove off Newman Road, and head back to the parking area.

• • • • • • • • • • • • • • • • • • • • • • • •

**GPS TRAILHEAD COORDINATES**  N42° 46.167'  W70° 51.436'

**DIRECTIONS**  From Boston, take US 1 N to I-95 N. From I-95, take Exit 54 and follow MA 133 E 4.5 miles. Turn left onto MA 1A N and drive 4.8 miles. Shortly after crossing Parker River, turn left onto Newman Road. The entrance and roadside parking for 10 cars are approximately 0.5 mile ahead on the left.

The open, grass-dominated marshland of Old Town Hill

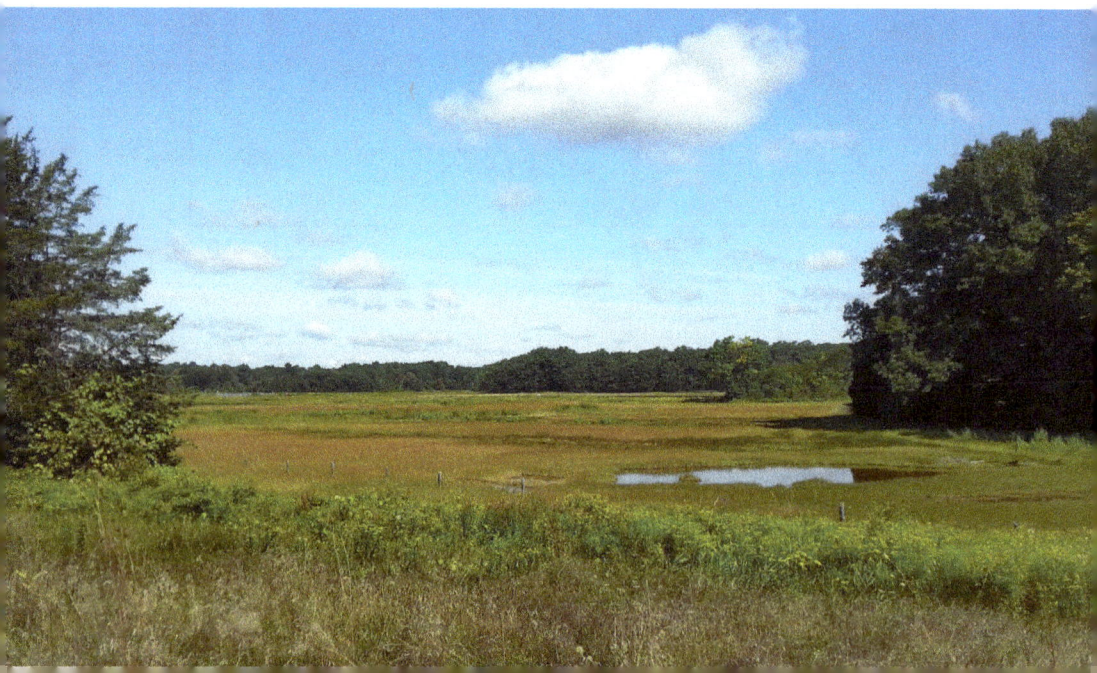

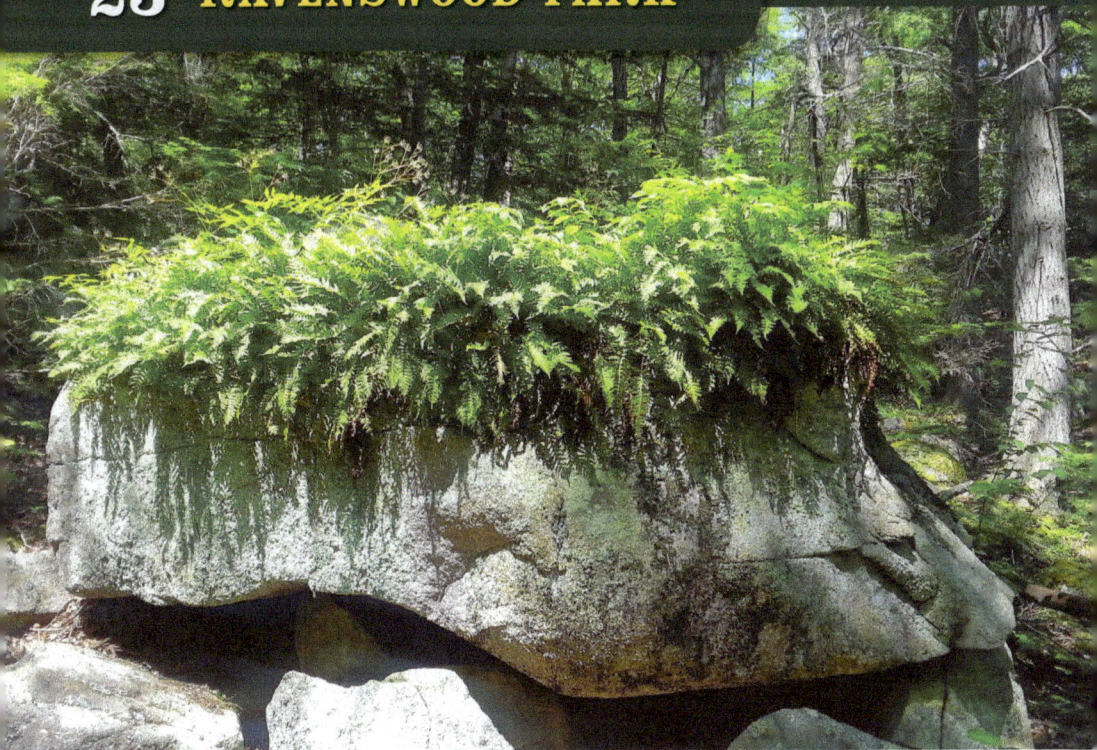

Ravenswood Park is a beautiful walk in the woods that features some fascinating rock formations.

**FOLLOWING CENTURIES-OLD FOOTPATHS,** carriage roads, and a boardwalk through a magnolia swamp, this hike rambles through woods to reach Fernwood Lake before passing the cabin site of "The Hermit of Ravenswood" and two granite quarries.

## DESCRIPTION

As rich in history as in rare and beautiful species of flora and fauna, these 600 acres have been maintained in their natural state thanks to the inspired vision and generosity of Gloucester businessman Samuel Elwell Sawyer.

From the parking lot, hike northwest on Old Salem Road—the gravel road that once bore stagecoaches traveling to and from Boston in the 1700s. Running parallel with stone walls, the path soon meets Magnolia Swamp Trail on the left. Follow this narrower trail west under hemlock boughs, uphill to start, then downhill as it winds southwest.

If hiking in June, you will likely see mountain laurel in full bloom. Heavy with white blossoms touched with pink, these elegant bushes dress the woods as if for a formal occasion. As the trail descends to wetland, the density of laurel increases.

125

**DISTANCE & CONFIGURATION:** 4.5-mile loop

**DIFFICULTY:** Moderate

**SCENERY:** Hemlock and hardwood forests, views of a lake and the ocean, historic quarry, magnolia swamp

**EXPOSURE:** Mostly shaded

**TRAFFIC:** Light

**TRAIL SURFACE:** The carriage roads are covered with finely crushed stone; all other trails are packed dirt with brief stretches of boardwalk.

**HIKING TIME:** 2 hours

**DRIVING DISTANCE FROM BOSTON COMMON:** 38 miles

**ELEVATION:** 137' at trailhead, 187' at highest point

**SEASON:** Year-round

**ACCESS:** Sunrise–sunset; free

**MAPS:** Posted at entrance

**WHEELCHAIR ACCESS:** The carriage roads are accessible, but the hiking trails are not.

**FACILITIES:** None

**CONTACT:** The Trustees of Reservations, thetrustees.org/places-to-visit, 617-542-7696

**LOCATION:** MA 127, Gloucester, MA

**COMMENTS:** The park's rare swamp magnolias bloom in early spring, making this an ideal time to visit.

Arriving at Magnolia Swamp, the trail transitions to boardwalk as it continues across the wetland. Lush moss grows on the edges of the narrow path, and thick shrubs close in on the sides. After taking you a fair distance through this wet zone alive with butterflies and frogs, the boardwalk terminates at the southeastern end of the swamp. Here you step onto earth again and continue along the granite ledge rimming the wetland.

A short distance ahead, the ledge gives way to a sizable chunk of granite protruding from the land. The only way around is to ford the swamp or take the boardwalk built to accommodate the rock's complex contours and the trees growing from its crevices.

Reconnecting with the ledge, the trail continues below hemlocks and beeches. Blue jays flit about in the foliage, loudly announcing their presence. Looking to your right, you may notice nylon netting enclosing a section of greenery. This fencing protects the tender shoots of sweetbay magnolia (*Magnolia virginiana*) from grazing deer. Easing north, the trail reaches a junction where the Magnolia Swamp Trail turns right and the Fernwood Lake Trail starts on the left.

Pick up the Fernwood Lake Trail, hiking northeast, and leave the wetland behind. Following blue blazes, this trail passes through property that is officially outside the borders of Ravenswood park.

Crossing short hills dotted with granite boulders of every shape and size, the trail passes through young beech groves varied by sassafras and laurel. Shortly the narrow path spills into a wide clearing where trails radiate in all directions. Looking across to the right, you will see a bold blue dot marking the way. Continue on the Fernwood Lake Trail to travel east on an old carriage road.

Passing abandoned farmland on the left now reclaimed by oaks and maples, the carriage road rolls on to soon reach a T intersection. Blue arrows painted on a beech

# Ravenswood Park

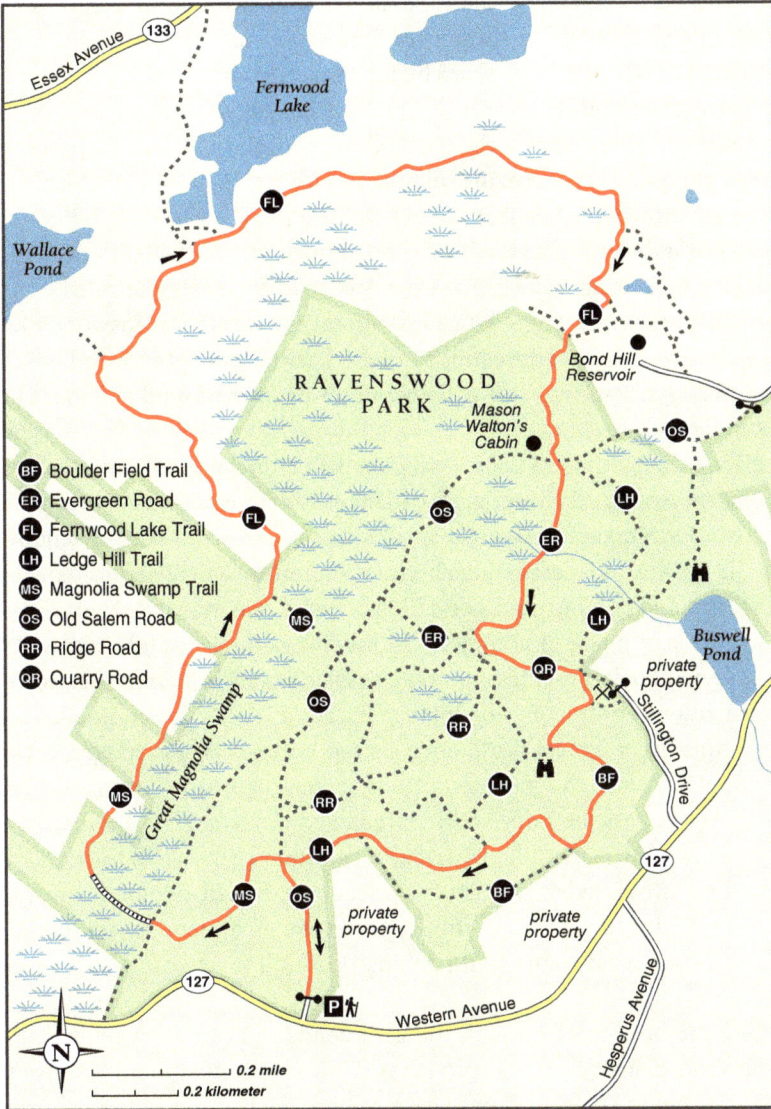

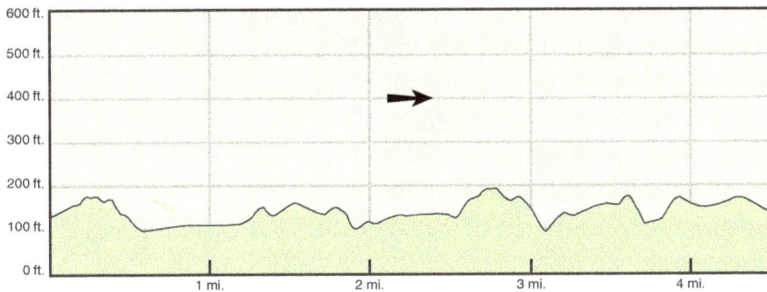

Essex Avenue
133
Fernwood Lake
Wallace Pond
FL
FL
Bond Hill Reservoir
OS
RAVENSWOOD PARK
Mason Walton's Cabin
OS
LH

**BF** Boulder Field Trail
**ER** Evergreen Road
**FL** Fernwood Lake Trail
**LH** Ledge Hill Trail
**MS** Magnolia Swamp Trail
**OS** Old Salem Road
**RR** Ridge Road
**QR** Quarry Road

FL
ER
MS
ER
LH
Buswell Pond
*private property*
QR
OS
RR
MS
Great Magnolia Swamp
RR
LH
BF
BF
LH
MS
OS
*private property*
*private property*
Stillington Drive
127
127
P
Western Avenue
Hesperus Avenue
N

0.2 mile
0.2 kilometer

tree point east and west. Follow the right-pointing arrow, and hike east. Through woods to the left, you will see the waters of Fernwood Lake. On this stretch of road, keep an eye out for exposed stone worn by the horse-drawn traffic back in the 1800s.

Turning east, the trail bends away from the lake, still visible on your left. Aside from some dips and short climbs, the trail follows a level route, usually paralleled by ramshackle stone walls. Several paths split off on either side, but follow blue markers to stay with the Fernwood Lake Trail. After passing a path that bears uphill to the left, you will notice that the trail is marked with both orange and blue. Don't worry about it.

Arriving at a clearing, hike left onto a dirt road to pass great piles of granite before crossing to the right where blue blazes point the way to Ravenswood's border. Back inside the park, the trail descends a hill thick with slender birch and beech saplings. Reaching lower ground, you will encounter patches of mud and giant lichen-covered boulders.

Before long the Fernwood Lake Trail comes to a four-way intersection where it meets Old Salem Road and Evergreen Road. This is where Mason A. Walton, better known as The Hermit, kept house in a small log cabin he built with the landowner's permission in 1884. A most gregarious hermit, Walton was highly educated. He welcomed all visitors and became quite good friends with Concord native Henry Thoreau. He and Thoreau had much in common, both being naturalists and writers. Two of Walton's published books are *A Hermit's Wild Friends* and *Proof That Animals Reason.*

From the intersection, continue hiking southeast on Evergreen Road. Like Old Salem Road, this broad gravel route once served horse-drawn carriages. Sweeping through hemlock woods, the path soon leads to Quarry Road. Turn left to take up this new route east. Pass the Ledge Hill Trail and continue a short distance to arrive at the long-abandoned, water-filled quarry and another entrance to the park.

Follow the narrow Ledge Hill Trail as it leads up the left side of this man-made pool and retreats into the woods to the south. At the next junction, marked 9, turn left to follow a somewhat vague trail running downhill through a puzzle of granite glacial waste.

Reaching the bottom of the hill, the trail bends right to head south. Here the trail becomes more distinct as it approaches the park boundary and a house to the left. When you come to marker 8, bear right to head back uphill. Winding north and northwest on this narrow path, you pass more gray boulders strewn carelessly about.

Soon the path joins the Ledge Hill Trail at a particularly massive rock. Turn left at this juncture to hike gently downhill. Following the route edged with small stones, you promptly come to a boulder that looks as soft and inviting as a worn sofa. Beyond this odd furnishing, the trail descends past a vernal pool. After rising again and easing by another small pond, the trail emerges from the woods at Old Salem Road just opposite the start of the Magnolia Swamp Trail. Turn left to return to the parking area.

## NEARBY ATTRACTIONS

Hammond Castle, one of Cape Ann's most celebrated attractions, is located almost immediately across the street (MA 127) from the entrance of Ravenswood Park at 80 Hesperus Ave. Built in the 1920s, this medieval-style castle offers self-guided and prearranged tours. It is open daily, 10 a.m.–4 p.m., June 23–Labor Day. Visit hammondcastle.org for a schedule of special programs and events. To book a tour, call 978-283-7673.

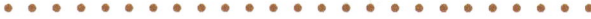

• • • • • • • • • • • • • • • • • • • • • • • • • • •

**GPS TRAILHEAD COORDINATES**  N42° 35.517'  W70° 41.900'

**DIRECTIONS**  From Boston, take US 1 N to I-95 N. Take Exit 14 (MA 133) and follow it 3 miles east toward Gloucester to MA 127. Turn right onto MA 127 and follow it 2 miles to the entrance.

The park is indeed a wonderful gift of the Sawyer family.

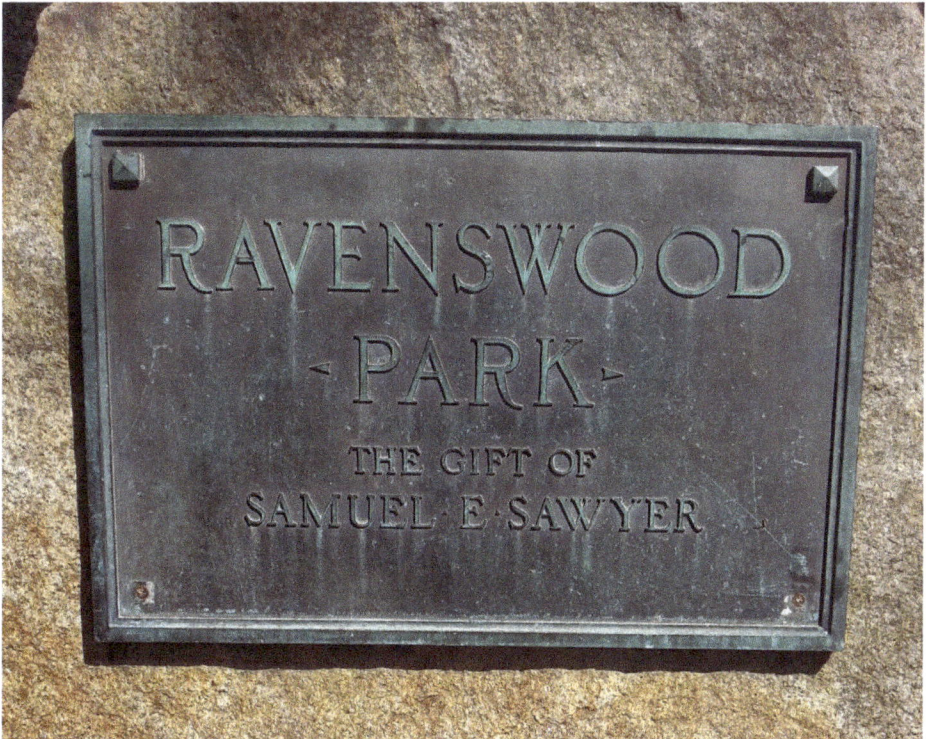

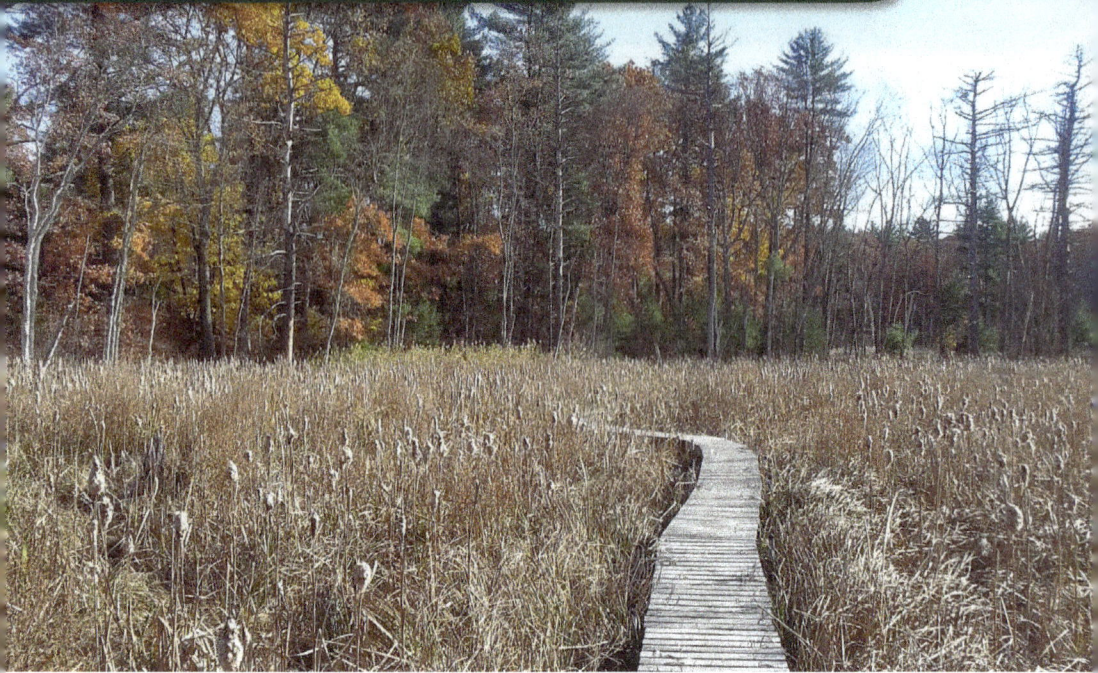

You start and finish your hike at the Skug River Reservation on this twisting, winding boardwalk.

**THIS HIKE STARTS** with a dramatic passage through swampland and takes you through a fascinating rock garden.

## DESCRIPTION

The trailhead for the Mary French Reservation (which abuts the Skug River Reservation) is marked on Korinthian Way with the modest square insignia of the Bay Circuit Trail. From this point, set out south on a narrow trail surfaced with clay dust. A kiosk posted by the Andover Conservation Commission greets hikers several yards into the woods. Dedicated to a former town selectman who was both a nature lover and a hiking devotee, the Mary French Reservation is a recent addition to Andover's share of the 200-mile Bay Circuit Trail.

A moment later, the path rolls out from under tree cover to reach a wetland tucked behind neighborhood houses but surrounded by a dense layer of shrubs. Where water floods to meet the forest, you'll come to a 1,000-foot boardwalk and follow it as it zigzags into the woods beyond. The Bay Circuit Trail reasserts itself with a marker on a pine tree where the boardwalk rejoins land. Here, in a shaded spot, a lovely sculptured bench overlooks a scene as poetic as any Monet masterpiece. This is a perfect spot to stop and relax for a moment.

**DISTANCE & CONFIGURATION:** 3.05-mile out-and-back with loops

**DIFFICULTY:** Easy–moderate

**SCENERY:** Wetlands, woodlands, dramatic glacial rock garden

**EXPOSURE:** Mostly shaded; exposed along the boardwalk

**TRAFFIC:** Light

**TRAIL SURFACE:** Firmly packed earth, exposed rock, lengthy sections of boardwalk

**HIKING TIME:** 2–2.5 hours

**DRIVING DISTANCE FROM BOSTON COMMON:** 23 miles

**ELEVATION:** 118' at trailhead, no significant gain

**SEASON:** Year-round

**ACCESS:** Sunrise–sunset; free

**MAPS:** Available at avisandover.org/maps /skughammond.pdf

**WHEELCHAIR ACCESS:** No

**FACILITIES:** None

**CONTACT:** The Andover Village Improvement Society, avisandover.org/skug.html

**LOCATION:** Andover, MA

**COMMENTS:** This gem of a hike crosses land managed by three distinct groups: the state, the Andover Conservation Commission, and The Andover Village Improvement Society (one of the oldest conservation groups in the country, founded in 1894).

Continuing on the Bay Circuit Trail, head south under a canopy of oak, beech, and hickory, brushing by fern fronds. Passing mammoth white pines, the trail bends southeast, bisects a stone wall, and mounts an earthen causeway built by farmers to create a watering hole for cattle and a source of ice for their iceboxes. Bear right at the stooped grandfather oak, and hike along the top of the heap of stones. Wooden bridges fill gaps now and again as the causeway spans varying depths of bog.

Arriving shortly at the causeway's end, the trail continues southwest over packed earth, navigating through and alongside lengths of lichen- and moss-dappled stone wall. Liberally marked with Bay Circuit Trail markers, the trail soon arrives at a junction. The path loops left here, but continue straight to cross mounds of submerged boulders and convex muddy spots often dimpled with the impressions of raccoon toes to reach Salem Street. Cross over here, and continue on the trail. If you have chosen to park here, it's well worth hiking back over the boardwalk then retracing your steps back to Salem Street.

After crossing Salem Street, you'll traverse several other short boardwalks. The trail cuts back into woods just past a brown saltbox house. Reminiscent of the old cart road it once was, the trail starts off wide and clear with stone walls on either side. Soon the border of the path changes to unruly shrubs and brambles. Forge on past a pile of brush to find a wide junction posted with AVIS and Bay Circuit Trail markers. Heed the AVIS arrow, and bear right onto the Bridge Trail, which, as a link in the Bay Circuit Trail, is also marked with white swatches. The trail here is hard-packed dirt, with occasional rocky uprisings.

Heading west, the trail quickly reaches mud and a boardwalk leading over the soggy bank of Skug River to a bench. The view upriver on a certain September day revealed the lithe trunks of flame-red maples leaning over a basin overflowing after a

**Skug River Reservation**

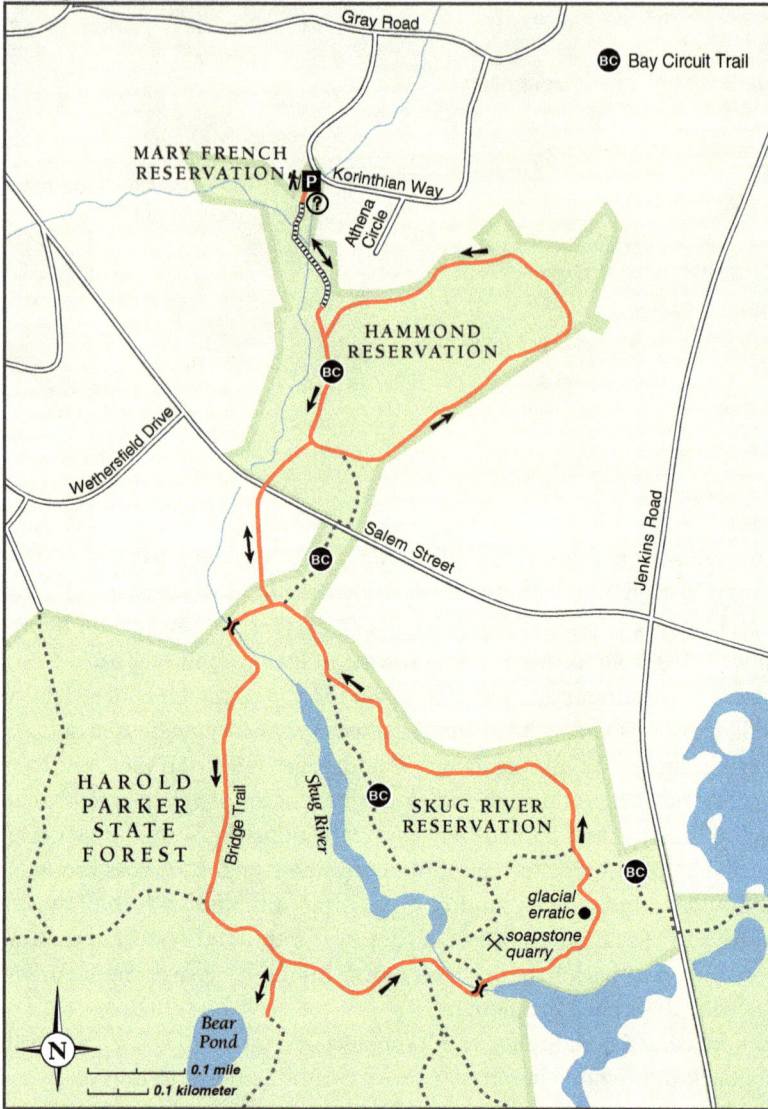

summer of heavy rain. Interestingly enough, the river's name—Skug—is an American Indian word for snake.

Hiking along the opposite riverbank, making use of the stone-wall border to keep dry, you'll reach a split in the trail at the boundary of Harold Parker State Forest. Take this right, leaving the river behind for now. An easy climb under pines on a southwest trajectory promptly ends at a T made by a second trail running parallel to the river. Bear left onto this wide cart road edged by a stone wall, and follow its even course southeast to where it crosses a path to Bear Pond.

From the intersection with Bear Pond, continue straight (southeast). Ahead, beyond a slight rise and rocky pitch, the trail rejoins Skug River. At a junction defined by stone walls, the trail splits abruptly. One route veers sharply right, and another pitches left through bushes. What lies beyond is William Jenkins's soapstone quarry and mill site. For a look at the site from atop massive stone walls built to control the water flow, take the left path. Afterward, return to the junction and follow the path to the right farther downriver. Keep an eye out for the first left, and follow a short, winding path down a rocky slope to a bridge.

Built where the turbulent water spills into a quiet pool, the solid bridge provides a peaceful vantage point. Blocks of stone cut and discarded, or left for a pickup that never occurred, lie partially submerged in sudsy water. In the country's first centuries, the soft, easy-to-work stone was popular for tombstones and hand-warming blocks.

To the right, beyond a narrow channel, the river empties into a sprawling wetland. Once across the bridge, take a path to the right marked with the white of the Bay Circuit Trail. Starting up a rough slope, the path passes a large soapstone slab lying swamp-side. Running along a ridge above the wetland, the trail broadens to the width of the carts that were used long ago to haul out stone. Gnawed maple stumps poking through debris confirm suspicions that beavers have moved in and are trying their best to reclaim the swamp.

Leveling out as it aims east, the trail proceeds through sparse woods grown in on old pastureland. It converges with a stone wall opportunistically propped against a glacial erratic of astounding proportions. Here since the last ice age, the boulder that was once just another stone in a wall is now popular with rock climbers. Keep looking around here, and you'll see a dramatic rock garden of massive boulders left by the retreating glaciers.

To reunite with the Bay Circuit Trail, circle the boulder counterclockwise, and head northwest. Progressing uphill amid glacial erratics lying about like giant hailstones, the trail nears a white house on the right. Pass this and the minor paths weaving in and out, and continue straight through a junction labeled with two white bars and a red marker.

The trail winds though the mostly open forest populated with oak, young pine, and the odd birch and beech. The red trail traces the edges of an obsolete pasture and eventually angles northwest to run back to the junction of Old County Road and the Bridge Trail. Having closed the loop, hike northwest back to Salem Street.

Returning to the Hammond Reservation, backtrack to where the trail splits, and bear right. Traveling east, the trail traces the periphery of an all but impenetrable wetland, passing suburban homes shrouded by tree cover. Near where the boardwalk begins, the Bay Circuit Trail detours right. Let it go, and continue north on the boardwalk, staying with the AVIS trail. Shortly this trail turns downhill and, heading west, reaches the causeway bordering the Mary French Reservation. Hike along this curious mound of stone and, when you arrive at the grand oak in the junction, bear right, and retrace the boardwalk back to the start.

## NEARBY ATTRACTIONS

The Addison Gallery of American Art, located at Andover's Phillips Academy (180 Main St., 978-749-4015, addison.andover.edu), offers a chance to see exciting art in a peaceful setting. Created by Thomas Cochran in 1913 to promote art appreciation and learning, the gallery is part of the Phillips Academy prep school but is free to the public. The gallery is open Tuesday–Saturday, 10 a.m.–5 p.m. (9 p.m. on Wednesdays), and Sunday, 1–5 p.m.

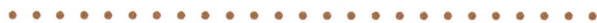

• • • • • • • • • • • • • • • • • • • • • • • •

**GPS TRAILHEAD COORDINATES**  N42° 37.783'  W71° 06.050'

**DIRECTIONS**  From Boston, take I-93 N 16.5 miles to Exit 41 and bear right onto MA 125. At 4.5 miles, turn right onto Salem Street and continue straight onto Gray Road. At 0.4 mile, turn right onto Korinthian Way. Park at the dip just before Athena Circle. Parking here is extremely limited. There's another parking area with more room on nearby Salem Street.

The boulder garden invites endless exploration.

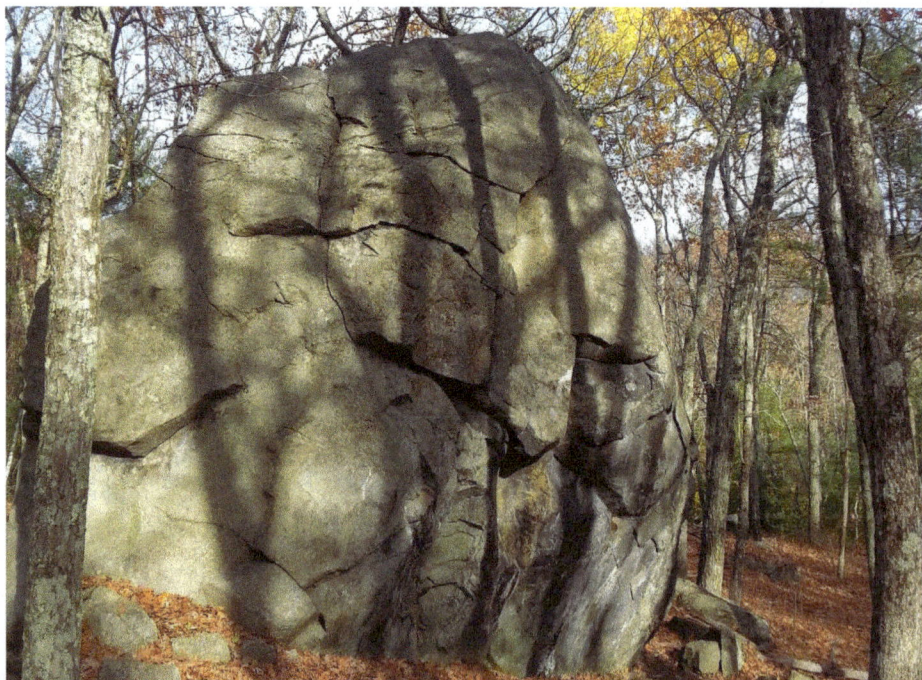

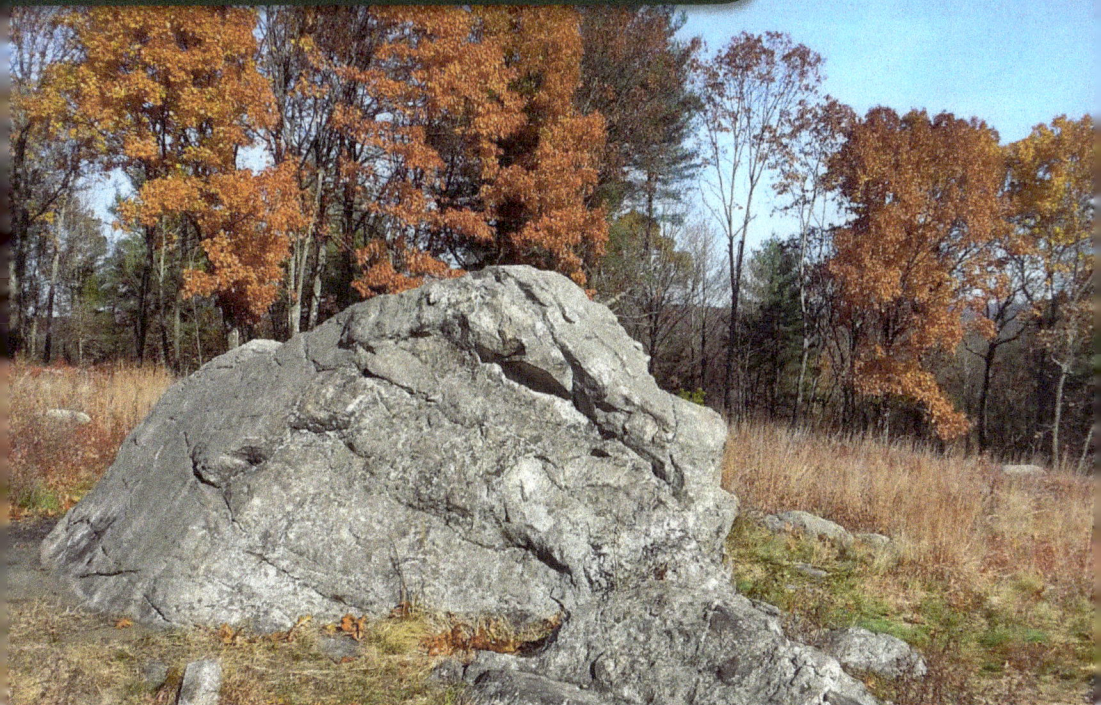

Elephant Rock presides over Boston Hill at Ward Reservation.

**TOURING A NEARLY** 700-acre parcel of former farmland and forest, this hike ascends Holt Hill for a view of the Boston skyline, leads around Cat Swamp and back to ascend Boston Hill, and then heads back toward the Ward farmstead.

## DESCRIPTION

Over the last several decades, nearly 40 parcels of land have been united and preserved to form what is now the Ward Reservation. The trailhead is easy to find: it's to the left of the kiosk at the end of the parking area. It was recently redirected, so follow the red blazes up a fairly steep, short, rocky pitch. Cross the road upon which you drove in, then bear right to climb along the edge of a sloping apple orchard. It's a spectacularly scenic start to your hike.

Toward the end of this side of the orchard, head left, continue through a wide gap in a stone wall, and cross the gravel drive. Continue across the grassland to a valley on the hill's eastern side. Here you're hiking through a column of tall, statuesque trees. Approach the edge of the woods and two trailheads. Head for the one farthest to the left, and follow this to another stone wall. Here you're following the yellow-blazed trail up Holt Hill. This is also part of the Bay Circuit Trail. The trail here is wide, firm, and smooth, like an old carriage road.

**DISTANCE & CONFIGURATION:** 4.7-mile loop

**DIFFICULTY:** Moderate

**SCENERY:** Farmland that has reverted to woods, centuries-old abandoned cart roads, an array of solstice stones, a rare quaking bog featuring concentric rings of floating vegetation

**EXPOSURE:** Mostly shaded

**TRAFFIC:** Light

**TRAIL SURFACE:** Mostly hard-packed, smooth dirt with grassy fields and an occasional boardwalk

**HIKING TIME:** 3–3.5 hours

**DRIVING DISTANCE FROM BOSTON COMMON:** 25 miles

**ELEVATION:** 293' at trailhead, 405' at highest point

**SEASON:** Year-round

**ACCESS:** Sunrise–sunset; parking $5, free for members of The Trustees of Reservations

**MAPS:** Available at entrance or tinyurl.com /wardreservationmap

**WHEELCHAIR ACCESS:** No

**FACILITIES:** None

**CONTACT:** The Trustees of Reservations, thetrustees.org/places-to-visit, 617-542-7696

**LOCATION:** Andover, MA

**COMMENTS:** The Ward Reservation has a wide variety of trails, providing myriad hiking options, depending on your time and energy.

At the wall, the orange trail splits to the right, and the Bay Circuit Trail continues straight on to the summit of Holt Hill. The Bay Circuit Trail arcs around Boston and is identified by white trail markers with the trail logo.

From the stone wall, the Bay Circuit Trail bends northwest toward a farmhouse built on a verdant cleft in the hill. Reaching an elevation level with the homestead, the trail arrives at a three-way junction distinguished by an epic birch tree. Parallel stone walls run due east from here, with two trails traveling in their shadows. The Bay Circuit Trail tracks the topmost wall briefly before veering north to girdle the hillside. Take this route as it curves through woods of monumental pines to approach Holt Hill, briefly winding east before taking the hill head-on. The well-trod grassy path is easy to follow, but the ascent is sudden and fairly steep.

Besides being a good test for the heart and lungs, Holt Hill's 420-foot elevation provides dramatic views of Boston and the Blue Hills. On June 17, 1775, settlers climbed to this vantage point to witness the raging fire in Charlestown set by British soldiers on orders of General Howe during the Battle of Bunker Hill.

At the top of the hill, you'll find Mabel Ward's solstice stones, arranged to mark the path of the sun on the longest and shortest days of the year—the summer and winter solstices, respectively—and the spring and autumn equinoxes. From the stones, hike 100 yards north to the imposing fire tower; then, following a stone wall on the right, locate a trail leading back into woods.

The trail here is much more like what you'd think of a hiking trail: narrower, winding, and a bit rocky in spots. The trail plunges straight down the hill's dark northern face toward Cat Swamp, so watch your footing, especially if there has been rain recently.

Upon reaching the swamp, the connector trail forms a T with the Sanborn Trail. Turn left and continue along the base of Holt Hill, heading west. The trail elevation

# Ward Reservation

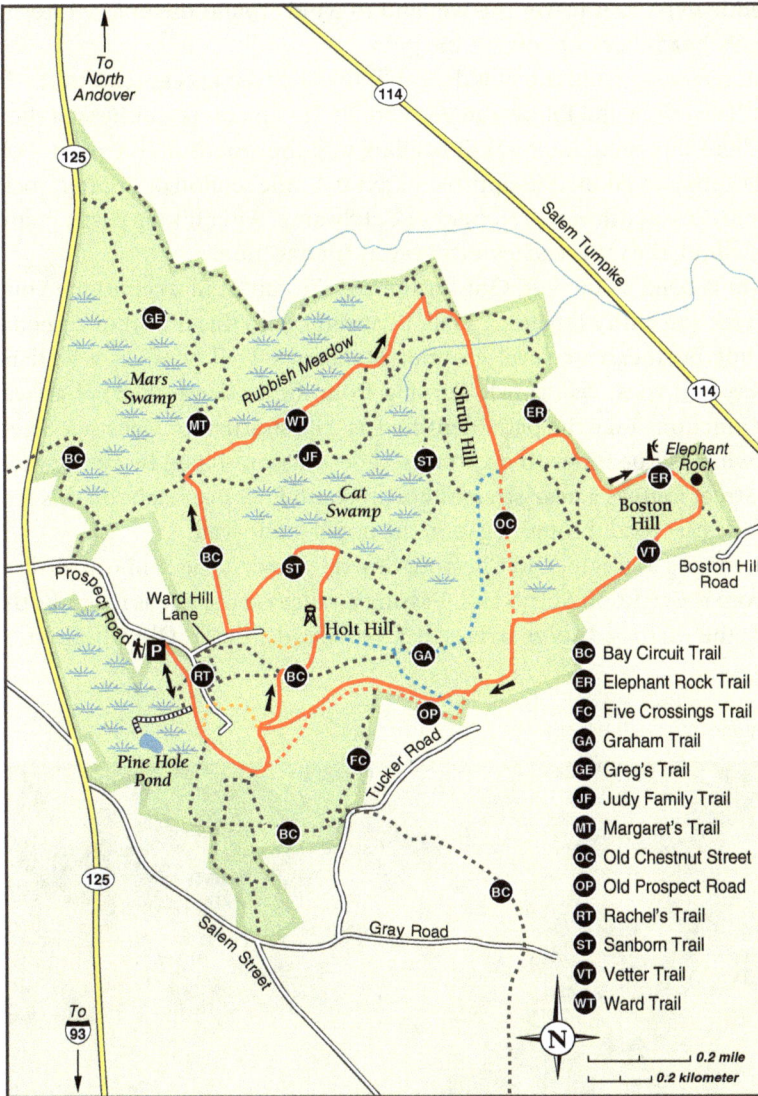

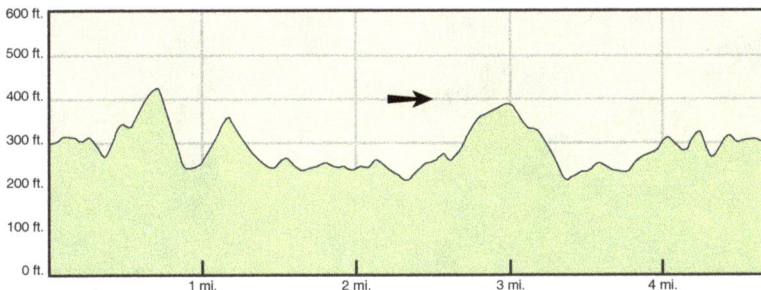

To
North
Andover

114

125

Salem Turnpike

114

GE

Mars
Swamp

Rubbish Meadow

MT

WT

BC

JF

ST

Shrub Hill

ER

Elephant
Rock

ER

Cat
Swamp

Boston
Hill

BC

ST

VT

Prospect Road

Ward Hill
Lane

Holt Hill

Boston Hill
Road

P

RT

BC

GA

Pine Hole
Pond

OP

FC

Tucker Road

125

BC

Salem Street

Gray Road

BC

To
93

| | |
|---|---|
| BC | Bay Circuit Trail |
| ER | Elephant Rock Trail |
| FC | Five Crossings Trail |
| GA | Graham Trail |
| GE | Greg's Trail |
| JF | Judy Family Trail |
| MT | Margaret's Trail |
| OC | Old Chestnut Street |
| OP | Old Prospect Road |
| RT | Rachel's Trail |
| ST | Sanborn Trail |
| VT | Vetter Trail |
| WT | Ward Trail |

N

0.2 mile

0.2 kilometer

**Elevation profile:** 600 ft. / 500 ft. / 400 ft. / 300 ft. / 200 ft. / 100 ft. / 0 ft. — 1 mi. / 2 mi. / 3 mi. / 4 mi.

is fairly gentle here, as it leaves the wetland to wind around the hill's western slope and gradually heads back up toward the peak.

As you reemerge from the woods, you'll find a paved access road to the hilltop reservoirs. Turn right and follow the Bay Circuit Trail markers southeast a short distance to where this route joins a trail heading into the woods on the right. Follow a stone wall northeast. Along this approximately 0.3-mile section of sloping, rocky terrain, the trail crosses the wet periphery of Cat Swamp. After hiking past a boardwalk and a brief climb, the trail reaches a three-way intersection.

Two trails bend to the left. Opt for the Bay Circuit Trail to continue your hike to the intersection with Margaret's Trail. Bear right onto this trail at intersection 22.

Traveling northeast on level ground, Margaret's Trail parallels a wetland rife with beavers and vocal waterfowl. Turning from the wetland, the trail arrives at a three-way junction. Take the path identified as "the shortcut to Chestnut Street" on the right, which serpentines to its promised destination. Lined by stone walls, Old Chestnut Street follows a near-straight north–south line. Bear right on this straight, smooth, wide cart road through a gap in the upper stone wall.

After crossing a stream, Old Chestnut Street intersects the Sanborn Trail, which drops in from the right off Shrub Hill. Passing a valley on the left as it climbs the side of this hill, the cart road soon arrives at a crossroads. Leave Old Chestnut Street,

The solstice stones atop Holt Hill

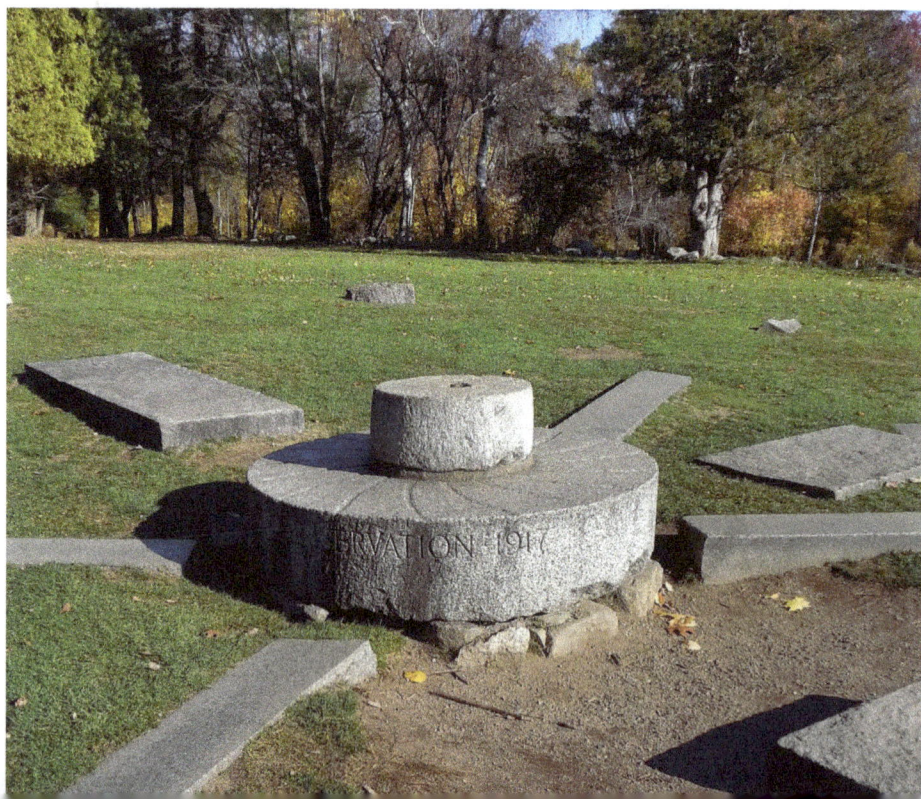

turning left onto Graham Trail at intersection 14 and hiking east toward Boston Hill. After turning here, the trail is narrower, rockier, and a bit steeper. At the next split in the trail, stay left on Graham Trail.

After climbing a bit farther to another junction, go right to continue your ascent. Stay on Graham Trail, following it southeast. Arrows eventually point the way to the top of Boston Hill. Curving around the top of Boston Hill, the trail passes a lovely vantage point above a meadow on the hill's western face. Continue east alongside a stone wall and a wire fence to a second meadow on the hill's eastern side.

Lying several yards ahead amid the fields of wild grasses and flowers is the curious glacial erratic named Elephant Rock. Angular yet rounded, the boulder does somewhat resemble an elephant basking in the sun. This is a great place to relax for a bit and take in the view of Boston to the south.

When you're ready to continue, hike down the hill, passing a service road, to a dense grove of birch saplings. Approaching the base of the hill edged by a stone wall, the trail meets another route merging from the right. The trail veers left to run along the outside of an abandoned, walled-in avenue.

Ahead, the trail crosses a broad stream via a boardwalk and, after navigating a series of stone walls, climbs gently to connect with Old Chestnut Street. Bear left on this familiar avenue, and continue several hundred yards to another trail, well marked with an arrow, that branches off to the right.

Pass another path that splits northward. Climbing away from the wetland, the trail skirts private property. Shortly, where it splits again, arrows point the way.

A few feet farther, at a junction, a trail sign directs you either right to head to the summit of Holt Hill or left to follow Old Prospect Road. Head left, easing southeast along the hillside that tapers downhill past a convergence of stone walls, to join an old cart road. Follow that trail back to the parking lot.

Established in 1940, Ward Reservation is a perfect example of landscape architect and conservationist Charles Eliot's ambitions to preserve New England's open spaces. Initiated by Mabel B. Ward's gift of 153 acres to The Trustees of Reservations, the reservation has grown to 700 acres as private individuals have made similar gifts over the years.

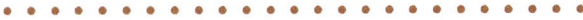

• • • • • • • • • • • • • • • • • • • • • • • • • • • • • •

**GPS TRAILHEAD COORDINATES**  N42° 38.433'  W71° 06.733'

**DIRECTIONS**  From Boston, take I-93 N to Exit 41. Exit onto MA 125 N and go 5 miles. Turn right onto Prospect Road and follow it 0.3 mile to the reservation entrance; there is a parking area on the right.

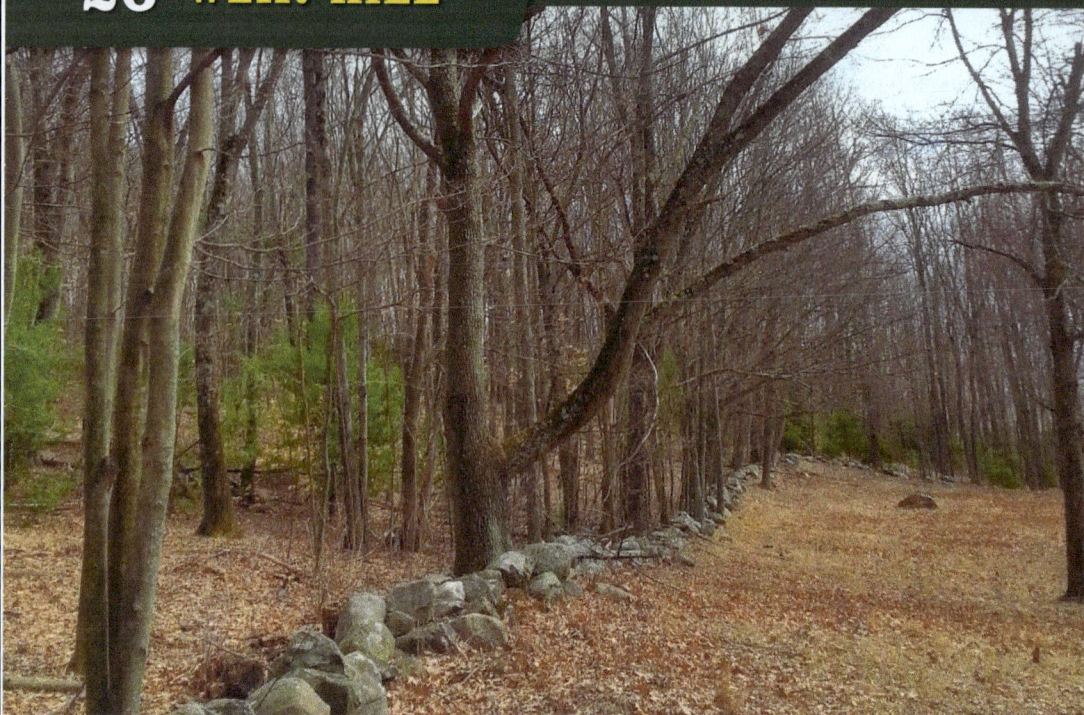

The Weir Hill hike takes you deep into woods, along the shores of a lake, and to sweeping hilltop views.

**TOURING LAND THAT** was once the estate of a 19th-century industrialist, this hike circles the base of a massive drumlin beside Lake Cochichewick and then climbs along its axis to reach a scenic vista atop a second conjoined drumlin.

## DESCRIPTION

From the information kiosk above Stevens Street, climb the grass-covered hill through a gap in a stone wall, and ease into the cool shade of woods, heading northeast. Trace the property's periphery along the base of Weir Hill. Stay left at each of the next two intersections to take up the gently arcing Edgewood Farm Trail. Watch for the next fork (it's less pronounced than the others), and bear left again to remain on this same trail as it descends to a streambed marked by skunk cabbage and mud the color of dark chocolate. A footbridge (and during wet season a few acrobatic leaps) will help you get to the other side without getting your hiking boots or sneakers too muddy.

Ahead, a trail entering from private property to the north interrupts Edgewater Farm Trail. Hike the wide path several yards south, and bear left again where Edgewater Farm Trail continues on its eastward tack through a stand of young birch trees. After being bisected one last time, Edgewood Farm Trail coasts downhill amid a blend of beech, pine, and birch to the shore of Lake Cochichewick. As currents of

**DISTANCE & CONFIGURATION:** 2.46-mile loop

**DIFFICULTY:** Easy–moderate

**SCENERY:** Hills, woods, open fields, hilltop views, views across Lake Cochichewick

**EXPOSURE:** Mostly shaded

**TRAFFIC:** Moderate

**TRAIL SURFACE:** Firmly packed dirt, although some sections can be muddy at times.

**HIKING TIME:** 1.5 hours

**DRIVING DISTANCE FROM BOSTON COMMON:** 27 miles

**ELEVATION:** 112' at trailhead, 302' at highest point

**SEASON:** Year-round

**ACCESS:** Sunrise–sunset; free

**MAPS:** Available at reservation while supplies last or at tinyurl.com/weirhillmap

**WHEELCHAIR ACCESS:** No

**FACILITIES:** None

**CONTACT:** The Trustees of Reservations, thetrustees.org/places-to-visit, 617-542-7696

**LOCATION:** North Andover, MA

**COMMENTS:** An ideal time to visit Weir Hill is 1–1.5 hours before dusk to reach the hike's scenic vista in time for sunset. From there, it's a short, simple walk back to the parking area.

air propel ripples of surf to land, small waves break against the edge of the woods, providing a constant soothing soundtrack.

Bearing south a foot or two from the water, the root-tangled trail soon arrives at a sort of beach beside a stone foundation. Now little more than an abstract form that excites the imagination, this pit edged with granite marks where the clubhouse of the North Andover Country Club once stood. Leaving this site, continue along the lake on what now becomes Cochichewick Trail. Hiking west around the base of the minor mound of glacial rubble that bumps shoulders with the more substantial Weir Hill drumlin, the trail crosses the watery gap between the two via a boardwalk. Then the trail heads south beneath the brilliant foliage of birch and hickory to where the tip of the great drumlin presses close to Lake Cochichewick's western bank.

It is likely that until Metacomet and allied tribes lost their war against colonial expansion, the Pennacook lived in settlements here. Archaeologists digging in the area in 1968 uncovered a campsite near where the lake narrows as it bends west toward Stevens Pond. The setting offered all that the native people needed: shelter from northern winds, woods full of game, and proximity to the alewife breeding grounds. The tribes set up woven traps fixed with wooden stakes just offshore to catch the coveted fish swimming from brook to lake.

The presence of the Pennacook and their use of the land are evident in the natural history of the hillside. Before the arrival of white settlers, American Indians altered the landscape almost as radically as did any subsequent farmer or timberman. To attract deer and facilitate hunting, the tribes practiced controlled burning. This had the immediate effect of clearing underbrush and promoting the growth of tender shoots and grasses—valuable fodder for grazing animals. Over the long term, the burnings affected the profile of the woodland by promoting tree and shrub species more resistant to fire.

## Weir Hill

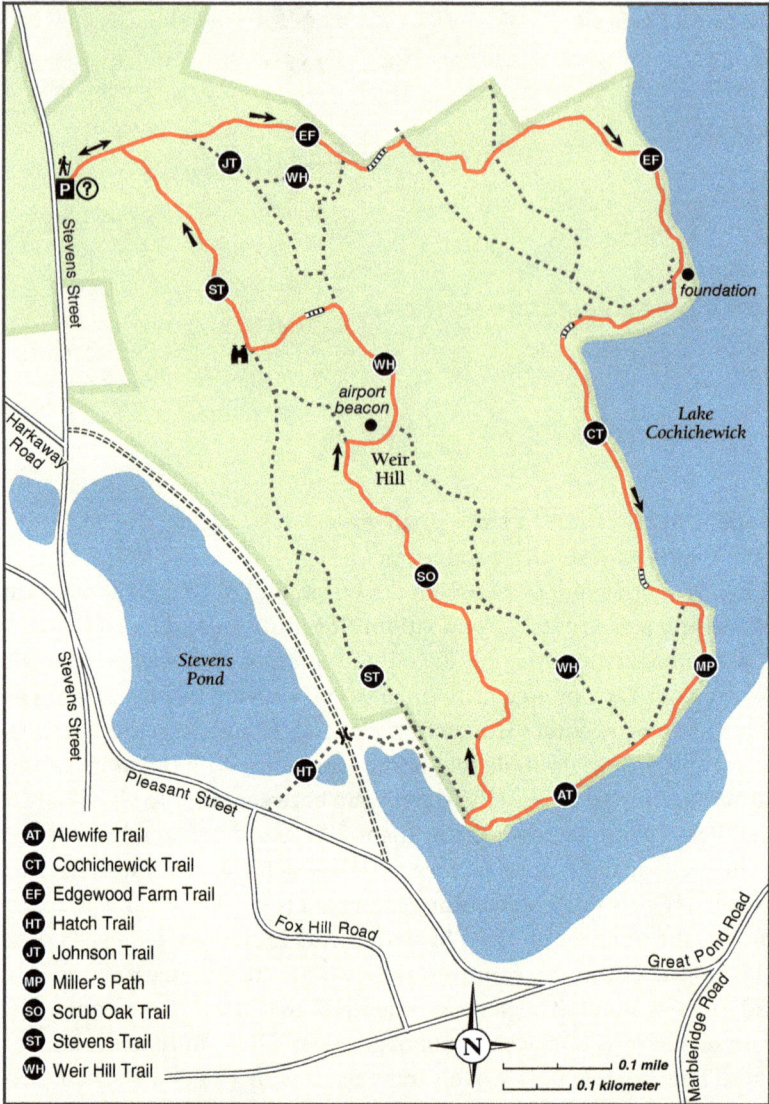

- **AT** Alewife Trail
- **CT** Cochichewick Trail
- **EF** Edgewood Farm Trail
- **HT** Hatch Trail
- **JT** Johnson Trail
- **MP** Miller's Path
- **SO** Scrub Oak Trail
- **ST** Stevens Trail
- **WH** Weir Hill Trail

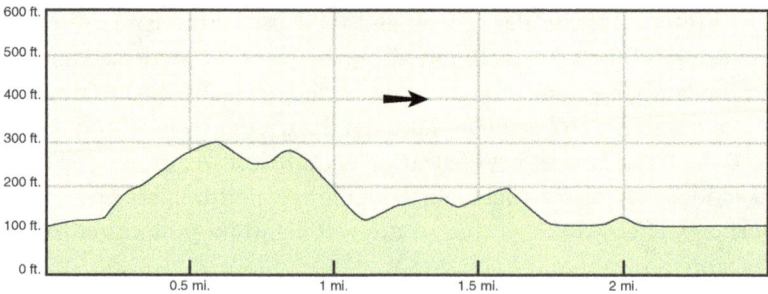

Like the Indians, the farmers and mill operators who once settled this area are gone, yet their mark on the landscape endures. Fragments of stone walls remain in the woods, and careful observation will reveal geometric patches of successional species telling which tracts were once pasture and which were timber lots. Many of the mill dams are gone, but the effect of human activity persists in the character of the area's ecology. In fact, the very name Weir Hill is said to have once been Wire Hill.

As a result of the property's complex history, several distinct types of plant communities grow on Weir Hill. Besides an uncommon 60-acre oak-and-hickory forest, the hill harbors several rare, protected species, including the white bog orchid (*Habenaria dilatata*), violet bush clover (*Lespedeza violacea*), and butternut tree (*Juglans nigra*).

At the tip of Weir Hill's blunt nose, Cochichewick Trail becomes Miller's Path. Remaining flush to the shore, the trail arches west, rising slightly to meet a path that emerges from woods below what appears to be former pastureland. Bear left to continue southwest along the foot of scruffy grassland dotted with scrub pine and oak. Improvised paths bleed off to the right now and again; ignore these and the (unmarked) Weir Hill Trail, and continue on level ground to where the lake curls north and a railroad trestle bridge comes into sight. Take the next trail here that bears north away from the water. Overall, the trails at Weir Hill are well defined, meaning you're not likely to wander off the trail, but they could benefit from being slightly better marked.

Looking something like a ski slope in summer pending a manicure by pruning crews, the southern face of Weir Hill—with its rangy blueberry bushes, ferns, and spotty oaks and pines—is a haven for bobolinks, goldfinches, bluebirds, and other bird species dependent on open meadowlands.

The first stage of the ascent ends at a junction well up the hill. To climb higher along the drumlin's middle, bear left. Rising and sinking into and out of deep swales, the trail reaches a tilted T intersection halfway up the hill. Turn left and continue northwest on Scrub Oak Trail. This trail winds between bristly oaks and graceful hickories on its approach to the hill's gentle summit.

Just as the trail starts down the hill's western slope, it meets a path entering from the right. Switch off here and head east briefly to pass an airport beacon erected amid trees at Weir Hill's highest point. When you come to the Weir Hill Trail immediately ahead, bear left and follow it as it descends north into a cleft formed by Weir Hill and its lesser twin.

Another trail diverts left, crossing a bog before mounting the eastern slope of the second hill. Follow this mud- and rock-laced detour to reap the reward of a magnificent view looking west from a gorgeous hillside meadow. The view from atop the hill looks much like it probably did when the area was first settled. Plan to reach this picturesque summit in time to take in the light effects of the setting sun. Whenever you're fully relaxed and ready, follow the Stevens Trail as it descends along the hill's axis to Johnson Trail. Bear left at this last junction to return to the reservation's entrance on Stevens Street.

## NEARBY ATTRACTIONS

If hiking Weir Hill sparks an interest in the American Indian history of the region, consider paying a visit to the Robert S. Peabody Institute of Archaeology, located at Andover's Phillips Academy (peabody.andover.edu). This museum, one of the country's most important repositories of American Indian archaeological collections, is located on the corner of Main Street and Phillips Street. The museum is open daily, and admission is free, but by appointment only. To arrange a visit, reach them at rspeabody@andover.edu or call 978-749-4490.

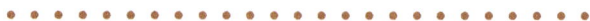

• • • • • • • • • • • • • • • • • • • • • • • • • • •

**GPS TRAILHEAD COORDINATES** N42° 41.840' W71° 06.653'

**DIRECTIONS** From Boston, take I-93 N to MA 125 N (Andover bypass) and proceed for 7.3 miles. At the traffic lights, merge left onto MA 114 W. At the traffic lights opposite Merrimack College (on the left), turn right onto Andover Street (MA 125) and follow it 0.2 mile. Turn right at the traffic lights (still on Andover Street) and go 0.6 mile. Bear right at the fork and continue 0.2 mile to the intersection at Old North Andover Center. Go straight another 0.1 mile, then make a left onto Stevens Street. Continue 0.8 mile to the entrance on the right. Park along the road.

Rest on the chunk of granite to enjoy the views from atop Weir Hill.

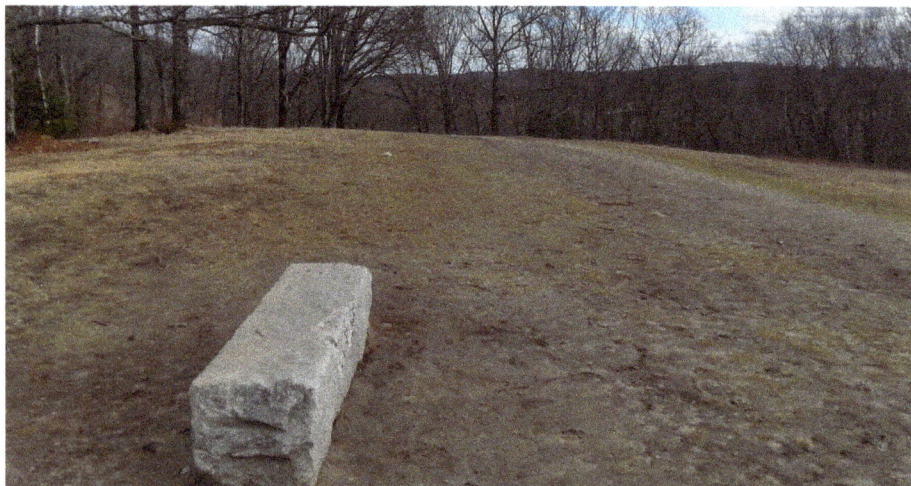

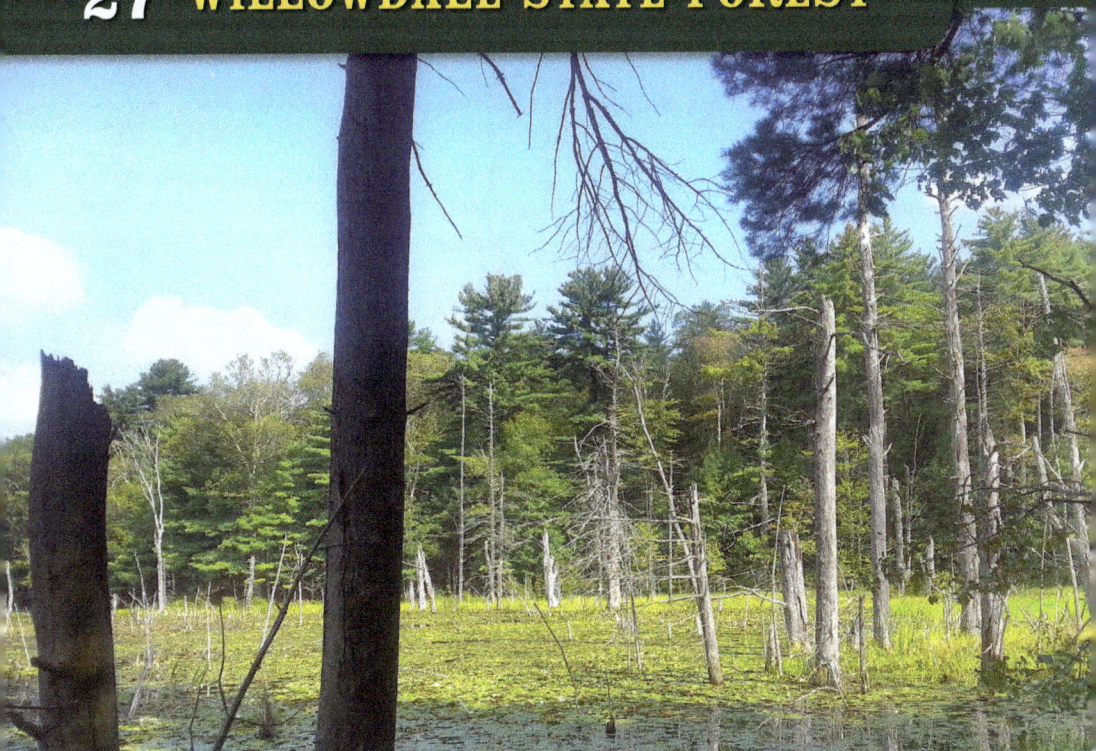

Willowdale State Forest winds through several marshlands.

**THIS HIKE EXPLORES** the pine swamp of the popular Willowdale State Forest, taking a detour halfway through to travel along the Ipswich River to a scenic 19th-century milldam.

## DESCRIPTION

From the Willowdale State Forest parking area on the side of Linebrook Road, navigate past the green steel fence, and hike south on the mowed path to the left of a cultivated strawberry field. Sloping to the edge of the farmland, the trail divides in two as it reaches shade.

Heed the white trail blazes for the Bay Circuit Trail, and enter the woods via a prominent esker bridging the wetland. Hardwoods, mostly oaks and hickories, frame the sides of the ridge. Except for the filtered sound of cars traveling on US 1 a couple of miles away, there is little to hear but buzzing insects, woodland birds, and the crunch of your own footsteps.

A stone wall follows along on the right, meeting the broad trail as it travels west, gently undulating to a triangular crossroads marked 24. Stay right, and continue hiking west to junction 25. Here, pick up a wide cart road heading southwest. By now the sound of cars is diminishing as you get deeper into the woods. Sloping to more

**DISTANCE & CONFIGURATION:** 7.6-mile loop

**DIFFICULTY:** Easy–moderate due to length

**SCENERY:** Woods, kettle ponds, vernal pools, Ipswich River, 19th-century milldam

**EXPOSURE:** Mostly shaded

**TRAFFIC:** Moderate

**TRAIL SURFACE:** Mostly packed dirt and gravel; some occasionally muddy areas

**HIKING TIME:** 3 hours

**DRIVING DISTANCE FROM BOSTON COMMON:** 29 miles

**ELEVATION:** 119' at trailhead, no significant gain

**SEASON:** Year-round

**ACCESS:** Sunrise–sunset; free

**MAPS:** Posted at trailhead or at tinyurl.com/willowdalemap

**WHEELCHAIR ACCESS:** No, but nearby Bradley Palmer State Park has wheelchair-friendly trails.

**FACILITIES:** None

**CONTACT:** Massachusetts Dept. of Conservation and Resources, mass.gov/locations/willowdale-state-forest, 617-626-1250

**LOCATION:** Ipswich, MA

**COMMENTS:** Deer ticks are common in these woods, so check yourself carefully after hiking. Also note that hunting is allowed in November and December.

wetland, the wide road flattens and narrows precipitously as it nears the next intersection. Choose the left route, and continue southwest, passing a scattered fragment of stone wall. Guided by parallel stone walls, the cart road passes through reforested farmland to reach junction 27.

Bearing right, the trail begins climbing, swings west, and keeps climbing to arrive at another junction. This intersection is marked 37.

The cart road exits to Old Right Road, which lies to the north. A lesser-used and narrower footpath splits off to the left. Take this route to continue south, hiking over rounded hillsides straight through junction 38. Ahead, a wetland basin rife with pine lies at the foot of upland. At junction 39, leave the primary trail, blazed with small blue and red markers, and hike left, bearing closer to the wetland. Rapidly filling in with frilly white pine saplings and bushy ferns, this moist enclave of formerly cleared land is an ideal environment for deer. Guided by a brook, the trail bends gradually northwest to reconnect with the trail from which it diverged earlier. At this unmarked juncture, descend a slight hill heading southwest to a causeway spanning the brook's overflow.

Atop the opposite rise, the trail arrives at junction 41. Continue straight to reconnect with the Bay Circuit Trail as it comes rolling in from the east on another broad cart road at junction number 10. Picking up with this long-distance trail, aim for its distinctive white and blue blazes posted across the way, and hike west through junction 11 to a large pond nestled in brush. Heading toward Hood Pond in Boxford, the Bay Circuit Trail rounds the swamp and directs itself to the Topsfield–Ipswich town line.

Depart this trail at junction 12, and hike south a few hundred yards to a broad four-way intersection that is missing a marker (but is likely number 29), and hike left. Following a stone wall up and over a modest hill, the route travels along a broad

## Willowdale State Forest

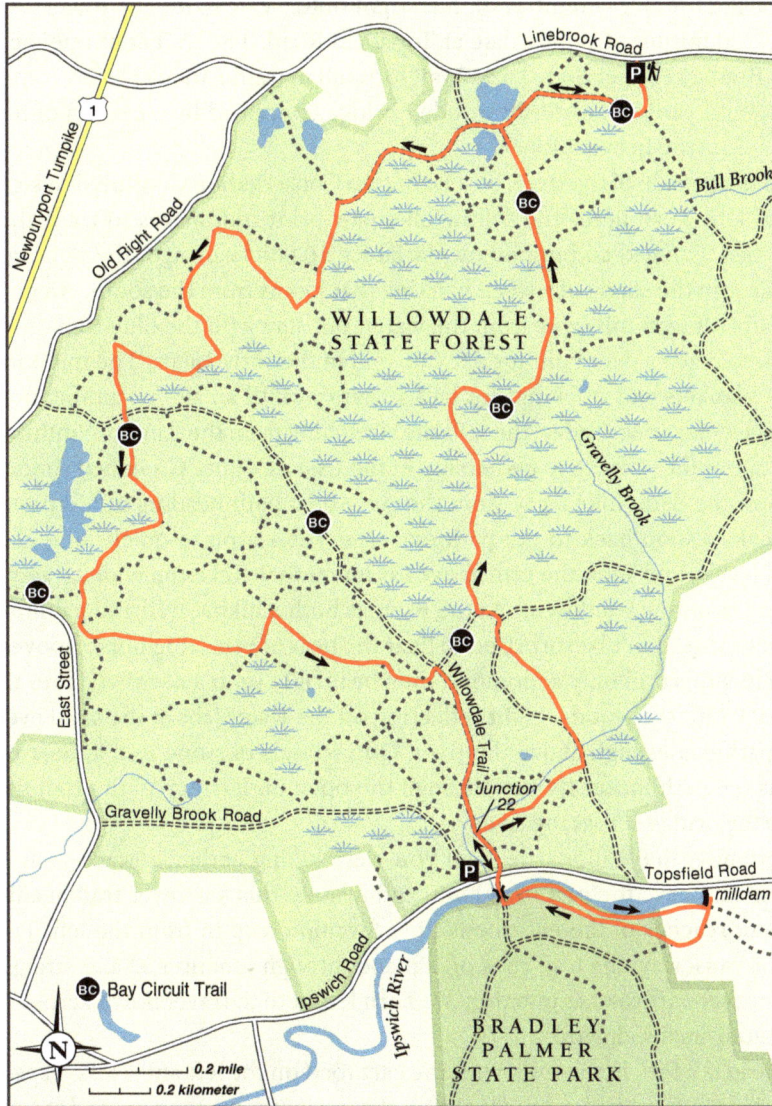

avenue through uncluttered woods of beech and pine to arrive at junction 45. Continue straight (east) through this crossroads and the next, gradually curving north to reach junction 33. Bear right, away from Pine Swamp, to follow an expansive trail edged with sweet-smelling ferns over a couple of small rises to junction 35. Deviate from this southeastern trajectory briefly to hike north. At this junction (6), the Bay Circuit Trail sweeps in from the northeast, jackknifes, and continues on its 200-mile journey around Boston.

Leaving the Bay Circuit Trail, turn right onto a cart road, and travel 0.4 mile to the western border of Willowdale at Topsfield Road. The trail continues across the road at Bradley Palmer State Park. Wait for a lull in traffic, then cross to continue the hike. Several yards in, a sturdy wooden bridge concealed by a curtain of hemlocks arches across the Ipswich River.

On the far side of the river, by a Hamilton Conservation Commission sign, a trail diverges left. Turn here, and follow blue paw-print trail blazes to trace the river's course east. Gouged and grated by glacial ice 10,000 years ago, the river lies like a black racer in the shade of a steep banking that looms from the south. An occasional path splits off to climb away from the water, but stay with the blue trail on its riverside run to reach a dam built for a textile mill in the early 1800s. The mill turned out woolen blankets and stockings for half a century until an all-consuming fire put an end to the enterprise. Today, the mill site stretching from the dam to Winthrop Street is held under the protective ownership of the Essex County Greenbelt Association.

From the dam, hike away from the river on a path heading uphill past marker 10 to make a loop back to the park entrance. After a pulse-quickening climb, the ground levels, and soon the trail arrives at junction 9. Take the wide, grassy avenue right and continue southwest. As the route is both a hiking trail and a jumping lane for equestrians, don't be surprised to hear the beat of cantering horse hooves.

Follow this trail only a moment, then bear right onto a narrower path that ventures back into the woods. Light reflecting off the water jabs at the staid evergreens as the path passes high above the river. Odd strands of stone wall appear now and again as the path makes its way through the open understory to the trail that leads back to the bridge across the river.

Resuming the Willowdale Trail you were hiking earlier, retrace your steps to junction 22. Leave the cart road here, and take up this narrower trail heading east. The outer reaches of the enormous Pine Swamp creep in from the left. Following a natural causeway, the trail runs on a plane through junction 32 and straight on to meet another cart road at junction 21. Turn left here to travel north across Gravelly Brook along its floodplain.

Ahead is a fork in the trail, with the cart road on the left and a less-traveled path on the right. A few hundred yards ahead, the two paths meet again, and the cart road continues to junction 20. At this slightly disorienting intersection, hike left and then straight at the next split to rejoin the Bay Circuit Trail, traveling north.

The trail crosses a culvert here and there and winds past pools teeming with life. Meandering west and then east, the trail navigates the swamp along several hillsides. The wide, flat path eventually straightens and climbs from the swamp. Ascending an extended gravel slope, the trail passes several others diverging from it, and finally returns to junction 24. Having come full circle, bear right and follow the familiar trail through the woods to the fields and Linebrook Road where you started.

## NEARBY ATTRACTIONS

After this long hike, you'll be ready for a bite to eat. Seek out The Clam Box at 246 High St. in Ipswich (978-356-9707, clamboxipswich.com). Custom built to resemble an actual clam box, the restaurant serves a full menu of fried freshly caught seafood. Their hours vary, so call before stopping by. Foote's Canoe Rentals (978-356-9771, footebrotherscanoes.com), located opposite the dam, has canoes to rent by the hour and by the day and will even organize overnight trips.

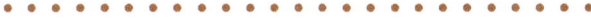

• • • • • • • • • • • • • • • • • • • • • • • • •

**GPS TRAILHEAD COORDINATES** N42° 41.100' W70° 53.833'

**DIRECTIONS** From Boston, take US 1 N toward the Tobin Bridge. Drive 15.1 miles and merge onto I-95 N. After 3.7 miles, take Exit 50 (toward Topsfield) to US 1 N. At 6.8 miles, turn right onto Linebrook Road. Continue about 1.3 miles. The parking area is on the right at the bottom of a hill just before Marini Farm Stand (259 Linebrook Road).

Stately mixed deciduous trees line the trail leading into the forest.

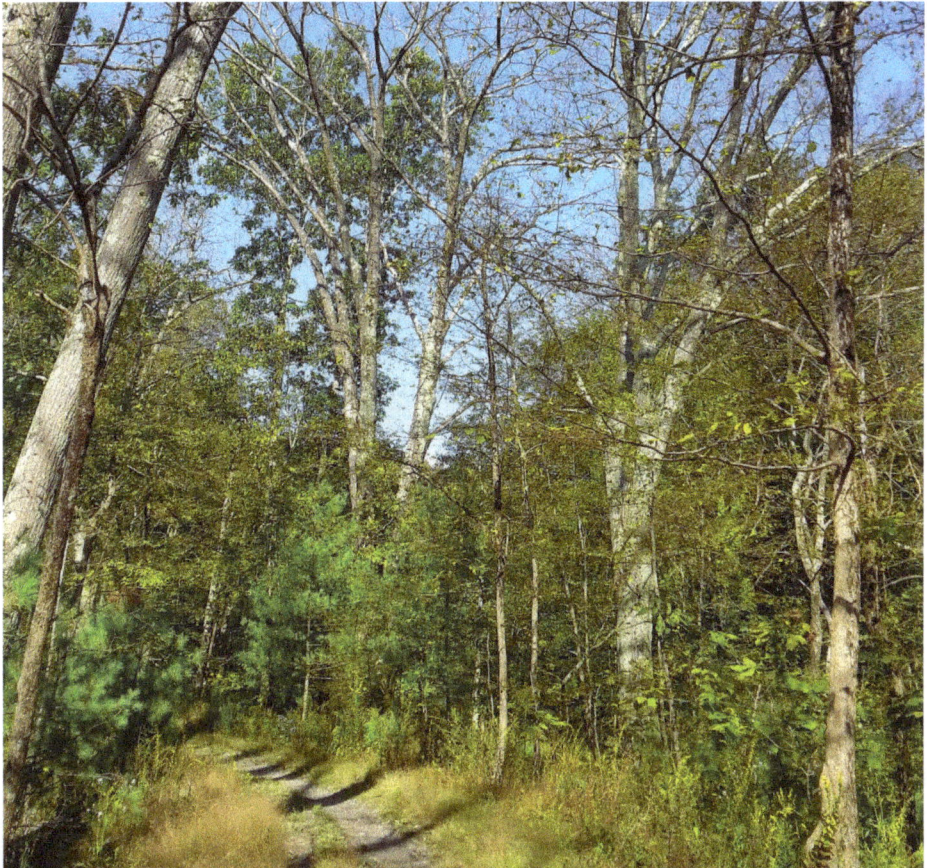

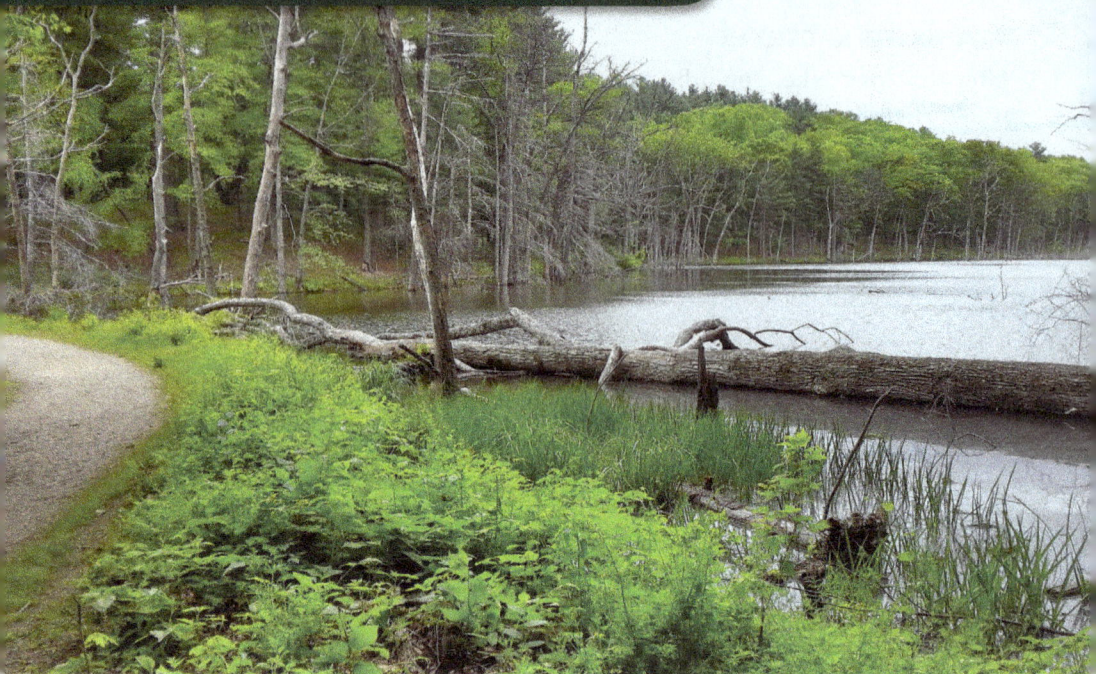

Winnekenni Park is a great hike for families with young kids.

**AFTER FIRST SURVEYING** the magnificent expanse of Kenoza Lake from a carriage road and footpaths, this hike climbs to a 19th-century castle built of fieldstone.

## DESCRIPTION

In 1861, chemist and agronomist James R. Nichols purchased the former Darling Farm and gave it the name Winnekenni, the Pennacook Indian word for "very beautiful." Two years earlier, poet and Haverhill native John Greenleaf Whittier had renamed Great Pond beside the farm Kenoza Lake, meaning "lake of the pickerel" in the same Indian tongue. Whittier was likely sincere in his sentiments when in his poem "Kenoza," he wrote:

> *Lake of Pickerel! Let no more*
> *The echoes answer back "Great Pond,"*
> *But sweet Kenoza, from thy shore*
> *And watching hill beyond.*
> *And Indian ghosts, if such there be,*
> *Who ply unseen their shadowy lines*
> *Call back the dear old name to thee,*
> *As with the voices of the pine.*

**DISTANCE & CONFIGURATION:** 5.6-mile out-and-back with 2 loops

**DIFFICULTY:** Easy

**SCENERY:** 2 lakes, woods, restored stone castle

**EXPOSURE:** Mostly shaded except for sun-exposed stretches along the banks of Kenoza Lake and on the grounds of Winnekenni Castle.

**TRAFFIC:** Moderate

**TRAIL SURFACE:** Packed earth

**HIKING TIME:** 3 hours

**DRIVING DISTANCE FROM BOSTON COMMON:** 38 miles

**ELEVATION:** 132' at trailhead, 243' at highest point

**SEASON:** Year-round

**ACCESS:** Sunrise–sunset; free

**MAPS:** Posted at the parking area; also available at tinyurl.com/winnekennimap

**WHEELCHAIR ACCESS:** The 2.5-mile Dudley Porter Trail that borders three quarters of Kenoza Lake is wheelchair-friendly.

**FACILITIES:** None

**CONTACT:** City of Haverhill, Conservation Dept., tinyurl.com/winnekennipark, 978-374-2334

**LOCATION:** Haverhill, MA

**COMMENTS:** Winnekenni Castle hosts many special events, including Haunted Halloween Nights in October.

After a decade of summering at his Haverhill farm, Nichols traveled to England and was struck by the country's great cathedrals and castles. He returned inspired and built a castle at Winnekenni of granite excavated from his hillside. In 1885, after 24 years at Winnekenni Castle, the doctor sold the castle and a parcel of land. A decade later, the City of Haverhill acquired the property and made Winnekenni its first public park.

Begin the hike heading north toward MA 110 on the path that runs wide along the bank of the Basin of Kenoza Lake. Shortly after passing a children's play area, the path cuts close to the road and dips into a wooded corridor. Emerging on the other side, stay right and continue south on a wide packed-earth path that leads between Kenoza Lake and the basin. Straight ahead, the woods end at a dam bridging the waters; cross here to arrive at the Dudley Porter Trail. Turn left at this junction and proceed east on the old carriage trail, edged by beech trees.

Keeping a fairly level grade, the carriage path rounds wide bends as it follows Kenoza's bank. About a quarter of a mile in, rhododendrons loom among the beech and oak. Ahead on the right, the trail approaches a monument erected in memory of the trail's namesake, Dudley Porter, who died in 1906.

Across the lake to the north, you will see an alluring forest of hemlock. Almost entirely devoid of deciduous species, these dark woods are at once forbidding and alluring. Ahead the trail arrives at a broad junction with a bench and a sign pointing east to the Castle Trail. Make a detour here for a quick trip to the castle, or hike on, staying with the Dudley Porter Trail, which winds around the eastern tip of the lake, forms a causeway, and crosses wetland as it heads north.

The trail turns away from the lake and ascends into woods. Once the water is out of sight, the trail arrives at a two-way split. Hike up the hill to find the ruins of a small gazebo or cabin poised on the edge of the path. Stop to have a look from this vantage point. Then follow the road into the hill's hemlock-shaded recesses. Following the

# Winnekenni Park

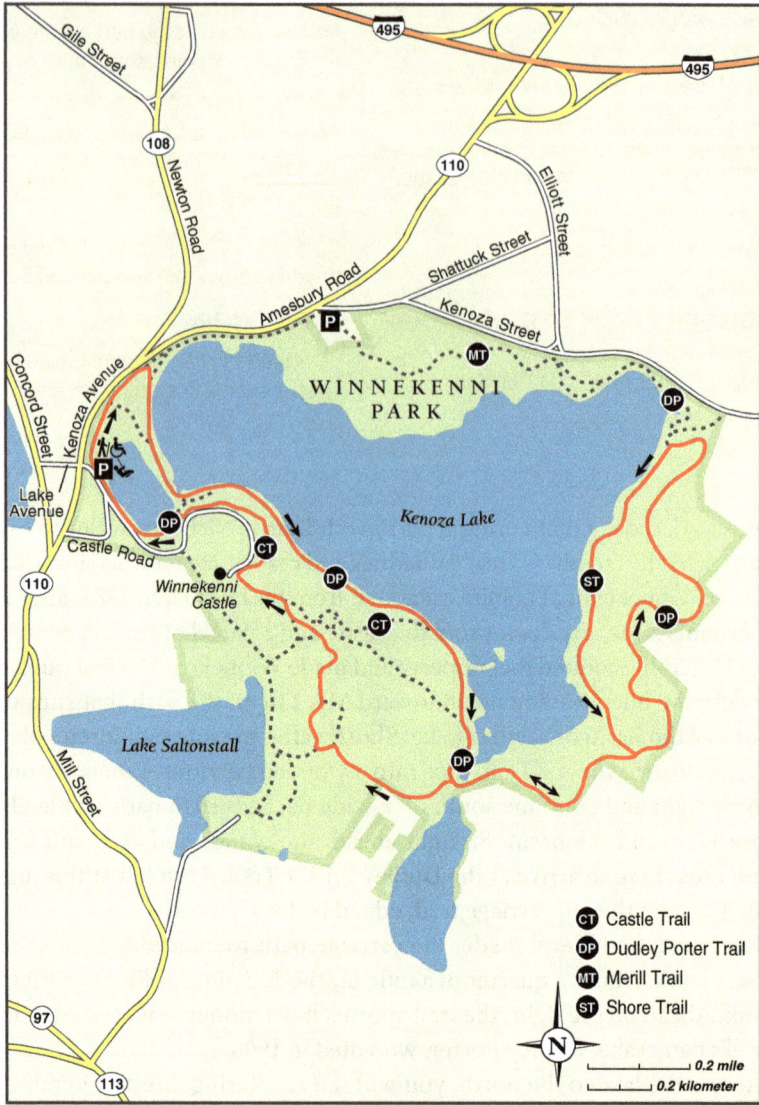

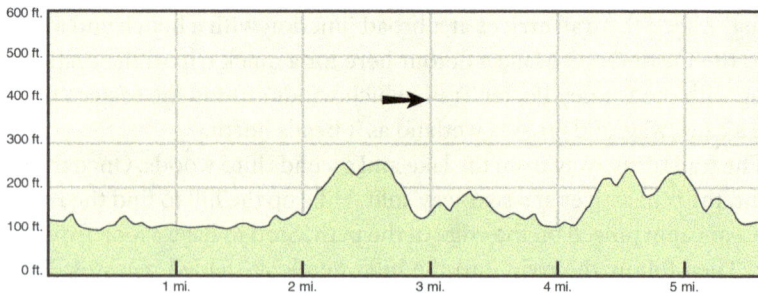

Castle Road

Winnekenni Castle

Kenoza Lake

Lake Saltonstall

WINNEKENNI PARK

CT Castle Trail
DP Dudley Porter Trail
MT Merill Trail
ST Shore Trail

N

0.2 mile
0.2 kilometer

pronounced contours of the land surrounding the lake, the trail bends this way and that as it gains elevation. Finally the path levels on a lofty plateau. Here the trail's left side falls away to a steep banking open to all but sunlight. Nothing but a few ferns and velvety silence fill the void beneath the hemlocks.

Passing a slender path that leads to a dome-shaped field beyond woods to the right, the trail weaves from the east to the west then north as it descends back to Kenoza Lake. After sloping to the water in an arc to the left, the trail levels at a junction. Pick up the Shore Trail, which runs southwest, to double-back to Winnekenni Hill. This path is littered with roots, rocks, and occasional muddy spots, so watch your step.

On the left, just past a birch with three trunks, the trail climbs away from the lake to meet the Dudley Porter Trail at an intersection passed earlier. Turn right and retrace your steps to the causeway. Look for a narrow trail marked with red blazes after crossing between the lake and the wetland. This trail will diverge from the carriage road. Follow this stony path southwest to another split. Stay with the red trail and continue uphill to a second junction. This time, choose the path to the right, changing course to follow a loose-stone wall running horizontal to the hill. The path is clear from use but otherwise poorly marked. However, where the direction gets sketchy, a light-blue arrow painted on a tree points the way. From the arrow on, light-blue dots appear with sufficient frequency.

At the next fork, bear left and hike downhill. Continuing in this direction leads you to Lake Saltonstall. Soon the path forks again. This time, take the trail to the right, and continue uphill on an old road surfaced with fractured asphalt disguised by moss and grass. At the top of the hill, on the left, you will spot the stone and brick foundation of a building and, a few feet higher on the hill, a second foundation with a crumbling tower. Offspring of trees cut centuries ago have returned the Darling Farm meadows to dense woods, obscuring this home's once-magnificent view of the lakes below.

Facing Kenoza Lake, find a path to the left of the homesite and follow it on its northwest course down the hill. Soon after it winds north to face the water, this path meets a crossroad. Turn left and continue several yards farther to join a carriage road to Winnekenni Castle. Because this road makes a rear approach, you will first see the outbuildings. The magnificent castle stands beyond these, overlooking Kenoza Lake. After taking in the castle and bronze elk statue, find the head of the Castle Trail on the edge of the woods to the right of the paved drive, and descend toward the lake. At the Dudley Porter Trail, turn left and hike to the trail's end at the entrance to the park.

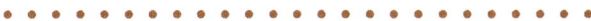

• • • • • • • • • • • • • • • • • • • • • • • • • • • •

**GPS TRAILHEAD COORDINATES**  N42° 47.450'  W71° 04.133'

**DIRECTIONS**  From Boston, take I-93 N 22.4 miles to I-495 N. From I-495 take Exit 52 to MA 110 W. Turn left onto MA 110/Kenoza Avenue. The park is 1.1 miles ahead on the left.

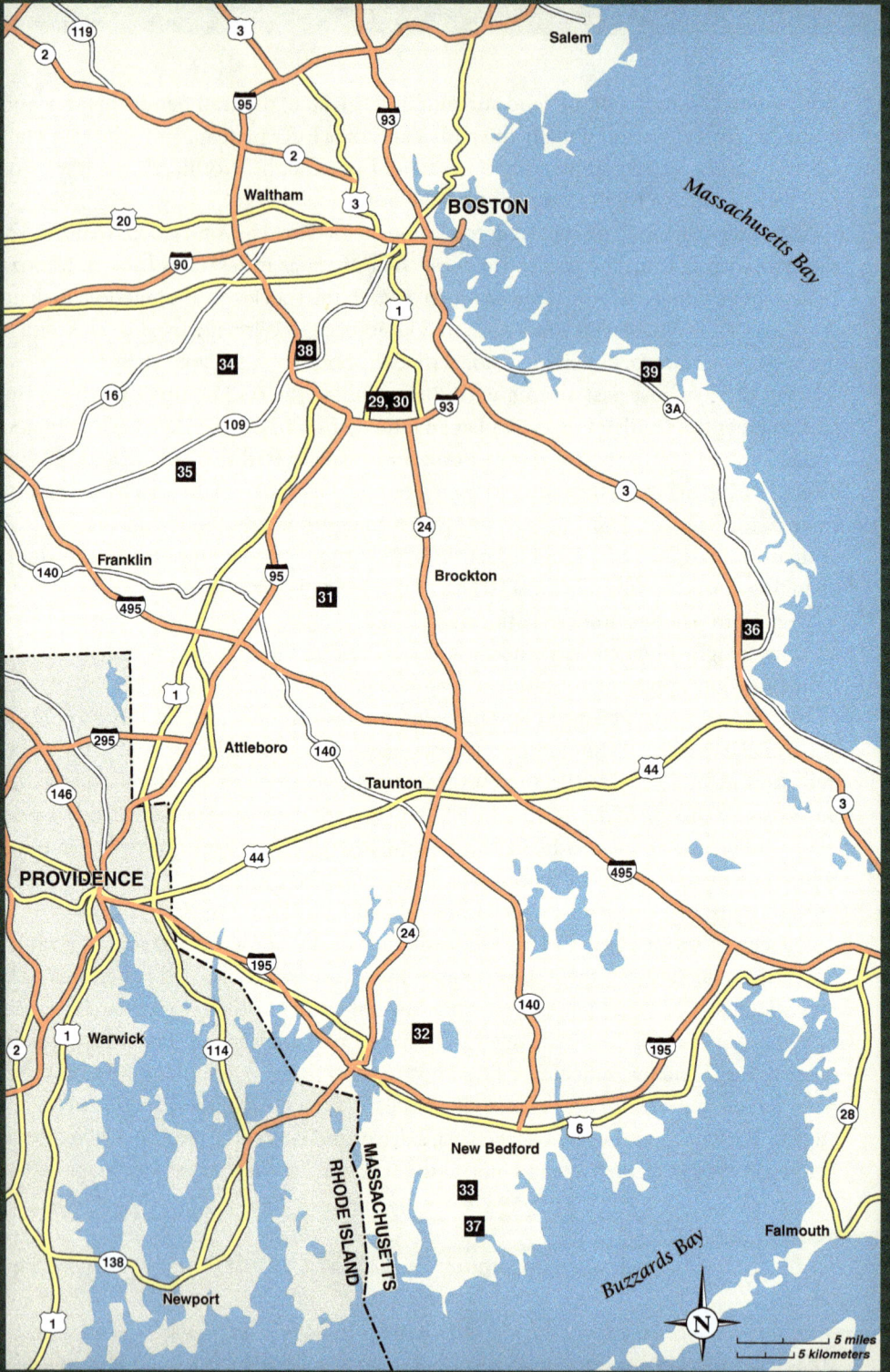

# SOUTH OF BOSTON

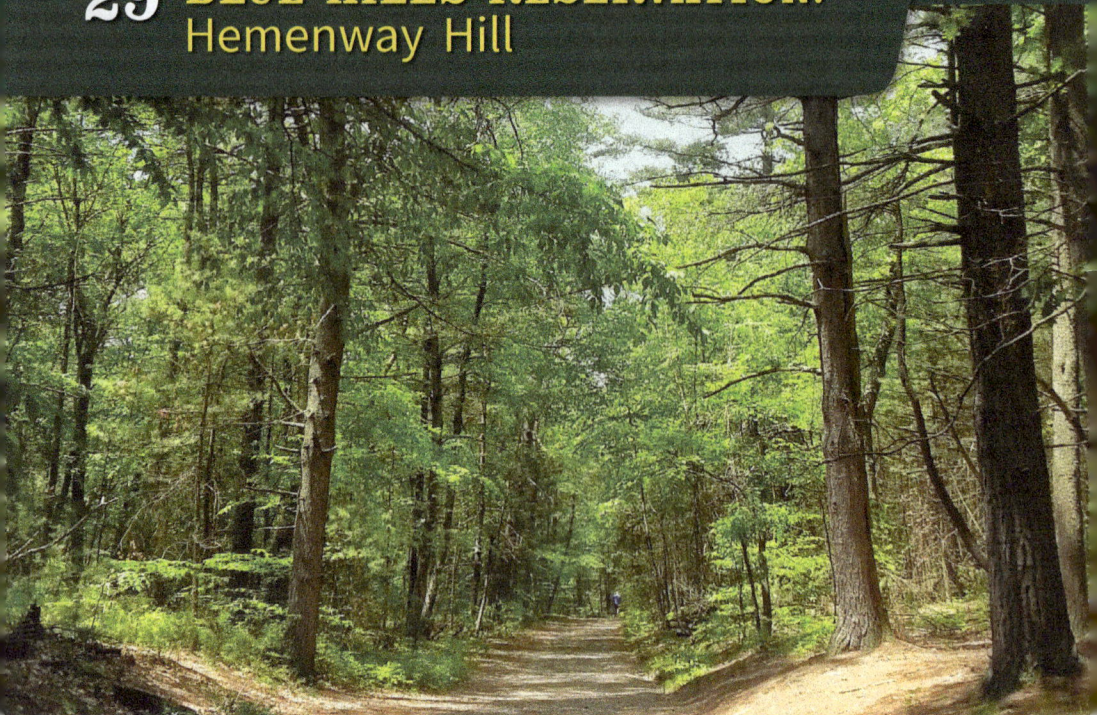

Blue Hills Reservation goes on for miles, so be sure to bring a map.

**LOCATED JUST SOUTHWEST** of Boston, the 7,000-acre Blue Hills Reservation offers a glimpse of the past and a sense of how the land may have looked before the city existed.

## DESCRIPTION

The Blue Hills Reservation is there today thanks in large part to landscape architect Charles Eliot, who campaigned hard for its creation in the late 1800s. A progressive visionary, Eliot knew that, "for crowded populations to live in health and happiness, they must have space for air, for light, for exercise, for rest, and for the enjoyment of that peaceful beauty of nature."

A refuge for deer, birds, amphibians, and a few footloose coyotes well versed in urban living, the Blue Hills—truly a stone's throw from the edge of the Boston metropolis—is a soothing woodland escape. Its woods of hemlock, beech, and oak spreading over hills of granite quiet the far-reaching sounds of the city and subdue them with birdsong and trickling streams. Old stone walls, like gray lines of slowed motion, divide the trees, casting the last shadows of Milton's farms.

Start the hike where the drive meets the woods just above the barn to the left of the office. Before long, the broad gravel trail picks up with a stream and a boggy basin to its left. When the climb eases, this trail joins another marked by a yellow

**DISTANCE & CONFIGURATION:** 3.9-mile loop

**DIFFICULTY:** Moderate

**SCENERY:** Woods, ponds, streams, wetlands, hills

**EXPOSURE:** Mostly shaded

**TRAFFIC:** Peaceful, though popular with horseback riders, mountain bikers, runners, cross-country skiers, and hikers

**TRAIL SURFACE:** Firmly packed dirt and stone; some spots are rough from erosion

**HIKING TIME:** 1.5 hours

**DRIVING DISTANCE FROM BOSTON COMMON:** 9 miles

**ELEVATION:** 204' at trailhead, 421' at highest point, with a considerable amount of rise and fall

**SEASON:** Year-round

**ACCESS:** Sunrise–sunset; free

**MAPS:** $3 at the Blue Hills Reservation Ranger Station near the trailhead or at tinyurl.com/bluehillsreservationmap

**WHEELCHAIR ACCESS:** No

**FACILITIES:** Restrooms at ranger station

**CONTACT:** Massachusetts Dept. of Conservation and Resources, mass.gov/locations/blue-hills-reservation, 617-626-1250

**LOCATION:** Milton, MA

**COMMENTS:** The trail may be wet in the spring and after heavy precipitation.

triangle. Take that trail, bearing right. From here, you will follow the yellow markers for the rest of the hike. While occasionally you may not see as many colored blazes on the trails, you can always confirm your location at the numbered intersections (of which there are many) as long as you've picked up a map at the ranger station.

The trail cleaves through the hill as it climbs. Red squirrels hustling acorns or fending off brothers and foes squabble amid the leaves. At the top of the rise, the trail surface smooths and the hiking becomes easier. The Skyline Trail, marked by blue signs, crosses the path here. Catch your breath as you walk past crags of granite humbled by moss and tenacious pine saplings rooted in their crevices. On an exposed face of this hill, blueberry bushes abound.

Soon the trail begins to descend. Though easy on the legs, here again the feet are kept busy by uneven ground. A short causeway elevates you above a stream before the trail dips and turns downhill once more. On this descent, you'll pass trails to the left and right. At the foot of the hill, turn left and hike east.

On this stretch, the trail undulates gently through the woods, keeping a straight trajectory. You will notice an assortment of oak species, pine, sassafras, hickory, and a few birch and beech. Only the occasional tree appears to be more than 25–50 years old. The generation of trees preceding these served as timber for fencing, boat hulls, and houses. Walking on, you'll encounter a slight downhill. A short way ahead, you come to another intersection, where an opening in the trees reveals a stream spilling into pools.

After crossing the stream, the trail meets a path leading from the road. Bear left, staying on the yellow trail. Vernal pools providing sanctuary to salamanders and hunting grounds for raccoons lie to the right, with hemlock-filled upland to the left.

## Blue Hills Reservation: Hemenway Hill

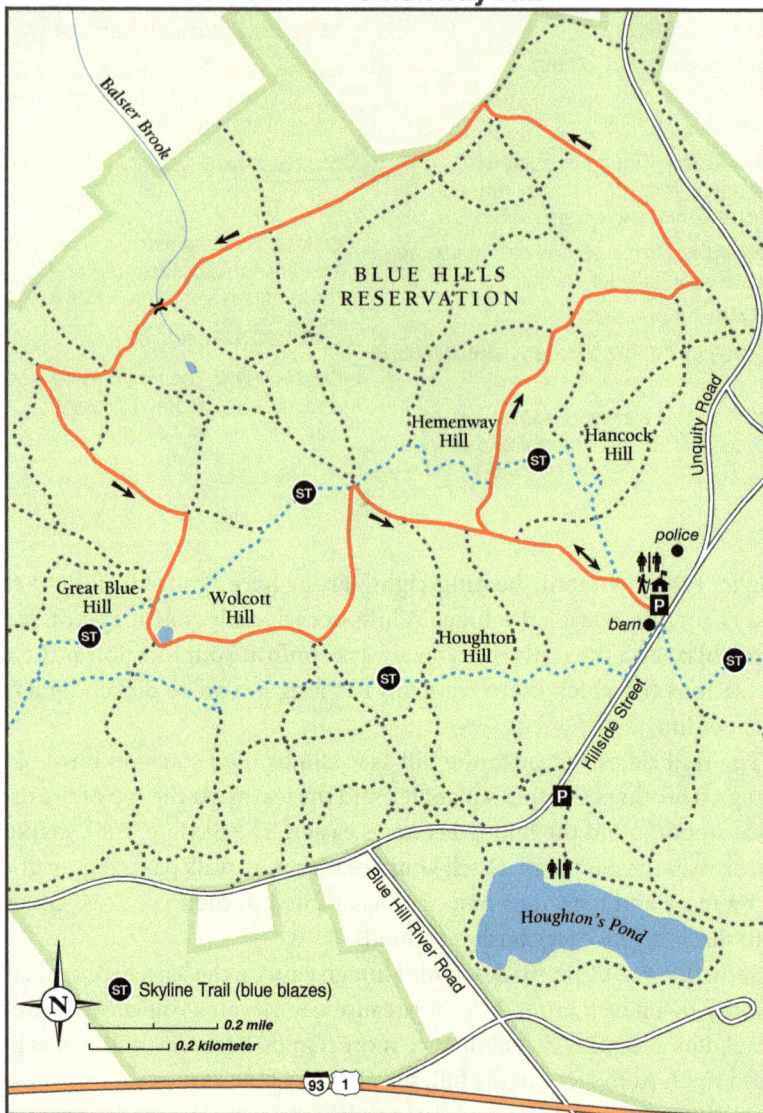

Balster Brook

BLUE HILLS
RESERVATION

Hemenway
Hill

Hancock
Hill

Unquity Road

police

Great Blue
Hill

Wolcott
Hill

Houghton
Hill

barn

Hillside Street

ST Skyline Trail (blue blazes)

N

0.2 mile

0.2 kilometer

Blue Hill River Road

Houghton's Pond

93 1

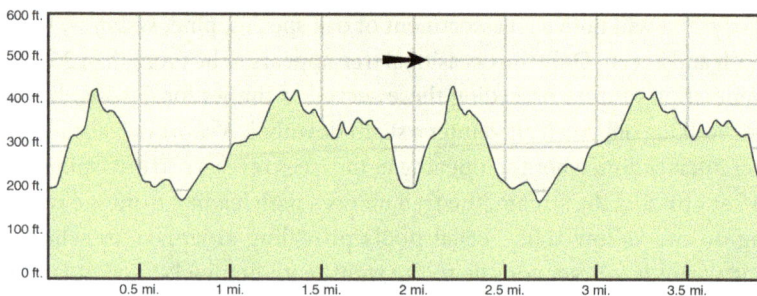

At the next junction, look for a sign for trail 1135 as well as a marker for the green trail. The yellow and green trails join and become one. Looking to the right, you can see a stone wall meandering through the woods on a parallel course.

Hemlocks cast dark shadows, shielding a sleeping great horned owl or two. An interlacing of well-fed streams trickles through this area most seasons. A wetland with springs feeding several small ponds supports an assortment of frog species. In the spring, the chirping of the peepers raises quite a racket, sounding like something between swirling ball bearings and the chilling soundtrack of a Hitchcock film.

As the trail continues, look to the right to see a red barn on private property abutting the Blue Hills Reservation. Behind the barn, a small meadow spreads to meet the woods beside the yellow trail. Though once common, fields such as this are now scarce and more vital than ever to bobolinks, bluebirds, and swallows.

You soon arrive at a point where the trail runs into a gravel road. As you turn right, markers confirm that the yellow trail and the green trail are still joined, even as they follow this road. Keep an eye out on the left for the point at which the yellow and green trails turn back into the woods. The trail veers left sharply, climbing into upland. At the fork, bear left. A small hill stretches your legs as the trail winds upward.

Keeping your eyes on the trail, you may see turkey footprints among the ubiquitous deer tracks. Turkeys have become common again in the region, and wherever there is an abundance of acorns, there is likely to be evidence of these magnificent birds. After leveling out, the trail descends again and arrives at a picturesque pond. A perfect kettle hole collared by a granite-studded ridge, this pond serves as a reminder of the glacial erosion that shaped the landscape in another age.

A trail cuts back into the woods on the pond's left. The yellow trail, however, continues along the near side of the pond, heading right. The trail jogs up an incline then quickly back down a gravelly pitch. Through a thicket to the left, you can just make out another pond that all but roars with bullfrog song in the summer.

A sign for the blue trail marks the yellow trail's departure to the right up a steep rocky slope. On the yellow trail, wetlands hug one side while, on the other, the land drops into a deep basin. The trail bends left away from a trail heading right. At the intersection with a trail marked 1120, markers indicate that the green and yellow trails are still conjoined. Head uphill again to an opening where the green and yellow trails meet the same gravel road you initially set out on.

Resume hiking on the gravel road, walking downhill. This final section leads back to the trailhead. For more information about the Blue Hills, visit the reservation's headquarters, located in the gray-shingled house on the hill to the right. A bulletin board on the porch outside presents a calendar of upcoming events, trail condition updates, and nature news. Visitors are invited to help themselves to maps for a contribution of $3.

## NEARBY ATTRACTIONS

Farther down Hillside Street on the left is Houghton's Pond. This recreation area offers swimming, fishing, and picnicking. Restrooms, picnic tables, and barbecue grills are provided free to the public. Also close by are the Trailside Museum, the Blue Hills Ski Area, and the Blue Hills Observatory and Science Center.

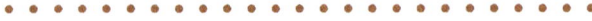

• • • • • • • • • • • • • • • • • • • • • • • • • • • • •

**GPS TRAILHEAD COORDINATES**  N42° 12.860'  W71° 05.622'

**DIRECTIONS**  From Boston, take I-93 S to the Ponkapoag Trail, Exit 3. Turn right onto Blue Hill River Road and drive 0.4 mile, then turn right onto Hillside Street. Continue 0.7 mile until you see the sign for the Blue Hills Reservation Headquarters. Parking is available on the other side of Hillside Street facing a gray barn. On busy days, you may have to seek alternate parking closer to Houghton's Pond. The trailhead is at the top of the drive beside the reservation's headquarters.

# 30 BLUE HILLS RESERVATION: Skyline Trail

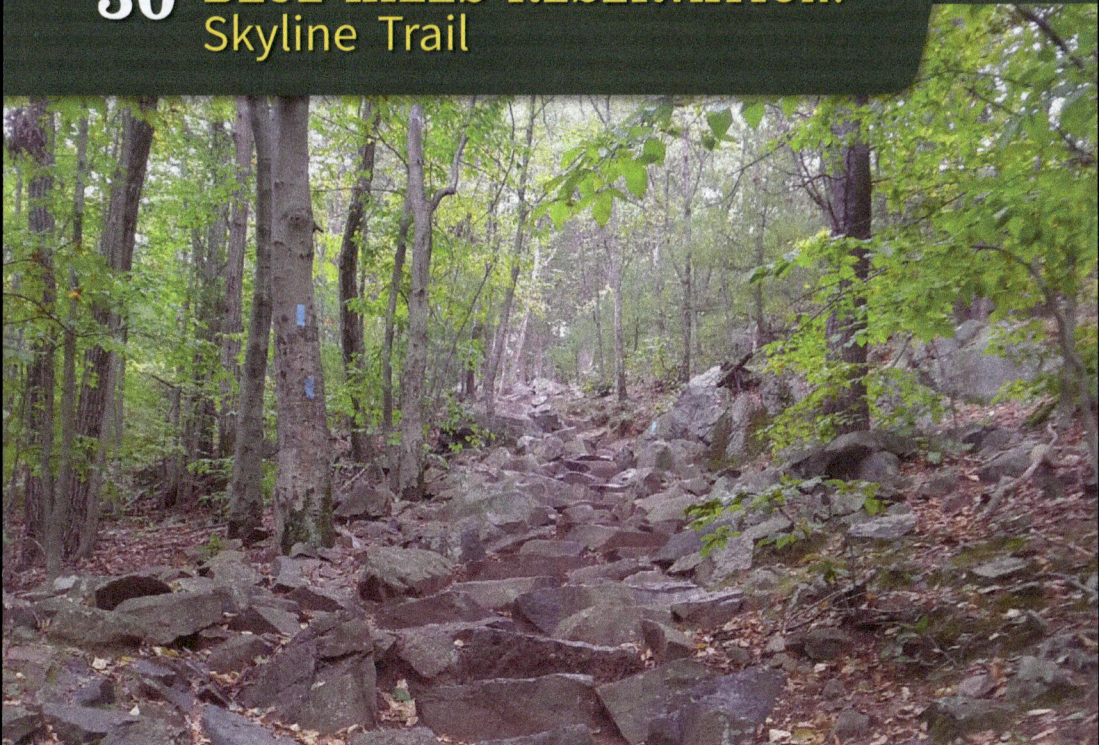

The Skyline Trail at Blue Hills Reservation will test your mettle.

**THERE ARE 125 MILES** of trails winding throughout the 7,000-acre Blue Hills Reservation. Trails take you over granite hillsides and through placid forests sheltering vernal pools and kettle ponds teeming with life. This hike follows the reservation's longest trail, which stretches from the town of Dedham to Quincy.

## DESCRIPTION

From the parking lot at Houghton's Pond, follow a path surfaced with clay that bears left (southeast), coasting downhill beside the sandy beach. Beyond a small bog on the left and a boathouse with public restrooms on the right, the path eases away from the pond and into the shade of woods. Just after a green trail marker on a tree to the left, look for a narrow dirt trail bearing away from the pond and take this brief path north to link with a paved service road. Continue north and merge with the Bugbee Path coming in from the west. Hiking east on a steep incline, you soon arrive at a broad turnaround. Head left to find Massachuseuck Trail, a route that ascends sharply uphill, quickly leaving the road behind. This point marks your first encounter with the rocky slopes of the Blue Hills.

The entire Blue Hills Reservation is well marked with numbered intersections. If you ever feel mixed up, just check the map when you come to any numbered

**DISTANCE & CONFIGURATION:** 13-mile loop

**DIFFICULTY:** Strenuous

**SCENERY:** Views from the peaks of the Blue Hills, woods, wetlands, several large ponds, wildlife

**EXPOSURE:** Mostly shaded, with sunny lookouts

**TRAFFIC:** Medium

**TRAIL SURFACE:** Variable—packed dirt, rocky, and root-covered in places

**HIKING TIME:** 7–8 hours

**DRIVING DISTANCE FROM BOSTON COMMON:** 15 miles

**ELEVATION:** 177' at trailhead, 609' at highest point, with a considerable amount of rise and fall along the trail

**SEASON:** Year-round

**ACCESS:** Sunrise–sunset; free

**MAPS:** Available for $3 at the Blue Hills Reservation Headquarters on Hillside Street in Milton or at tinyurl.com/bluehillsreservationmap

**WHEELCHAIR ACCESS:** No

**FACILITIES:** Restrooms and picnic tables at Blue Hills Reservation Headquarters and Houghton's Pond

**CONTACT:** Massachusetts Dept. of Conservation and Resources, mass.gov/locations/blue-hills-reservation, 617-626-1250

**LOCATION:** Milton, MA

**COMMENTS:** To enjoy this hike to its fullest, plan to start early. Bring plenty of water and food, and wear sturdy hiking boots.

intersection. That will give you your precise location. Pass junction 2094, traveling east to reach wetland. The Massachuseuck Trail follows the wooded rim of an overgrown pond. Dense underbrush conceals shallow waters teeming with amphibians. Varieties of hickory and oak mix with beech and evergreens. The trail leaves the wetlands and makes its way up the side of Buck Hill. Stay with the trail's eastward course about 0.5 mile longer to reach Skyline Trail, marked with blue. Descend the stone-riddled bank, passing through junction 2210 to the base of the hill, where MA 28 cuts a swath through the reservation.

The Massachuseuck and Skyline Trails pick up again on the other side of MA 28. The two trails travel north together parallel to the road before diverging. Where they split, switch to Skyline Trail. From the intersection at 3042, follow the blue markers to begin your ascent of Chickatawbut Hill. It's a fairly strenuous climb to the 517-foot peak.

Upon reaching the top, the trail eases as it navigates between the peaks of two lesser hills, Kitchamakin and Nahanton, situated beside Chickatawbut. Short of the summit is a sunken plateau where the hills meet. Here you will find a monstrous boulder resplendent with fern fronds. For a brief respite from the physically demanding Skyline Trail, follow yellow trail markers west to Chickatawbut Tower. Otherwise, forge on to the ridge of Nahanton Hill.

Skyline Trail drops steeply down the eastern face of Nahanton to the foot of Wampatuck Hill. The trail continues to rise and fall dramatically, twisting and winding its way through the forest. The trail surface continues to be rough, rocky, and rooty, so watch your footing. Across Wampatuck Road, Skyline Trail rolls on, leading you over tumbling granite rubble to the peak. Coming down the northern side of the hill, you soon arrive at an old granite quarry, now a deep pool fed by trickling springs.

# Blue Hills Reservation: Skyline Trail

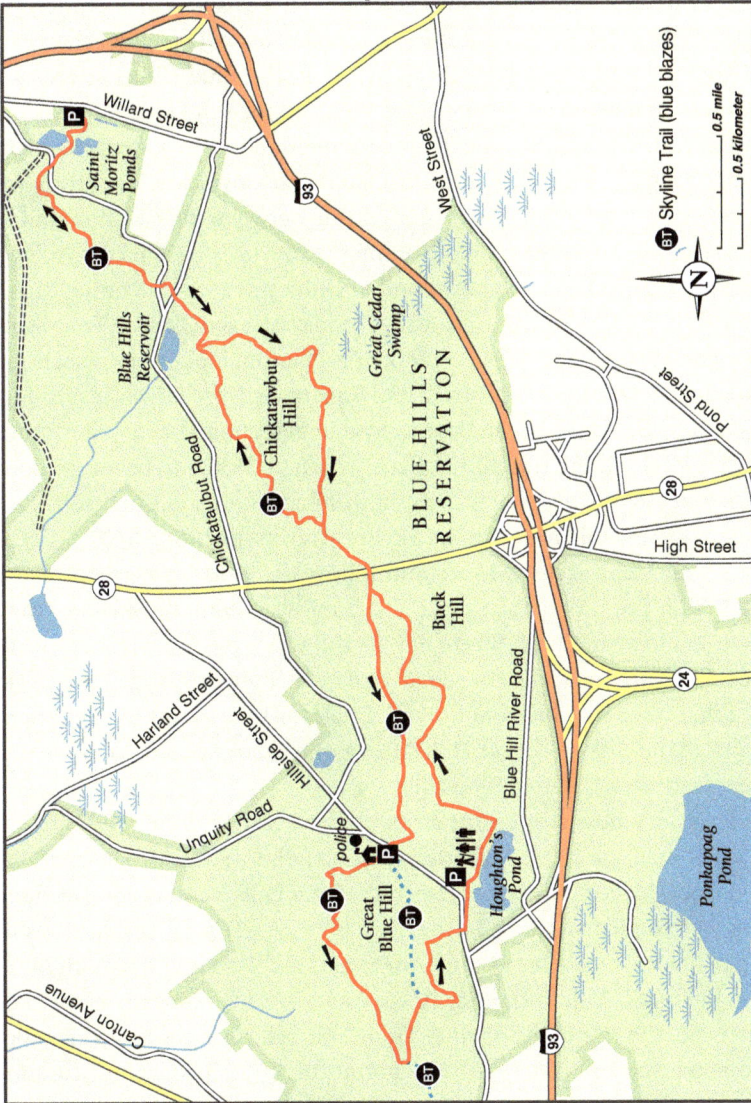

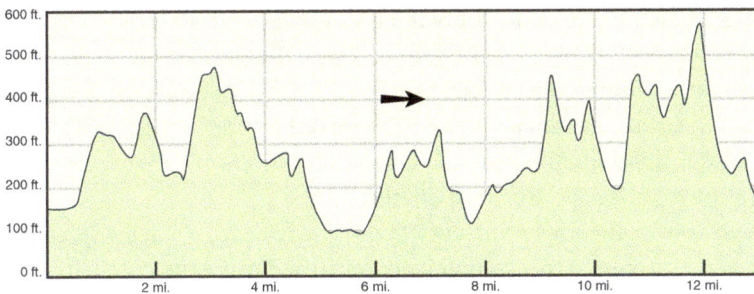

Willard Street

P

Saint Moritz Ponds

93

West Street

BT Skyline Trail (blue blazes)

0.5 mile
0.5 kilometer

N

Pond Street

BT

Blue Hills Reservoir

Great Cedar Swamp

Chickatawbut Hill

BLUE HILLS RESERVATION

28

High Street

Chickataubut Road

BT

28

Buck Hill

Blue Hill River Road

24

Harland Street

Hillside Street

BT

BT

Unquity Road

police

P

P

Houghton's Pond

Ponkapoag Pond

BT

Great Blue Hill

BT

Canton Avenue

93

BT

600 ft.
500 ft.
400 ft.
300 ft.
200 ft.
100 ft.
0 ft.

2 mi.    4 mi.    6 mi.    8 mi.    10 mi.    12 mi.

After Wampatuck Hill, the path levels out slightly. The last elevation on this eastern side of Blue Hills is called Rattlesnake Hill. This hill is milder than its name suggests. Timber rattlesnakes are known to live in the Blue Hills but are rare and reclusive. If you do happen to see one, keep your distance and take some pictures.

From Rattlesnake Hill, Skyline Trail continues about 0.5 mile to Saint Moritz Ponds. Cross Wampatuck Road and head southeast down a wide, sandy path to the twin ponds rife with pond lilies. After cutting between the two, the trail curves south up a hemlock-shaded banking. Continue a short distance farther to arrive at the trail's end in the peaceful neighborhood of Quincy near Shea Skating Rink.

Resuming your hike from Saint Moritz Ponds, take the Skyline Trail back over Rattlesnake and Wampatuck Hills. Ascending Nahanton, look for intersection 3144. Turn left off Skyline Trail and hike south into Squamaug Notch. Foliage envelops you as you descend this less used route. Bear right at intersection 3143 to join Curve Path, marked with red. Soon the trail turns sharply right at 3130 and becomes Bouncing Brook Path. Skirting the bases of Nahanton, Kitchamakin, and Chickatawbut Hills, this route runs west 1 mile to rejoin the Skyline Trail at junction 3042.

Retrace your steps across MA 28 and follow the blue markers up the rugged face of Buck Hill. From this open peak at the midway point of Skyline Trail, look south to see Ponkapoag Pond. Stretching to the west, the Skyline Trail leads you down a steep drop to a peaceful tree-shaded plateau, then drops again to a root- and boulder-riddled pitch in a lowland hollow. Look for blue blazes to lead you out of the quagmire to the side of Tucker Hill. After a quick, strenuous trip to the top, you reach a clear view west to Great Blue Hill.

Wind your way downhill again, crossing the green trail before merging with Bugbee Path at junction 2054. Turn right and take this paved road a short distance to Hillside Street. Make your way across to the Blue Hills Reservation Headquarters next to the state police station and the gray barn. A gateway beside the shingled headquarters marks the trailhead. Enter here and make an immediate right to start back on Skyline Trail. This is another steep, rocky incline, but it is well marked and well defined, like the rest of the Skyline Trail. The trail zigzags first up Hancock Hill and then Hemenway Hill. The trail throughout this stretch is narrow, twisting and winding, and fairly rocky, so take your time and watch your footing.

Coming off Hemenway Hill, you will cross the green trail. Enjoy level ground for the few yards that lead you to the foot of Great Blue Hill, then begin your final and highest peak. Granite steps laid by the Civilian Conservation Corps in the 1930s make the arduous climb a bit easier. Press on, up another steep rise, then lift your eyes to the stone monolith directly ahead called Eliot Tower, named for the renowned Boston landscape architect Charles Eliot.

Have a look from the tower and a celebratory snack and, when ready, walk south toward the weather observatory to find junction 1066. From here, turn left to pick up

Skyline Trail's southern branch, and head east back downhill along a stream. At junction 1094, leave Skyline Trail and take up Wildcat Notch Path, running off to the right.

Far less traveled than Skyline Trail, this path of firmly packed leaves and dirt descends gradually. At junction 1093, turn left to travel east on Half Way Path to cross two small hills split by a stream. Pass straight through junction 1110 to reach Coon Hollow Path a bit farther on. Take this next right, and walk along the deep hollow toward the road. Cross Hillside Street on a diagonal to find the yellow trail on the west side of Houghton's Pond. Follow this trail east, keeping the pond to your right to return to the parking lot.

## NEARBY ATTRACTIONS

Once you have discovered the Blue Hills, you'll want to come back. Rock climbers are drawn to the Quincy granite quarries accessible by car, public transportation, or hiking trail just over 0.5 mile from Saint Moritz Ponds in Quincy. Now linked to the Blue Hills Reservation, the quarries are open to the public for climbing and various programs run by the Department of Conservation and Recreation year-round.

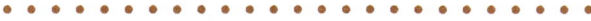

• • • • • • • • • • • • • • • • • • • • • • • •

**GPS TRAILHEAD COORDINATES**  N42° 12.533'  W71° 05.967'

**DIRECTIONS**  From Boston, take I-93 S 13 miles to Exit 3, the Ponkapoag Trail, toward Houghton's Pond. Turn right onto Blue Hill River Road; continue 0.4 mile and turn right onto Hillside Street. The parking lot for Houghton's Pond is 0.7 mile ahead on the right.

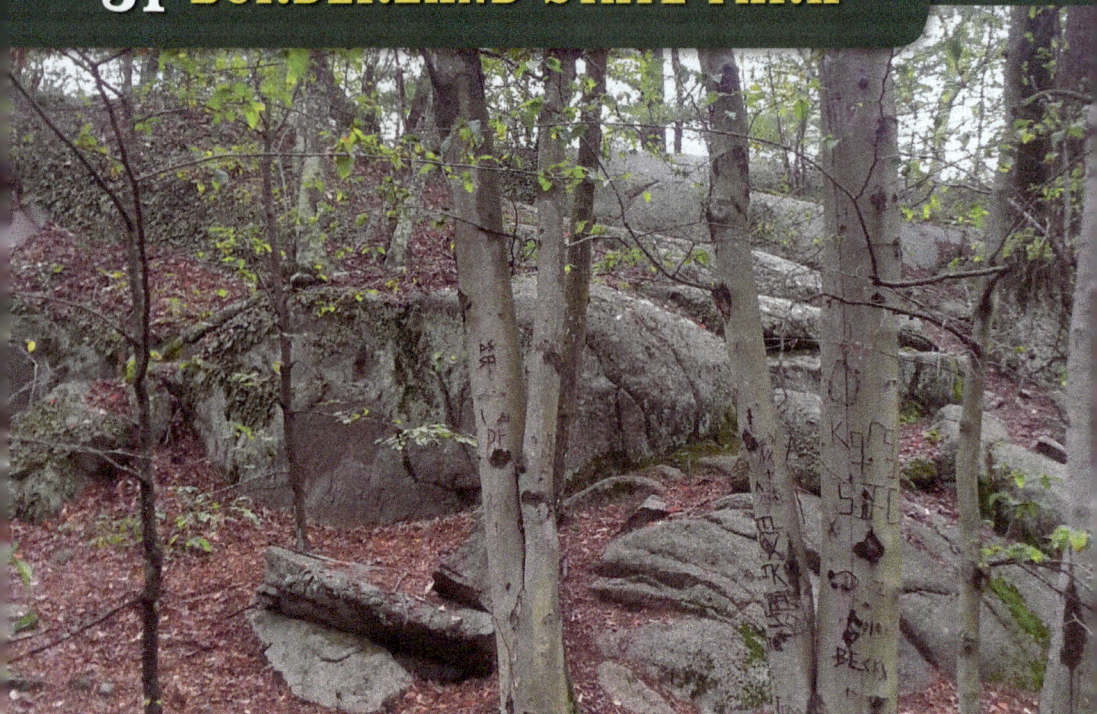

Borderland State Park may be a busy place, but it's also big enough for you to find some solitude.

**BORDERLAND STATE PARK** is often fairly busy and can be crowded, but there are plenty of corners of the park and more-remote trails where you can have the forest to yourself.

## DESCRIPTION

This hiking route through Borderland State Park provides a varied tour of Borderland's northern reaches. The trailhead lies not far from the edge of the parking lot, just beyond the visitor center. Begin walking on the gravel road, bearing left. This path turns through woods briefly before arriving at the stone cabin on Leach Pond. After pausing at the cabin, continue on the gravel road. Just ahead on the left, you will see a sign for the West Side Trail. Take this trail, leaving the pond behind. You'll find the trails well marked for the most part, but take a map with you just in case.

The West Side Trail is entirely different from the wide gravel path. This narrow trail climbs gradually into dense woods scattered with large chunks of granite dispensed by the retreating glaciers. As the trail surface is quite rugged, the West Side Trail leaves crowds and commotion behind.

A few minutes along the route, the trail forks where it meets the French Trail. The West Side Trail veers west. Follow the French Trail east instead. Ahead the trail

**DISTANCE & CONFIGURATION:** 6.25-mile loop

**DIFFICULTY:** Moderate

**SCENERY:** Woods, ponds, streams, granite boulders, historic Ames Mansion

**EXPOSURE:** Mostly shaded, with exposed lookouts

**TRAFFIC:** Light, except the first 0.25 mile

**TRAIL SURFACE:** Variable, including a gravel multiuse path, soft level ground, rocky footing, and wooden bridges spanning streams

**HIKING TIME:** 3 hours

**DRIVING DISTANCE FROM BOSTON COMMON:** 27 miles

**ELEVATION:** 207' at trailhead, no significant gain

**SEASON:** Year-round

**ACCESS:** Sunrise–sunset. Parking is $5 for MA residents, $6 for nonresidents.

**MAPS:** Available at the visitor center or at mass.gov/eea/docs/dcr/parks/trails /borderland.pdf

**WHEELCHAIR ACCESS:** No—the recommended route for wheelchair users is the Pond Walk trail that circles Leach Pond.

**FACILITIES:** Visitor center with restrooms; many picnic tables

**CONTACT:** Massachusetts Dept. of Conservation and Resources, mass.gov/locations /borderland-state-park, 617-626-1250

**LOCATION:** North Easton, MA

**COMMENTS:** Besides offering miles of hiking, Borderland State Park welcomes anglers, horseback riders, and disc golfers. For a schedule of mansion tours and special events, visit friendsofborderland.org.

threads through a glacial stones then arrives at a massive boulder. The effect of this glacial granite garden is quite dramatic.

The trail winds and weaves enough to be tricky to follow at times. Keep an eye out for painted blue blazes on rocks and trees to stay on track. At the next intersection, where the French Trail meets the Northwest Trail, stay left to switch to the Northwest Trail. The terrain remains stony and undulating as you head north, passing numerous vernal pools and ponds. At streams and perpetually wet spots, wooden planks help you pass through without getting your feet wet or further eroding the trail. Through the woods to the left, you can see a pond surrounded by dense underbrush. In the warmer months, red-winged blackbirds enliven the forest with flashes of red and wild chattering.

Here the trail levels out and briefly widens as it passes an imposing wall of stone before reaching an intersection with the Ridge Trail. Leave the Northwest Trail at this point, and bear right. Immediately ahead you will see another large pile of granite glacier debris.

The Ridge Trail continues, passing scores of pools on either side. The footing remains rocky and rough but level, except where the trail encounters the occasional monstrous boulder. On several sections of the hike, the trail cuts through gaps in stone walls, reminders that all this was once farmland. You might notice at this point that the trail markers you were following earlier are no longer blue but white, designating the Ridge Trail.

After weaving through grassy forage land, the trail leads to a crossroads where the Ridge Trail meets the Quarry Loop Trail. To pay a visit to the Moyle's Quarry on

167

## Borderland State Park

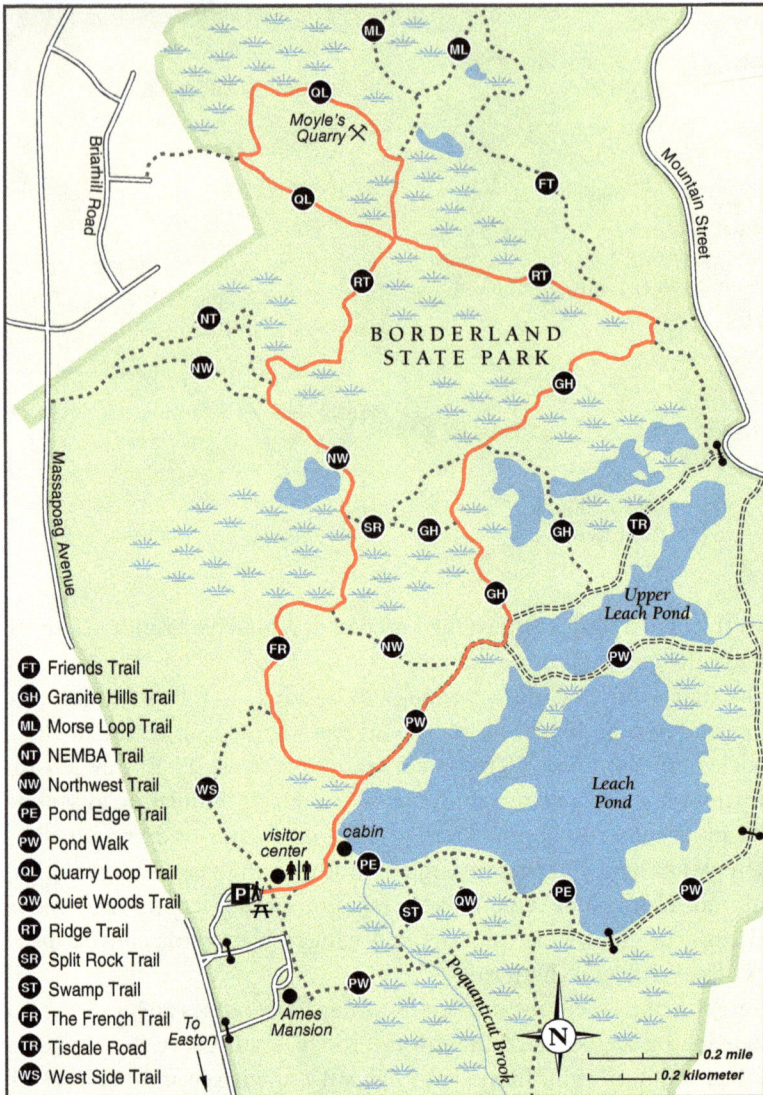

FT  Friends Trail
GH  Granite Hills Trail
ML  Morse Loop Trail
NT  NEMBA Trail
NW  Northwest Trail
PE  Pond Edge Trail
PW  Pond Walk
QL  Quarry Loop Trail
QW  Quiet Woods Trail
RT  Ridge Trail
SR  Split Rock Trail
ST  Swamp Trail
FR  The French Trail
TR  Tisdale Road
WS  West Side Trail

this circuit, you can go clockwise or counterclockwise. If you prefer counterclockwise, take the path straight ahead. Otherwise, bear left and head northwest. Almost immediately, you will cross a wet bog via a small bridge. A bit farther along, the trail passes through a grove of young white pines.

Where the Quarry Loop Trail reaches its northern tip, continue right and stay on the Quarry Trail. Heading east, and soon southeast, the trail leads past a steep-faced granite monolith. Weathered holes drilled into it tell of the hard labor of the quarrymen who years ago cut blocks from the wall of stone. Rounding a bend, the now narrow trail opens to the site of the Moyle's Quarry. The cavity left by excavators is ringed by a wall of granite that provides a grand acoustic backdrop like a sound stage. Shortly after the quarry, the trail passes the tail end of the Morse Loop Trail. Stay right to complete the Quarry Loop Trail. Arriving back where the loop began, bear left to rejoin the Ridge Trail, heading east.

Ahead you'll find the remains of a vehicle abandoned many storms and sun-scorching summers ago. Now reduced to flaking rust, its style and vintage is anyone's guess at this stage. It may have last been driven when the quarry was still actively working.

On this stretch of trail, you will pass by dense underbrush. If you're making the trek in July and August, you just might discover some blueberry bushes. Not long after meeting the Friend's Trail, the Ridge Trail jogs abruptly right. Be on the lookout for this turn. Although not well marked, this elbow is a part of the Ridge Trail. From here, the trail winds south, heading downhill much of the way. After passing more boulders and crossing a wooden bridge, look for a pond through the woods to the left. Finally you'll see a sign confirming that you are on the upper Granite Hills Trail. At the end of a long boardwalk, the trail eases right.

After crossing more wetland and climbing uphill, the trail reaches a fork. To the right is the Split Rock Trail; however, take the Granite Hills Trail, which continues left. Before long, this meandering trail breaks from tangled thickets to rejoin the more civilized gravel path that hugs the banks of Leach Pond. To head back to the visitor center and parking lot, follow this road right. The sight of water rushing over the lip of a dam that divides Leach Pond may cause you to divert left at the split ahead. Once you have had a look, return to the gravel road and follow it west to the visitor center.

Until 1971, the grounds of Borderland State Park were actually the estate of Blanche and Oakes Ames, a prominent and intriguing couple in New England history. Oakes was revered as an expert on orchids and was a professor of botany at Harvard University. Blanche—an artist, an inventor, a suffragette, and a graduate of Smith College—was the daughter of Brigadier General Adelbert Ames (no relation to Oakes), the provisional governor of Mississippi under Abraham Lincoln. The 20-room granite mansion Oakes and Blanche built has been preserved and is available for tours and functions.

## NEARBY ATTRACTIONS

If it's strawberry, blueberry, or apple season, don't miss a chance to stop at Ward's Berry Farm (781-784-3600, wardsberryfarm.com), at 614 S. Main St. in Sharon, just 6.34 miles up the road from Borderland. Besides offering seasonal, pesticide-free produce grown on its 150 acres, Ward's has friendly farm animals, a sandbox for kids, and gourmet delights for sale year-round.

**GPS TRAILHEAD COORDINATES**  N42° 03.750'  W71° 09.867'

**DIRECTIONS** From Boston, take I-93 S toward I-95/Dedham, then merge onto I-95 south (Exit 1) toward Providence, Rhode Island. Travel 5.3 miles to Coney Street (Exit 10) and head toward Sharon/Walpole. Stay on Coney Street 1.6 miles before turning onto Norwood Street. Turn left onto Upland Road/MA 27. Continue on Upland 0.5 mile to Post Office Square. Drive 0.1 mile and turn right onto Pond Street. At the roundabout, take the first exit onto Massapoag Avenue. The entrance to Borderland State Park is 3.8 miles ahead.

Most of the trails in the state park are gentle enough for younger hikers.

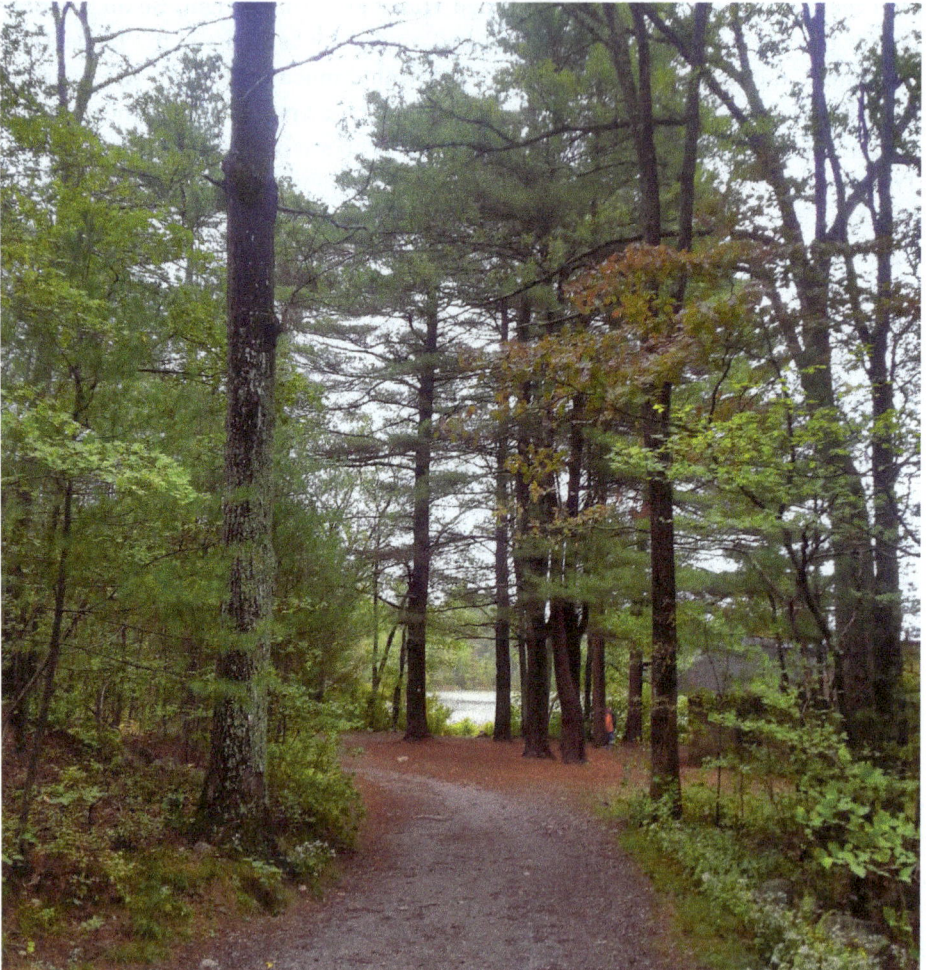

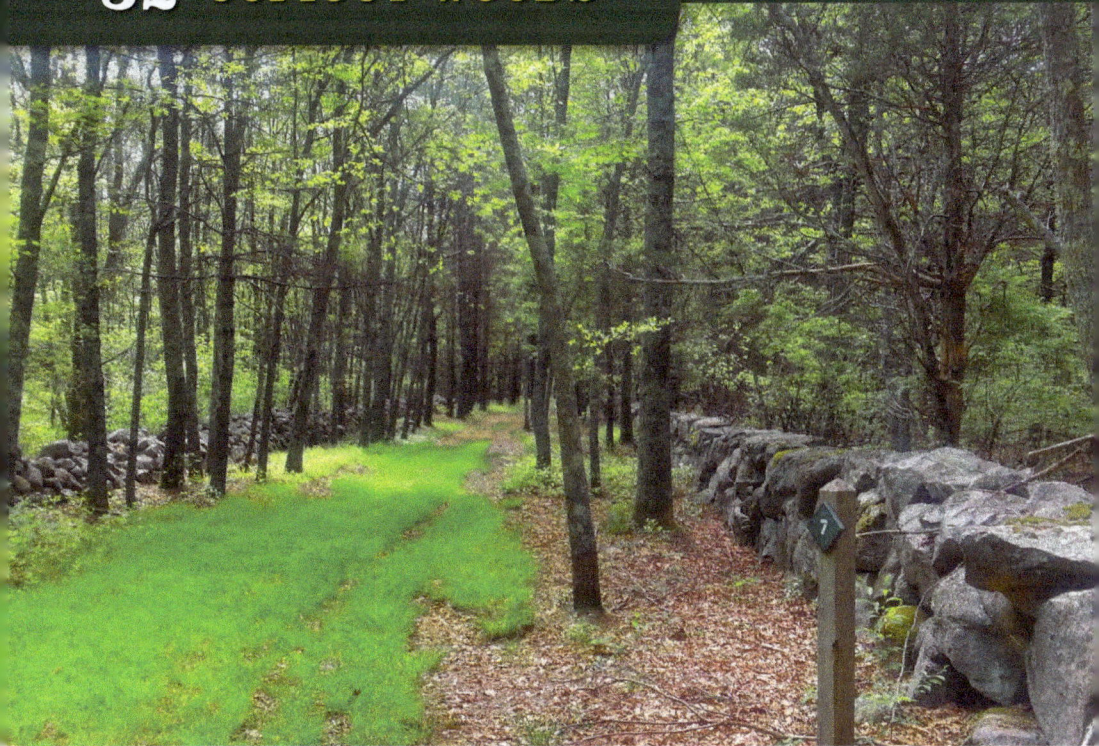

Copicut Woods is a refreshing wilderness right near the busy city of Fall River.

**YOU'LL EXPLORE THE** well-preserved woodland haunts of the Wampanoag and America's first generations of English settlers, including some fascinating stone foundations.

## DESCRIPTION

Copicut is the Wampanoag word for "deep, dark woods." This 516-acre property was farmed over the course of several lifetimes. Today, successional growth has nearly returned the land to its original wooded state, but among the trees, blueberries, and other shrubs, there are several intriguing artifacts of human industry.

Walk across Old Indian Town Road from the parking lot to the trailhead on the other side of the road. Enter at the green gate beside a sign for Copicut Woods, and begin hiking along the slender path that weaves southeast through a mixed forest of beech and pine trees. Downtown Fall River is 10 minutes away by car, but there's little here to stir the silence but chattering chipmunks and red squirrels.

After descending a slight grade, the trail reaches a barely paved road that looks more like a logging road than anything else. Continue across to pick up the trail where it resumes on the opposite side. This junction is marked as number 2. From here, hike northeast alongside wetland shrouded by tangled understory. Sifting

**DISTANCE & CONFIGURATION:** 3.4-mile loop

**DIFFICULTY:** Easy

**SCENERY:** Ecologically rich wetlands, vernal pools, abandoned farmstead, 150-year-old scenic cart path

**EXPOSURE:** Mostly shade

**TRAFFIC:** Light

**TRAIL SURFACE:** Mostly packed dirt, some grassy sections

**HIKING TIME:** 2 hours

**DRIVING DISTANCE FROM BOSTON COMMON:** 56 miles

**ELEVATION:** 263' at trailhead, no significant gain

**SEASON:** Year-round

**ACCESS:** Sunrise–sunset; free

**MAPS:** Available at tinyurl.com/copicut woodsmap

**WHEELCHAIR ACCESS:** No

**FACILITIES:** None

**CONTACT:** The Trustees of Reservations, thetrustees.org/places-to-visit, 617-542-7696

**LOCATION:** Fall River, MA

**COMMENTS:** Copicut Woods is linked to the 13,600-acre Southeastern Massachusetts Bioreserve.

through the trees, you'll note the first of the property's impressive stonework. This long wall of stacked stones represents hundreds if not thousands of hours of labor.

Bending gently left, the trail opens to an intersection marked 3. Up the trail to the left is another gate across the trail before it again intersects Old Indian Town Road. Hike to the right to an intersection marked 4. Cross the wide carriage road to reenter the woods on a newer, narrow trail heading northeast.

Winding through wetland dense with brush, the trail soon leads to a brook with a unique and rustic log bridge. This thick single log outfitted with a handrail provides a slightly precarious passage over the gurgling waters. Keeping on high ground, the path dead-ends at a small kettle pond a few feet farther on.

From the pond, backtrack to the brook and pick up the trail heading east. The trail isn't all that well marked but is moderately well defined. Follow this route as it turns northeast. After meeting a stone wall to the left, the path continues through a parting in another. This point also marks a transition from woods of swamp oak to lighter forest of white pine.

Up ahead, the trail intersects with another perpendicular trail. At this juncture, turn right and continue east on a moss-lined trail bordered by a stone wall and a crowd of pines standing in an old pasture. Turning south, the path promptly leads to a post-and-beam shelter built by volunteers for the Trustees.

Several paths radiate from this spot. One to the right leads to a junction marked 5. Choose the route between this path and the shelter and continue southeast. A few feet along, the trail passes a particularly remarkable stone wall assembled from massive stones.

The path runs on its southeastern course past meadowland reclaimed by oaks, cedars, hickories, and beeches until it reaches a broad crossroads marked 7. The expansive, grassy avenue running straight ahead is Miller Lane, a cart path built 150

## Copicut Woods

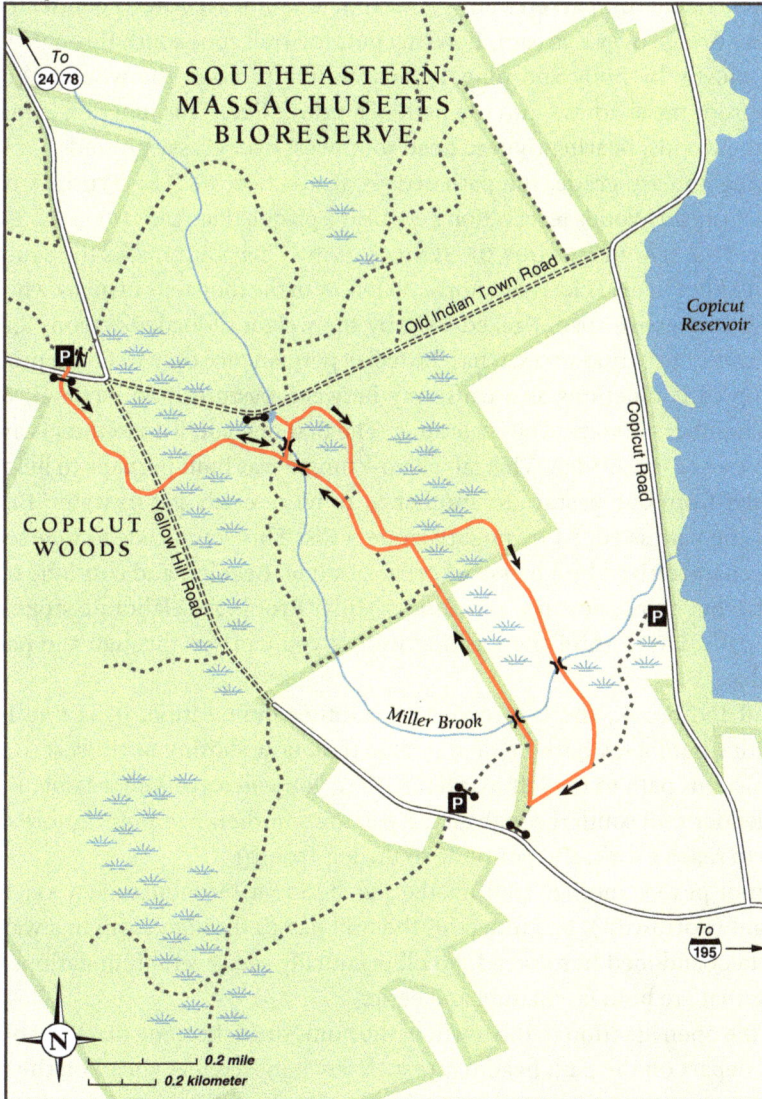

years ago. Stone walls straight as a plumb line and high enough to fence in spirited horses border the path on either side.

Take the wide path to the left of Miller Lane, and hike east, straight along the path of another stone wall. The trail descends on a slight incline to another junction, this one marked 12. At this split, bear right onto a scrappy trail heading southeast. Paralleling another wall, this one less intact, the trail crosses meadowland, giving itself up to opportunistic shrubs and saplings. Hollies and ancient fruit trees overrun by bittersweet vines stand over the bramble-ridden grassland.

Continue on this unmarked trail as it meanders southeast down a gentle slope to a small stone bridge over a stream. Leveling out, the trail runs south through woods populated mostly by holly and pine. After traveling through the woods, the trail soon spills from the shadows into the path of a power line. This junction is marked 11. Leave the woods, bearing right to head southwest over grassy ground.

Climbing an easy grade, the path arrives at junction 10. The Trustees have a sign for the Copicut Woods reservation here near a plaque that reads MILLER'S BROOK CONSERVATION AREA, IN MEMORY OF BENNY COSTA. This point marks the southernmost end of Miller Lane. Hike right, north, to follow in the footsteps of many who have trodden this impressive road. Packed solid by the weight of loaded wagons and the tonnage of cattle and workhorses, it has the feel of permanence only wear can produce.

Built up so it functions as a causeway between pastures and wetland, Miller Lane has a number of interesting structures. The first one you'll encounter is an odd tunnel known as a dry bridge. This tall narrow tunnel was built perhaps to help livestock wander from one pasture to another or to more easily get to water. Bearing northwest, the path is edged by mighty stone walls. This soon leads to intersection 9, which is characterized by a massive corner of stone. Bear left and continue north.

A bit farther along, the lane encounters Miller Brook. An elaborate stone grate keeps the path dry, despite the gushing waters you can see through the parallel granite slabs.

Beyond the brook, the lane comes to another intersection. This one is not marked with a number. Continue on the same trail, now shifting northwest to reach an inconspicuous path to the left marked 8. Here you will leave Miller Lane. Follow this new slender trail south through an old pasture smothered in pine. Ignore divergent paths to reach a fork, and continue to the left (south).

This trail passes another trail on the left beside a birdhouse. Stay on track, bearing right (northwest). In a moment, the trail passes through a gap in a wall and arrives at an abandoned homestead. You'll eventually see several foundations lying in the grass that are both fascinating and eerie.

From the open junction to the north of the homestead, keeping marker 6 behind to the left, depart on the path heading west. A few hundred feet ahead on the right, this broad avenue passes the foundation of a barn. Farther still, the trail reaches junction 5, marking the path leading back to the post-and-beam shelter. About 0.1 mile later, the trail arrives at another familiar junction. The path to the right leads to the wood duck pond, and the one to the left leads back to the parking lot.

## NEARBY ATTRACTIONS

If you would like to do some sightseeing after your hike, consider Tiverton Four Corners, Rhode Island (tivertonfourcorners.com), just 11 miles away. Listed on the National Register of Historic Places, this rural village offers something for everyone, including antiques shopping, gourmet food, crafts, equestrian centers, beach access, and unspoiled open space excellent for hiking and biking. To get there, take I-95 east 1.2 miles and merge onto MA 24 S at Exit 8A. Continue 4.2 miles to Exit 6. Turn left onto Fish Road. Continue 1.4 miles and turn right onto Bulgarmarsh Road (RI 177). After 1 mile turn left onto Main Road (RI 77). Continue 3.4 miles to arrive at Tiverton Four Corners.

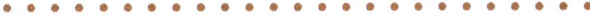

• • • • • • • • • • • • • • • • • • • • • • • • • • • •

**GPS TRAILHEAD COORDINATES:** N41° 42.533'  W71° 03.900'

**DIRECTIONS**  From Boston, take I-93 to Exit 4 and join MA 24 S toward Brockton. Continue 33.4 miles. From MA 24, take Exit 7 to merge onto MA 79 south toward North Fall River/Somerset, and continue 4 miles to the I-195 E exit toward New Bedford/Cape Cod on the left. From I-195, take Exit 9 (Sanford Road) and turn left to pass under the highway. Sanford Road bears right and becomes Old Bedford Road. Turn left onto Blossom Road and follow it 1.3 miles. Bear right onto Old Indian Town Road and follow it 1.7 miles to the parking area on the left.

This unique single-rail bridge brings you across a stream.

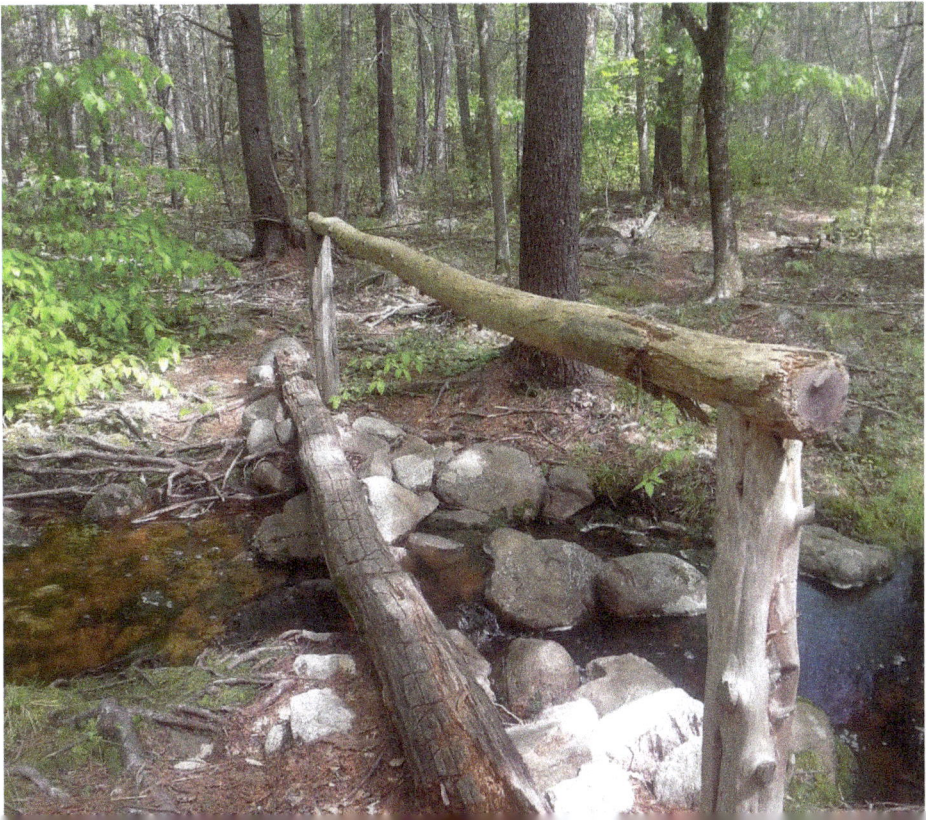

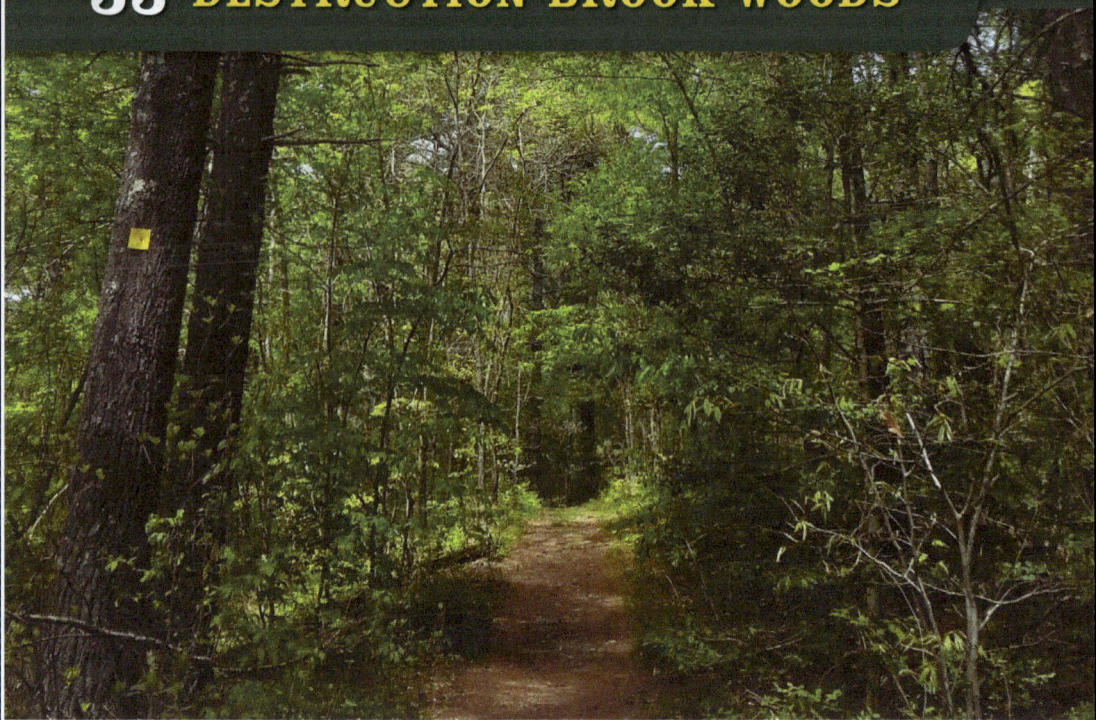

The deep and dense woodland of Destruction Brook Woods

**LOCATED UPSTREAM FROM** Dartmouth's historic Russell Mills, this hike takes you on a tour of land preserved much as it was in the 1600s, when the area was first settled.

## DESCRIPTION

Destruction Brook Woods trailhead access and parking is tucked just off the road. Once you're on the trail, head southwest, away from the road. You'll see it marked by the Dartmouth Natural Resource Trust (DNRT) sign. A hundred yards or so in from the road, the trail leads to a kiosk displaying a map of the reserve. Continue from here along the yellow trail to reach a three-way intersection. At this junction, turn left to hike east along the yellow trail. This trail runs roughly parallel to Fisher Road, which you can occasionally see through the loose forest of pine, oak, and maple.

Ahead where the yellow trail meets the blue trail, bear left to hike southeast behind houses on Fisher Road. Then, turning away from backyards, follow blue trail markers to the uneven terrain of a weathered esker. At the next split, bear right, switching back to the yellow trail to retreat into the deeper woods.

Becoming narrower as it runs under a canopy of trees, the trail dips and climbs then merges with another trail. Continue following the yellow trail markers. At a slightly confusing intersection, follow the path to make almost a hairpin turn and

**DISTANCE & CONFIGURATION:** 4.07 miles, 2 linked loops

**DIFFICULTY:** Easy

**SCENERY:** Millworks first built in 1690; holly woods and abandoned farm established in 1853, American beech and Atlantic white cedar

**EXPOSURE:** Mostly shade

**TRAFFIC:** Light–moderate

**TRAIL SURFACE:** Packed dirt

**HIKING TIME:** 2.5–3 hours

**DRIVING DISTANCE FROM BOSTON COMMON:** 63 miles

**ELEVATION:** 92' at trailhead, no significant gain

**SEASON:** Year-round

**ACCESS:** Sunrise–sunset; free

**MAPS:** Available at kiosk by the trailhead and online at tinyurl.com/destructionbrook woodsmap

**WHEELCHAIR ACCESS:** The red and yellow trails both offer limited wheelchair access.

**FACILITIES:** None

**CONTACT:** Dartmouth Natural Resources Trust, dnrt.org/destructionbrook, 508-991-2289

**LOCATION:** Dartmouth, MA

**COMMENTS:** Destruction Brook Woods is one of 40 reservations managed by the Dartmouth Natural Resources Trust, which has helped preserve more than 4,000 acres.

head north to stay on the yellow trail. Continue downhill off the ridge to reach another junction. Stay left and follow the wide yellow trail over level ground. The trail passes by a stream and scattered birch groves. Bear left again at the next fork to follow the yellow trail as it swings south. Snaking through the forest, the trail soon leads to a bench on a banking overlooking Destruction Brook and remnants of the millworks first established here around 1690.

From this spot, descend the banking, and turn left onto the red trail, which traces the route of the brook. Shortly this route joins the yellow trail, and the two continue as one. Passing a gate to the left, the trail curves south and crosses a wide bridge. On the opposite bank, the trails separate. Stay with the red trail, and continue hiking south.

The trail eases west to pass a white house sitting among pines on the left. Just beyond this, the trail reaches another intersection. The path to the left leads to an alternate parking spot for the reservation, and a path straight ahead leads to an open meadow. Steer away from these and stay with the red trail, bearing right. A moment later, a red arrow at knee level redirects the trail left, back on a westward course.

Here knobby American holly trees (*Ilex opaca*) punctuate the woods otherwise dominated by red oak and white pine. Many of the unique tree species have small signs marking them and explaining their scientific name and classification. Keep hiking, and up ahead the land to the left dips to a valley, while on the right it remains even with the trail, which now eases north. At the next two forks, stay left on what remains of the red trail, which is scarcely marked through here.

Dipping beside wetland on the left, the trail swings on several compass points but continues generally north. Holly trees grow more thickly along this avenue, mixing with maple, beech, and omnipresent oak and pine. At one point, the trail passes

## Destruction Brook Woods

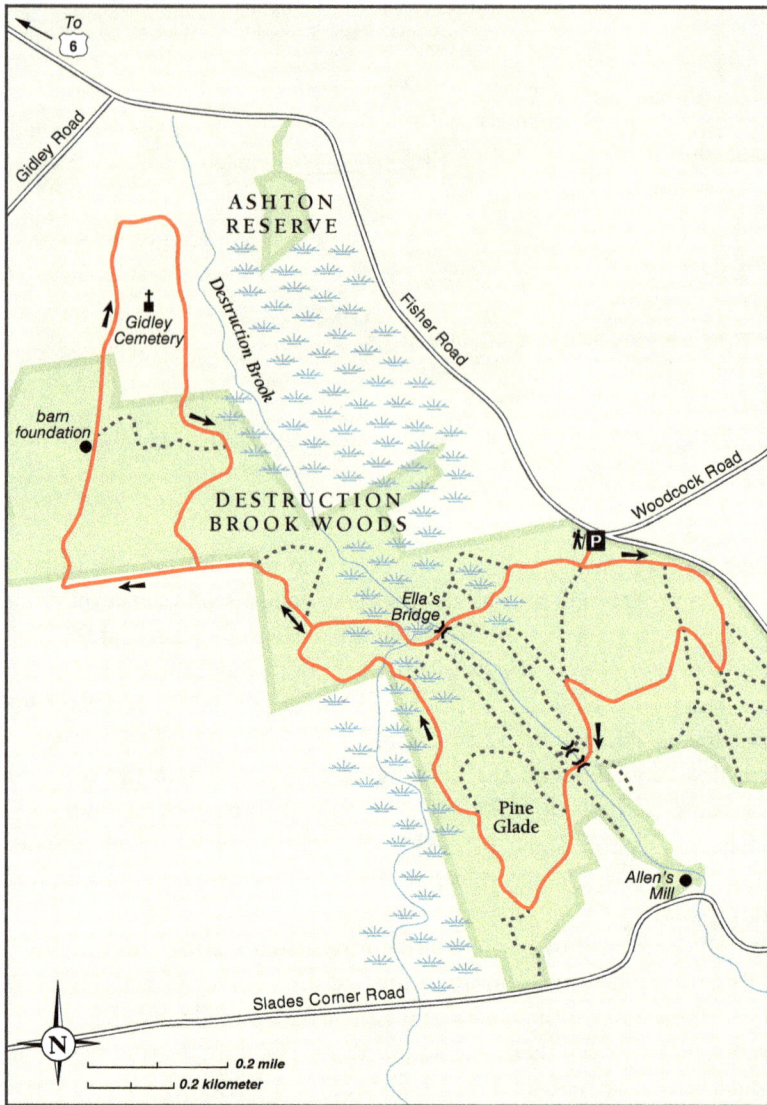

a magnificent beech tree growing flush to an equally magnificent oak. They make an interesting pair.

Weaving through wetland, the red trail eventually heads northwest to intersect the green trail. This junction is marked both with the letter *D* on a stone and a sign that reads START OF GREEN LOOP. Leave the pine-thick red trail here, and continue northwest down a slight grade on the green trail. Thick woods and a stone wall lie to the right. A few hundred yards ahead, where the trail forms a T, turn left and continue west toward a house neighboring private property. Where the trail forks a few feet farther on, bear right to hike north, tracking a stone wall built in the mid-1800s, when a farm was established on the 90 acres encircled by the green loop.

Along this section of former cart road, boughs of giant hickory trees arch overhead. Though nearly retaken by nature, the place has not yet fully given up its former self. It has been years since this land was a working farm, but midway down the path on the right, there is still a foundation for what was once a great barn.

A short distance farther, the path reaches a point where the DNRT reservation ends. The green trail continues ahead, emerging from the woods briefly as it passes privately owned land lying to the west. Watch to the east for a path leading into a thicket of pines to the Gidley Cemetery, where several who lived on this land are buried.

Trust the trail as it forges north. The way is clear, though momentarily bereft of markers. Coming to the end of the avenue draped voluminously with vines, the trail arrives at a junction. NO TRESPASSING signs rule out the paths to the left and center, leaving two paths to the right. Of these, choose the soft right, and hike southeast down a pitch. A sandpit lies ahead on the left and, in it, the carcass of a sedan pinned between two pine saplings. The trail cuts sharply away from this wreck and runs into woods of cedar and holly. Looping around the eastern side of the wetland, the trail splits briefly upon reaching an esker. For the sake of the view, bear left to ascend the 30- to 50-foot skeletal mound of glacial debris.

As the esker subsides, the land on the right falls away to a deep glade. Having the hushed feel of a room just made empty by a crowd, this natural basin held grazing cows. Scrappy trees have grown in over time, but none look as though they will ever achieve the height and girth of the tremendous oak that stands at the center.

From this old meadow, the barely marked green trail continues southeast through swales and over bumps until, bending west, it returns to the start of the loop. To complete the hike, return to the junction where the green and red trails meet, and bear left onto the red trail, heading east. Running wide and flat through wetland thick with maples, this trail is easy to follow. Plentiful red markers guide the way to Ella's Bridge, which lies just ahead at Destruction Brook.

Upon crossing to the opposite bank, quit the red trail, pick up the yellow trail once more, and continue straight ahead. Weaving through woods draped with curtains of bittersweet, the trail soon reaches a vibrant pine grove. Look for where the trail splits left to return to the start at Fisher Road.

## NEARBY ATTRACTIONS

The Lloyd Center for the Environment (430 Potomska Road, Dartmouth; 508-990-0505; lloydcenter.org) has five walking trails over 55 acres of oak/hickory forest, freshwater wetlands, estuary, and salt marsh. From Destruction Brook Woods, drive southeast on Fisher Road 4.3 miles. Turn right onto Russell Mills Road, then turn left onto Rock O' Dundee Road. Turn right onto Potomska Road, and continue 1.2 miles to the Lloyd Center.

• • • • • • • • • • • • • • • • • • • • • • • • • • •

**GPS TRAILHEAD COORDINATES** N41° 34.800' W71° 00.950'

**DIRECTIONS** From Boston, take I-93 S 12 miles, then take Exit 4 on the left to merge onto MA 24 S toward Brockton. Drive 38.1 miles to Exit 4 to merge left onto I-195 east toward New Bedford. Continue 4.6 miles and take Exit 11 toward Dartmouth. Head south on Reed Road. After crossing US 6, turn left on Beeden Road. Turn right on Old Westport Road/Fisher Road, then left to stay on Fisher. Just before the fork with Woodcock Road, look for the DNRT sign for Destruction Brook Woods on the right. Park off Fisher Road near the sign; there is room for approximately six cars.

It's certainly easy to find Destruction Brook Woods.

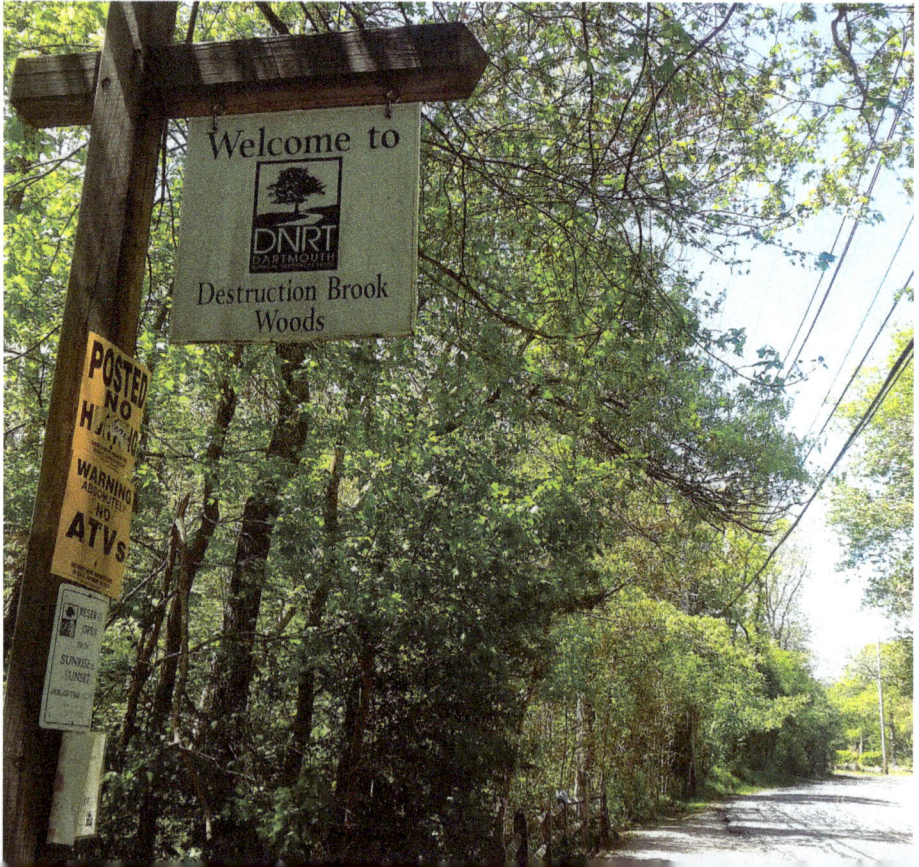

# 34 NOANET WOODLANDS

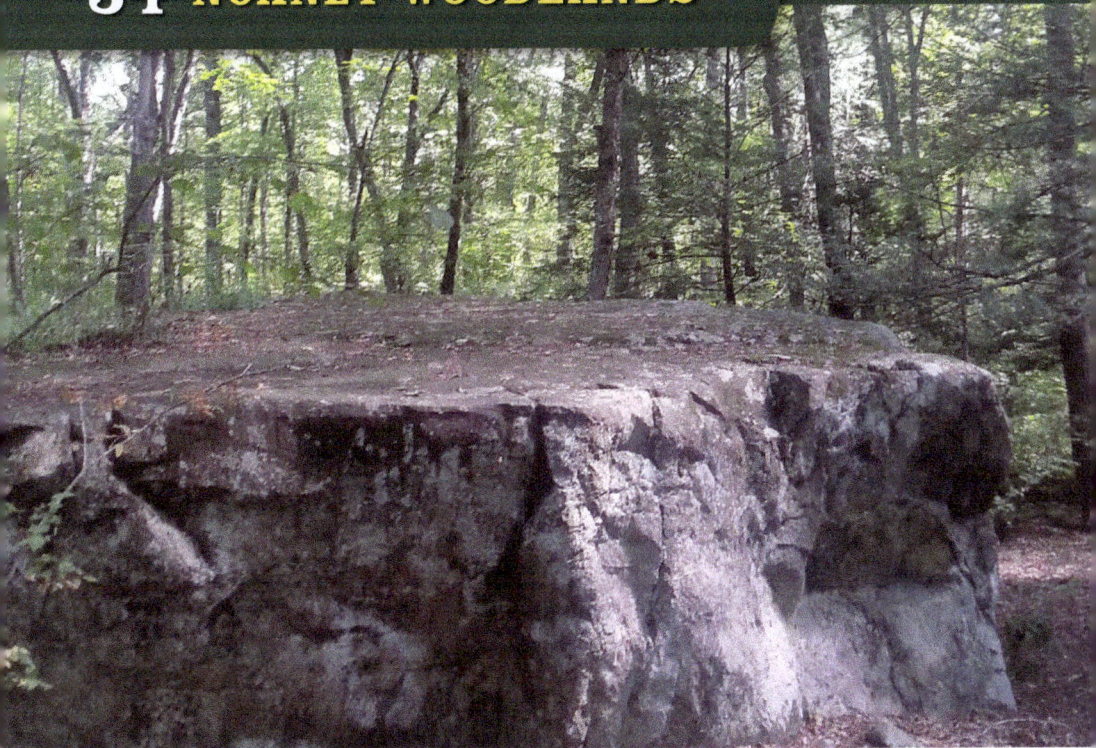

The pancake rock at Noanet Woodlands

**THIS HIKE TRAVERSES** undulating woodlands named for Noanet, a chief of the Natick tribe who was well known among Dover's first white settlers. Circling the ravine carved by Noanet Brook, the trail diverts to the reservation's highest point, Noanet Peak, then passes near the site of a 19th-century mill.

## DESCRIPTION

The acres within the Noanet Reservation were first farmed by colonial settlers during the 1700s. Much of the credit for discovering and preserving Dover's history goes to Amelia Peabody, who, in 1923, purchased the first of what, over the course of 60 years, grew to be a nearly 800-acre estate.

The hike begins at the trailhead to the right of the ranger station at Caryl Park, near the former home of Reverend Benjamin Caryl. To reach the red-blazed Caryl Loop Trail, follow this short clay path southeast to its end at a dirt road. Bear right at this junction and proceed on this winding road past a composting site on the right and an unmarked path on the left. Beyond a sign reading TO NOANET WOODS, the trail bends southwest to cross a stream. Several yards farther, it encounters a junction marked 2 and then reaches junction 3, where it meets the Larrabee Trail (marked by orange blazes) and Peabody Trail (marked by blue blazes). For a quick hike to the mill

**DISTANCE & CONFIGURATION:** 5.11-mile loop

**DIFFICULTY:** Easy–moderate

**SCENERY:** Woods, ponds, views of Boston from Noanet Peak

**EXPOSURE:** Mostly shaded

**TRAFFIC:** Moderate

**TRAIL SURFACE:** Firmly packed dirt with some more-rugged areas of loose gravel and exposed rock

**HIKING TIME:** 2.5–3 hours

**DRIVING DISTANCE FROM BOSTON COMMON:** 21 miles

**ELEVATION:** 148' at trailhead, 370' at highest point

**SEASON:** Year-round

**ACCESS:** Sunrise–sunset; free

**MAPS:** At the trailhead or at tinyurl.com /noanetwoodlandsmap

**WHEELCHAIR ACCESS:** No

**FACILITIES:** Restrooms open seasonally

**CONTACT:** Trustees of Reservations, thetrustees .org/places-to-visit, 617-542-7696

**LOCATION:** Dover, MA

**COMMENTS:** The Noanet Woodlands is dog-friendly, but dogs are not allowed in the parking lot at the adjoining Caryl Park.

site, opt for the Peabody Trail. Otherwise, you can continue south on the Noanet Peak (marked with yellow blazes) and Larrabee Trail to take a full tour of the reservation. Like most Trustees of Reservations lands, the trails are overlapping loops. You can follow the prescribed hike here, or arm yourself with a map and go exploring.

At junction 6, the Noanet Peak Trail shoots west and soon thereafter jackknifes to head southeast to reach junction 7. From this turn, the Noanet Peak Trail straightens, allowing for a full gallop to junction 9, overshooting Noanet Peak and intersecting with the Larrabee Trail. Hikers wanting a view from the high point should continue on the Noanet Peak Trail at junction 8 and bear left to head to upland. At the next junction, turn right and climb southeast to reach the pinnacle of Noanet Peak. Tree-covered except for an outcrop of granite, the hilltop provides a perfect view of Boston's skyline.

To continue on the Noanet Peak Trail, locate a path several feet downhill from the peak marked with a white square, and follow it southwest over roots and stones to the base of the hill. Join this bridle trail and continue on level ground through junction 9, traveling southwest on an easy downhill slope. At junction 10, the orange-blazed Larrabee Trail crosses the blunt swath of a gas line. Having reached the reservation's boundary, the trail swings southeast at junction 11.

After pitching down a rocky slope, the trail steadies on the shoulder of a hill overlooking wetland. Upon leaving a burly oak stand, the character of the woods changes abruptly from deciduous to primarily evergreen. The sudden appearance of a well-built stone wall explains the transition, as the acres contained within it were once cleared pastureland.

Once around the tip of the wetland, the Larrabee Trail traces the reservation's southern border, running parallel to the fencing of a private farm. To briefly break away from the border, bear left at junction 16 to hike on glacial debris mounded

# Noanet Woodlands

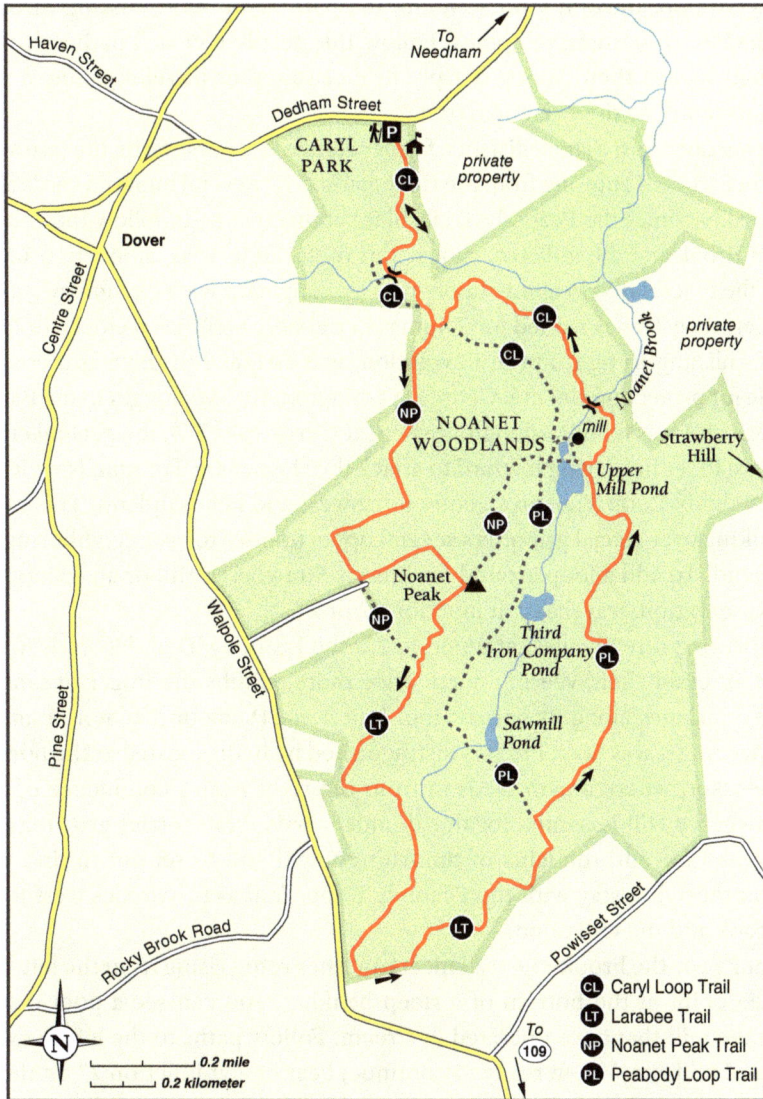

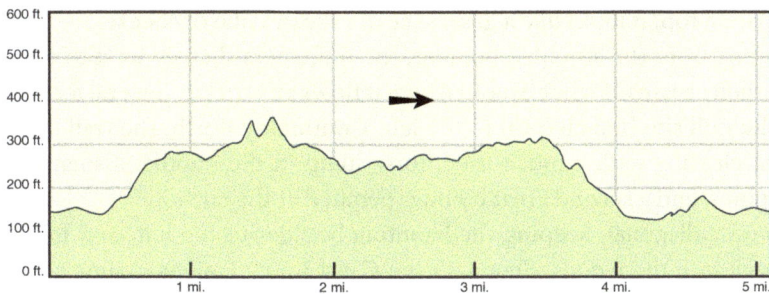

Haven Street

To
Needham

Dedham Street

**P**

CARYL
PARK

*private
property*

Dover

CL

Centre Street

CL

CL

CL

Noanet Brook

*private
property*

NP

NOANET
WOODLANDS

mill

Strawberry
Hill

*Upper
Mill Pond*

NP

PL

Noanet
Peak

Walpole Street

NP

*Third
Iron Company
Pond*

PL

Pine Street

LT

*Sawmill
Pond*

PL

Powisset Street

Rocky Brook Road

LT

**CL** Caryl Loop Trail
**LT** Larabee Trail
**NP** Noanet Peak Trail
**PL** Peabody Loop Trail

To
109

**N**

0.2 mile
0.2 kilometer

| | | | | | |
|---|---|---|---|---|---|
| 600 ft. | | | | | |
| 500 ft. | | | | | |
| 400 ft. | | | | | |
| 300 ft. | | | | | |
| 200 ft. | | | | | |
| 100 ft. | | | | | |
| 0 ft. | 1 mi. | 2 mi. | 3 mi. | 4 mi. | 5 mi. |

around the swamp. Beyond a horse jump, the path bends east, passing through a clearing shaded by looming red pines. Follow this deeply recessed path as it meanders through woods then climbs sharply to meet another traveling along a ridge. Bear right to return to the Larrabee Trail.

Traveling northeast a short distance farther alongside a horse farm, the trail swings north onto a cart road entering from the right marked 17. Several hundred yards ahead, this cart road becomes the Peabody Trail (blue) at marker 18. To follow the course of the Noanet Brook and the millrace, choose this route. Otherwise, at junction 18, bear right onto the blue-blazed Peabody Loop Trail to complete a wide circumnavigation.

The Larrabee Trail is named for Thomas Larrabee, a well-loved citizen of Dover, who, after enlisting to fight in the Revolution, was assigned to the guard company responsible for protecting General George Washington. He both fought in the Battle of Ticonderoga and was with Washington when, at Christmas 1776, the general crossed the Delaware River in a raging blizzard to attack the Hessians at Trenton, New Jersey.

The Peabody Loop Trail arcs gently northwest and heads upland. This section of easy walking over glacial grit offers several opportunities to visit neighboring conservation land. To add a loop around Larrabee's Strawberry Hill or an excursion to the Hale Reservation, travel east at junction 22 or 24.

After bearing directly west at junction 22, the Peabody Trail descends to meet the end of an esker then, veering north once more, climbs the finger of sand and gravel and continues along its narrow top. Junction 24 may or may not be marked (as of this writing it was not), but it is distinguished by being located at the northern end of the esker, where a path feeds in from the right near a confluence of stone walls. Strawberry Hill is named for the abundant wild strawberries growing on its slopes. If it is June and thoughts of the fruit compel you to set out to find them, bear right; otherwise, stay with the Peabody Loop Trail as it switches west toward Noanet Brook and the mill pond.

Drawing near the brook, the trail meets another route rising from the left. From this vantage point at the bottom of a steep banking, you can see a pool that was shaped by the mill that once operated upstream. Follow paths to the left to explore the pond and mill site. When ready to continue, bear east at junction 27 on the red-blazed Caryl Loop Trail. Around a bend sits a massive glacial erratic; being almost perfectly flat on top, it looks like a giant slice of cake or cube of cheese.

Departing from the stranded boulder, the trail veers sharply west to parallel a stone wall then crosses Noanet Brook, where it flows at a trickle. Several feet farther, a trail to the mill site branches off to the left. Continuing north, the trail leads to a wide, open clearing with a much-used horse jump in the middle, a smattering of imposing pines, and a second great boulder perched at the far side.

Cross on a diagonal, keeping the haunting boulder to the left, and follow red markers back into the woods. Stay with the Caryl Loop Trail as it aims northwest and then, bending like an elbow at marker 33, bears southwest, traveling uphill to junction 3, where the yellow and red trails converge. Continue on the Caryl Loop Trail, bear right and follow it north to the parking lot.

## NEARBY ATTRACTIONS

The Dolphin Seafood Restaurant is just 5 miles away at 12 Washington St. in downtown Natick (508-655-0669, dolphinseafood.com). This eatery is open seven days a week for lunch and dinner. From Caryl Park, follow Dedham Street west, and bear right onto Haven Street. After 1.2 miles, turn right onto Main Street and left onto Pleasant Street, which becomes Union Street. After 1.5 miles, turn left onto East Central Street (MA 135), and at 0.2 mile turn right onto Washington Street.

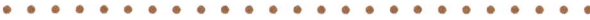

• • • • • • • • • • • • • • • • • • • • • • • • • •

**GPS TRAILHEAD COORDINATES**  N42° 14.900'  W71° 16.150'

**DIRECTIONS**  From Boston take I-90 W to Exit 15 (I-95/MA 128) toward Waltham/Dedham, and merge onto I-95 S/MA 128 toward South Shore/Cape Cod. After 6.8 miles take Exit 17 to MA 135 toward Needham/Wellesley. Turn left onto MA 135/West Street. Continue 0.6 mile, then turn left onto South Street. After 1.8 miles, South Street becomes Willow Street. Turn right onto Dedham Street and continue 0.3 mile to Caryl Park.

There are several small ponds and an old mill site within Noanet Woodlands.

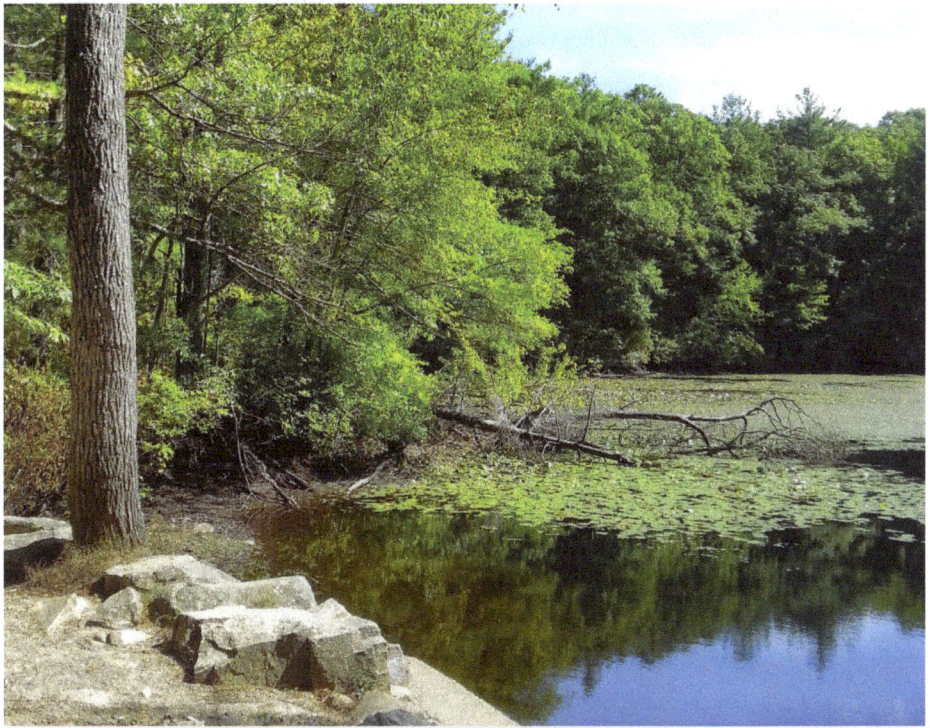

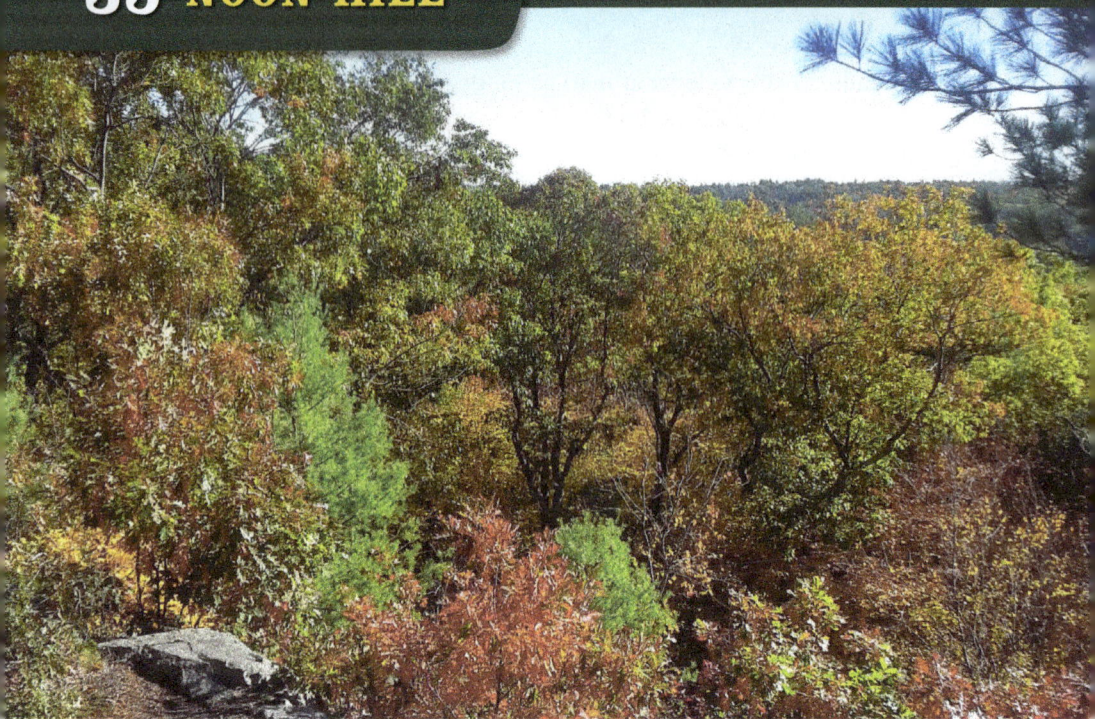

Noon Hill's trails wind through a dramatic, dense mixed forest of deciduous and coniferous trees.

**THIS SECLUDED RESERVATION** provides 204 acres of peaceful hiking, with trails suitable for horseback riding, mountain biking, and cross-country skiing. Miles from the busy Charles River esplanade in downtown Boston, this location provides an opportunity to experience the river in its natural state.

## DESCRIPTION

Like most of the land of Massachusetts, the wooded acres of Noon Hill were once open pasture enclosed for generations by stone walls. The oak, beech, birch, and hemlock have grown in over the last century. From the parking area, set off uphill, heading southeast. Pass the sunken remains of an old foundation, continuing straight as the path tapers back downhill and enters the woods. The trail passes through a mix of hardwoods and evergreens before reaching a sign bearing the number 1 and, shortly thereafter, a second marked with the number 2. Here you have the choice of following a fork to the left on a new trail or continuing straight with the trail identified as a part of the Bay Circuit Trail. Continue straight on the Bay Circuit Trail, which is red-blazed like the trail to the left.

At the next intersection there's a path to the right, but continue straight, up what is the start of Noon Hill. Not much farther along, the trail splits again. Instead of following the yellow-blazed trail, keep right on the red-blazed trail and proceed

**DISTANCE & CONFIGURATION:** 4.6 miles; loops around Noon Hill and Holt Pond, with an extension to an overlook on the bank of the Charles River

**DIFFICULTY:** Easy

**SCENERY:** Views include forest wetlands, the Charles River, Holt Pond, and a panoramic overlook from the top of Noon Hill

**EXPOSURE:** Mostly shaded

**TRAFFIC:** Moderate

**TRAIL SURFACE:** Packed dirt with some areas of gravel

**HIKING TIME:** 3 hours

**DRIVING DISTANCE FROM BOSTON COMMON:** 23 miles

**ELEVATION:** 167' at trailhead, 337' at highest point

**SEASON:** Year-round

**ACCESS:** Sunrise–sunset; free

**MAPS:** Available at the trailhead or online at tinyurl.com/noonhillmap

**WHEELCHAIR ACCESS:** No

**FACILITIES:** Picnic tables

**CONTACT:** The Trustees of Reservations, thetrustees.org/places-to-visit, 617-542-7696

**LOCATION:** Medfield, MA

**COMMENTS:** Noon Hill is a link in the Bay Circuit Trail; the latter connects green space in 43 towns in Eastern Massachusetts, from Newburyport to Duxbury and Kingston.

slightly downhill. From here, the trail, still level and wide, winds southwest in easy curves through the woods.

Arriving at marker 5, turn off and climb southeast on a slender, more rugged path through a grove of young white pines. In the first week of May, the woods are bright with half-sprung leaves in vivid shades of green—and red, in the case of some oaks and maples. After winding around a granite ledge, the trail noses north to meet another trail. Hike right, rounding the curve of the hill. Follow the blue markers to take the detour marked 8A.

This new trail gradually ascends over a track of packed pine needles to the peak of Noon Hill at 370 feet. Explore the hilltop's nooks and crannies as the view opens and the trail becomes obscure momentarily, then continue southwest, traveling downhill to reach an intersection with a trail marked 7. Turn left and ascend southeast a short distance to a scenic overlook. Ahead a mass of exposed granite serves as balcony seating for viewing Boston's skyline. Retrace your steps from the overlook back to marker 7 and continue downhill. At the next intersection, number 6, turn right to head northwest. A bubbling spring makes for a wet zone, but for the most part, the trail provides easy, dry passage as it winds through wetland.

Pass marker 5 and continue northeast on a piece of trail traveled earlier. Beyond marker 4, where the trail reaches another intersection, turn left to head southwest. You will come to a granite boulder off to the side and, farther on, to a bridge across a rushing stream. The trail along this part makes many twists and turns as it narrows. The woods are peaceful here. The trail is not all that well marked, but it is clearly defined and easy to follow.

A seemingly forgotten small gray shack sits off the trail to the left, where the trail eases northwest. Continuing, pass through a gap in a stone wall and walk down

## Noon Hill

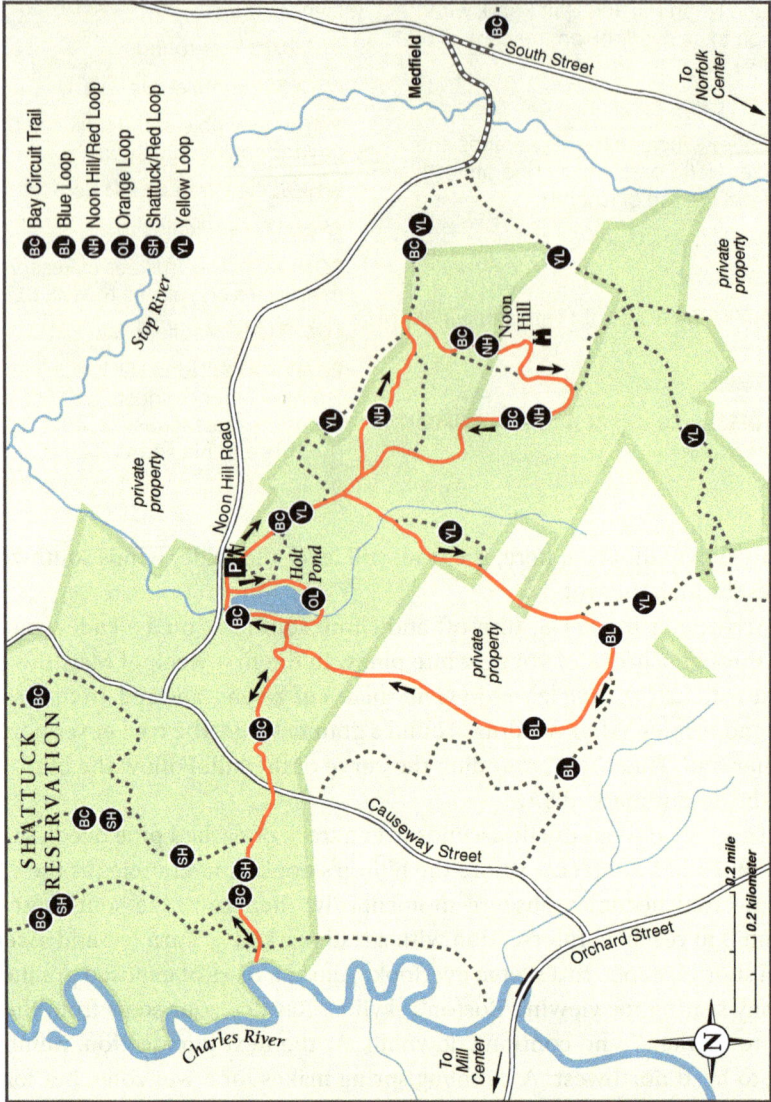

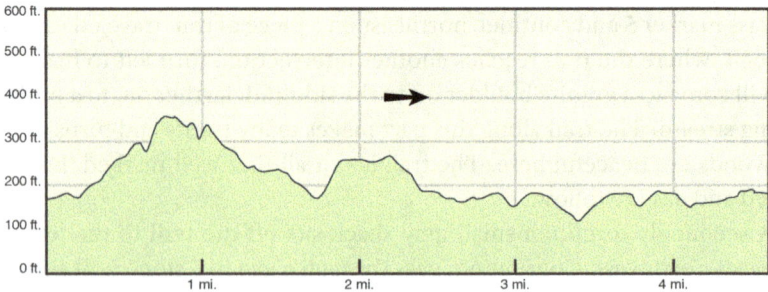

a long avenue between two stone walls. Keep an eye out for forget-me-nots and less-friendly poison ivy growing along the edge of the grassy way.

Stay with the trail, heading northeast. Passing a trail on the left, you will shortly come to a dirt driveway. Cross here and continue on through more woods to a junction. Turn left and left again at the next split, which is marked as intersection 12. Follow this new path as it twists and turns westward. Beyond a small wooden bridge and another stone wall, the path bisects Causeway Street and arrives at marker 14.

Aim for the well-concealed river on this wide, pine needle–strewn path by bearing left at the next two forks. As the land begins to slope to the Charles River, you will see marker 17 posted on a tree. By now you will be able to see the Charles River through the tangle of trees and shrubs growing along its banks. The path ends at a gorgeous spot beside a massive oak.

When you are ready to leave this idyllic scene, follow the trail back to the junction at marker 12. From here, take the path heading left. This less-used route leads through a grove of young pines to Noon Hill Street. Emerging from the woods, turn right and walk briefly on the pavement to Holt Pond. On spotting a path alongside the road, reenter the woods, following the path over a footbridge, then head right to circle the pond.

Holt Pond was formed in 1764 when the nearby Sawmill Brook was dammed to provide power for a mill. In the next century, the woods surrounding the pond were cleared and fenced for pasture. Once you're around the southeastern bend of the pond, a second trail branches off, banking to the right. Take this turn and follow the path uphill to a boulder. Press on through bushes concealing the path to find a more pronounced trail. To make your way back to the parking area, hike left then left again at a wide junction.

In 1676, 1,000 warring Wampanoag tore through this area, setting fire to 32 houses, two mills, and a slew of barns. Having lost patience with the English settlers, Wampanoag chief Massasoit Sachem (or Ousamequin) instructed his fighters to eliminate them.

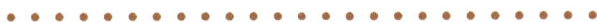

• • • • • • • • • • • • • • • • • • • • • • • • • •

**GPS TRAILHEAD COORDINATES:** N42° 09.900' W71° 19.083'

**DIRECTIONS** From Boston take I-93 S to Exit 1. Go south on I-95 S 7.3 miles. At Exit 9 merge onto US 1 S. Turn right onto Old Post Road; soon after, turn slightly left onto Common Street. After 1.8 miles Common Street becomes Elm Street. Stay straight on Elm Street/MA 27 and follow MA 27 for 2.6 miles. At the intersection of MA 27 and MA 109, take MA 109 W 0.1 mile, then take an immediate left onto Causeway Street. Follow it 1.3 miles and turn left onto Noon Hill Road. The entrance and small parking area are 0.2 mile ahead on the right.

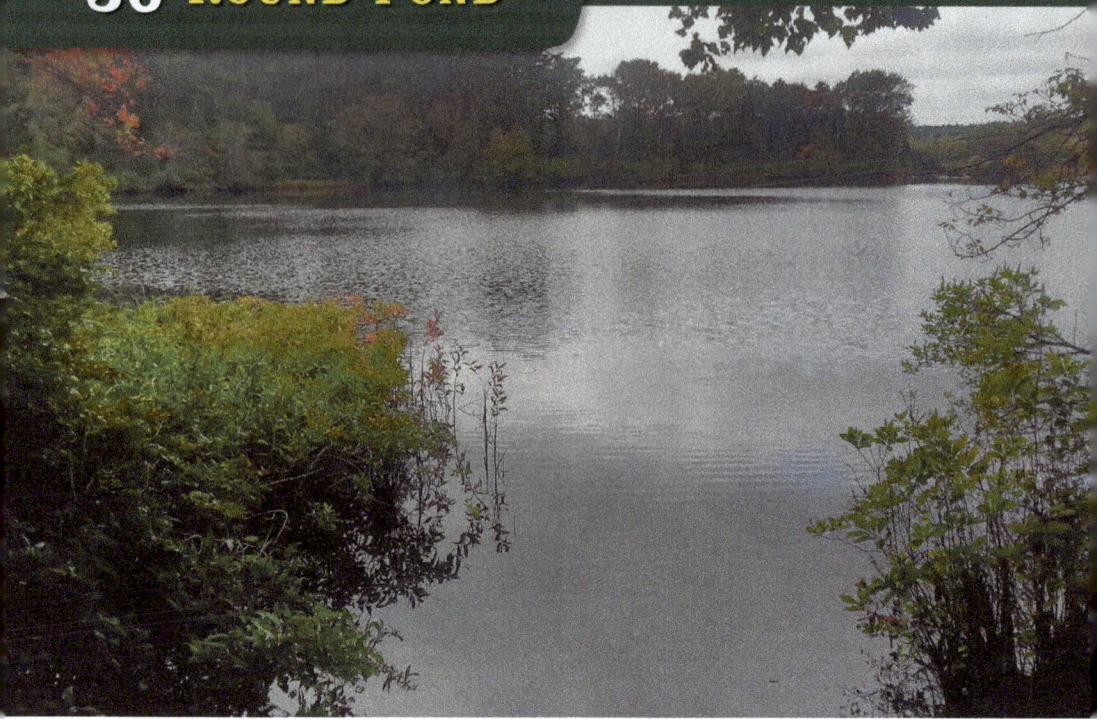

The Round Pond hike is fairly gentle and winds past ponds and cranberry bogs.

**THIS LOOP TAKES** you through a landscape of cranberry bogs, kettle ponds, and peaceful woodland.

## DESCRIPTION

This land was originally used only for crops during the growing season, but inevitably the green pastures to the north lured families away from Plymouth for good. After successfully petitioning Plymouth officials for permission to build their own church, the ruddy *Mayflower* captain, Myles Standish; passengers William Brewster and John Alden; and others officially founded their new village, which Standish named Duxbury after his family's estate in Chorley, Lancashire, England. The hulls and masts for more than 643 ships were built of wood cut from Duxbury's old-growth forests.

Starting the hike from the parking area on Mayflower Street, set out on the Yellow Trail, heading west through sparse woods of white pine and red oak. At about 0.2 mile, the trail converges with the Bay Circuit Trail and bends south, passing a shade east of Round Pond.

Ahead, where the Bay Circuit Trail diverts west, continue on the Yellow Trail to reach a T intersection, where Old Meetinghouse Road runs east and west. Located beside the Old Burial Ground, the meetinghouse is a 2-mile walk from this spot.

**DISTANCE & CONFIGURATION:** 2.33-mile loop

**DIFFICULTY:** Easy

**SCENERY:** Oak and pine forest, several ponds, cranberry bog

**EXPOSURE:** Mostly shaded

**TRAFFIC:** Moderate

**TRAIL SURFACE:** Packed dirt with roots and rocks and some sandy areas

**HIKING TIME:** 1–1.5 hours

**DRIVING DISTANCE FROM BOSTON COMMON:** 34 miles

**ELEVATION:** 56' at trailhead, no significant gain

**SEASON:** Year-round

**ACCESS:** Sunrise–sunset; free

**MAPS:** Available at Duxbury town hall (878 Tremont St.; follow Mayflower Street east to its end, and turn left onto Tremont; the town hall is ahead on the left). Hiking trails leading to Round Pond and North Hill Marsh are accessible immediately behind the town hall.

**WHEELCHAIR ACCESS:** No

**FACILITIES:** None

**CONTACT:** Duxbury Rural and Historical Society, tinyurl.com/roundpondmap, 781-934-6106

**LOCATION:** Duxbury, MA

**COMMENTS:** This hike is easily extended into longer hikes by linking to trails in Duxbury Town Forest and North Hill Marsh, or by using it to access the Bay Circuit Trail, which leads south approximately 2 miles to Bay Farm on the edge of Duxbury's Kingston Bay.

Bear left to briefly follow this route worn by the footsteps of the Pilgrims, then bear right at the next intersection to resume hiking south on the Red Trail. Dipping in elevation, the trail passes over increasingly sandy terrain. Chickadees, tufted titmice, the occasional flock of cedar waxwings, and other forest birds flit and sing among the pines and understory of lowbush and dryland blueberries, ferns, teaberry, and lady's slippers.

Opening to a pronounced dune after winding west, the trail swings south again to pass a trail to the right. Continue to the next junction, then bear left, leaving the Red Trail for a narrower path sloping east into wetland, where species including red maple, aspen, black cherry, alder, sagebrush, summersweet, highbush blueberry, sweet pepperbush, and native azaleas grow in humus-rich soil. At the bottom of the hill, the trail spills out to one of Duxbury's many cultivated cranberry bogs.

Although called *ibimi* by the Pequot people, folklore has it that the Pilgrims saw in the cranberry's small pink blossoms the head and bill of a sandhill crane and hence renamed the native fruit "crane berry."

Partial to the unique and highly acidic conditions found in glacier-formed peat bogs, cranberries were harvested exclusively from the wild until 1816. Skirting the cranberry bog, the trail traces woods to reach a drive running parallel to Island Creek Pond. Bear right passing a pump house, and at the southern end of the bog loop, head west to hike along a causeway that divides the bog in two.

Arriving at a crossroads where the Bay Circuit Trail swings in from the north and drops south, take up this epic trail and continue west into the woods. In a short time, the Bay Circuit Trail winds north and, after a stretch through sometimes wet lowland, gains elevation on nearing the southeast shore of Pine Lake.

## Round Pond

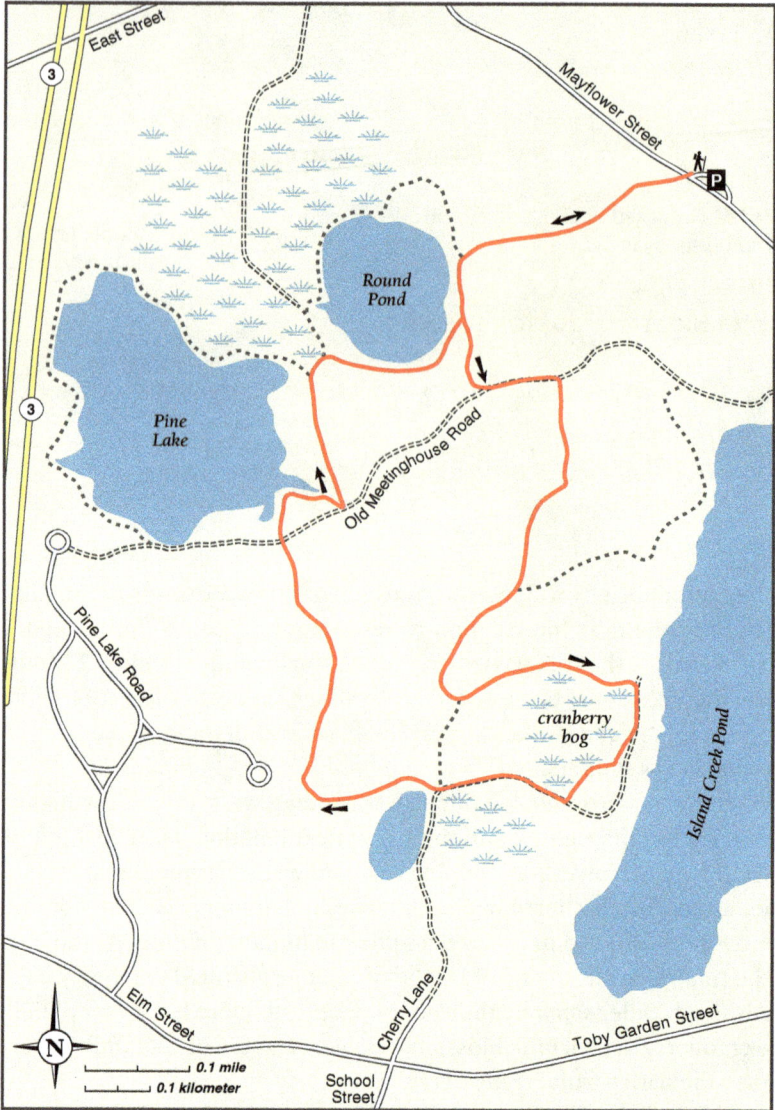

Together with the cranberry bogs lying farther north and Round Pond ahead to the east, Pine Lake attracts a full spectrum of wildlife. In the early morning and evening hours, raccoons and opossums descend from trees and upland haunts to forage at the waterside. Deer and foxes dash in and out like apparitions, and overhead, when the wind obliges and the light is right, osprey course in to swipe at schooling fish.

Follow the trail as it hugs the bank of Round Pond, pauses at a lookout, then arches northeast. Where it meets the Yellow Trail, bear right and finish your hike by heading back to the parking lot.

## NEARBY ATTRACTIONS

The town's beauty is reason enough to prolong your visit, but if you enjoy history, two of Duxbury's historic homes provide a ready excuse to do some sightseeing. Visit Alden House Museum Historic Site (105 Alden St., just off MA 3A; 781-934-9092; alden.org). Built in 1653 on property deeded to the Alden family in the 1620s, this remarkable house has never been owned by any other family. Unlike other historic houses, Alden House has never been updated. Admission is $5 for adults (age 18 and over) and $4 for children (ages 3–17). There is a $1 discount for AAA members. The museum is open to the public mid-May–Columbus Day, Monday–Saturday, noon–4 p.m.; the last tour begins at 3:30 p.m. Off-season hours are generally 10 a.m.–1 p.m., but it's best to call ahead to be sure.

King Caesar House (20 King Caesar Road; 781-934-6106; duxburyhistory.org) is a second historic house worth visiting. It's open July–August, Wednesday–Sunday, 1–4 p.m., and in September, Saturday and Sunday, 1–4 p.m. From Mayflower Street, drive northeast to Lincoln Street. At the rotary, take the first exit onto MA 14. MA 14 becomes St. George Street. After 1 mile, turn left onto Washington Street, which becomes Powder Point Avenue. Turn right on King Caesar Road.

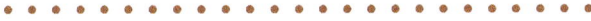

• • • • • • • • • • • • • • • • • • • • • • • • • •

**GPS TRAILHEAD COORDINATES**  N42° 02.133' W70° 42.783'

**DIRECTIONS**  From Boston, take I-93 and merge onto MA 3 S. Take Exit 10 off MA 3 S and bear right. Follow MA 3A to the Duxbury Fire Station. Turn left onto Mayflower Street. Parking for Round Pond is about 1 mile past the Duxbury transfer station, on the left.

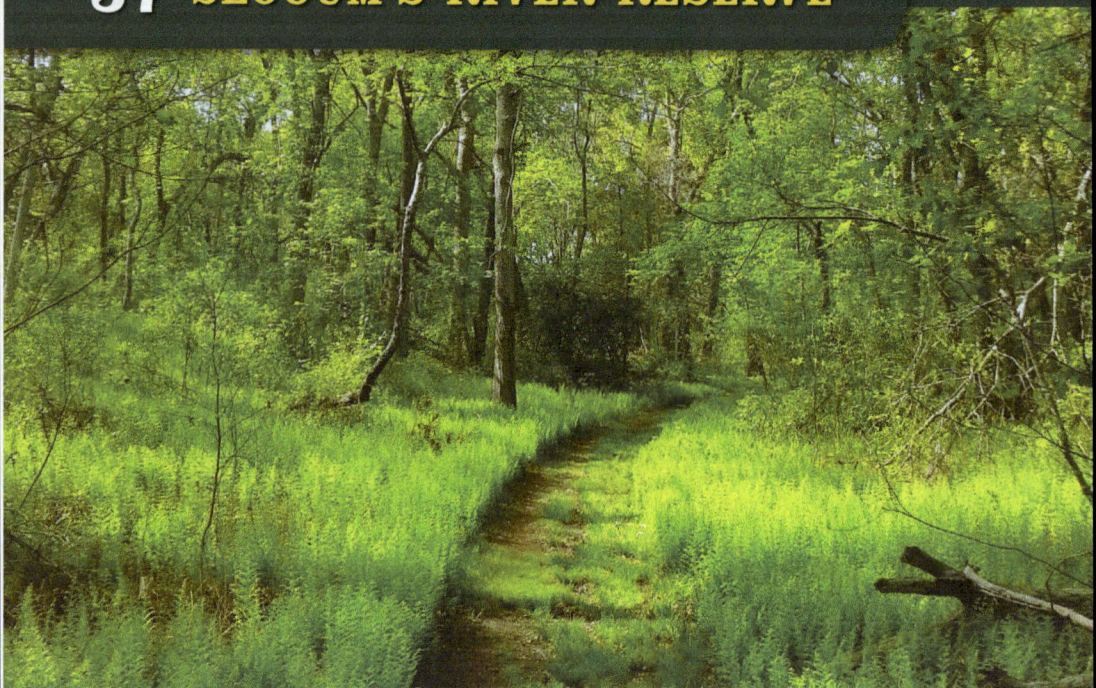

Slocum's River Reserve is a relatively short but incredibly scenic hike.

**NO PLACE IN MASSACHUSETTS** is more beautiful than this reservation set on a hillside overlooking the picturesque Slocum's River. Following easements across privately owned farmland, this hike explores a quintessential New England landscape as lovely now as it was centuries ago.

## DESCRIPTION

Whether the river was named for Anthony Slocum in the 17th century or his descendant Joshua Slocum in the 19th century depends on whom you ask. Either man is worthy of the honor.

The hike begins at the far end of the parking lot beside a Trustees of Reservations kiosk. Once you can stop gazing across the fields to the river, set out along the easement that runs east between a formidable stone wall and a field planted with young fruit trees.

As you leave the fields and stone wall behind, you'll see a Trustees sign marking the true boundary of the reserve. Enter the woods here and continue east, following the trail as it leads slightly right and then downhill beside another stone wall partially concealed by bittersweet vines. Step through first one gap in the stone wall then another, bearing left to hike to the river over upland grown in with hearty oaks, hickories, and sassafras. As the trail descends closer to sea level, the view clears and the south-flowing waters of Slocum's River seize center stage.

**DISTANCE & CONFIGURATION:** 3.87-mile loop

**DIFFICULTY:** Easy

**SCENERY:** The magnificent Slocum's River, woods, wetlands, nursery, agricultural fields

**EXPOSURE:** Mostly shaded

**TRAFFIC:** Light

**TRAIL SURFACE:** Grass, firmly packed dirt with some muddy areas

**HIKING TIME:** 2 hours

**DRIVING DISTANCE FROM BOSTON COMMON:** 58 miles

**ELEVATION:** 74' at trailhead, no significant gain

**SEASON:** Year-round

**ACCESS:** Sunrise–sunset; free (donation appreciated)

**MAPS:** At kiosk in parking area while supplies last or at tinyurl.com/slocumsriverreservemap

**WHEELCHAIR ACCESS:** No

**FACILITIES:** None

**CONTACT:** Dartmouth Natural Resources Trust, dnrt.org/slocumsriver, 508-991-2289

**LOCATION:** Dartmouth, MA

**COMMENTS:** Dogs are welcome but must be leashed. Water-resistant boots—or all-weather sandals—are recommended when the weather is warm and wet. The Dartmoor Farm Wildlife Management Area portion of the hike remains open, but the trail is no longer managed or maintained.

The trail winds free of the woods and opens to a field stretched flat beside salt marsh buffered by a thin screen of trees. To get a good look at the river, follow one of the several short paths that cut through to the windswept marsh. Step carefully to avoid running into any poison ivy.

When you're ready to continue, follow the trail as it traces the field's periphery counterclockwise to its southwest corner, where the trail diverts back into the woods. Take it slow to allow a chance sighting of a dazzling bluebird or oriole, an acrobatic flycatcher, or a wild turkey hen with hatchlings. For a good long look, take a seat on the granite bench placed among daisies and Indian paintbrush at the center of the field.

From the edge of the field, hike west, bearing right at a junction to continue north through the woods. Here the trail is still firm and relatively flat. It also cuts through a dense carpet of ferns. When you emerge on the edge of privately owned farmland, bear right where the trail makes a T, and follow the wide, grassy avenue spotted with wild strawberries past a small meadow ensconced in trees to a Trustees' sign pointing left to Dartmoor Farm. Turn here and track the reservation's northern boundary via a mowed path that leads back to Horseneck Road.

To continue the hike, navigate the iron gate on Dartmoor Farm's drive, and travel north along the west side of Horseneck Road, following a mowed path running between an electric fence and a wooded buffer on the farm's northern boundary. There are few trail markers; however, birdhouses with hay spilling from their circular openings line the way, and pastel-colored beehives stationed on the route indicate the easement's halfway point.

Beyond a large barn set back behind Dartmoor Farm's many rows of ornamental trees and shrubs, the trail darts north, leaving solid footing for the forested wetland of the Dartmoor Farm Wildlife Management Area. Because this portion of the hike is no longer managed or maintained by the Trustees of Reservations, the trail will be

## Slocum's River Reserve

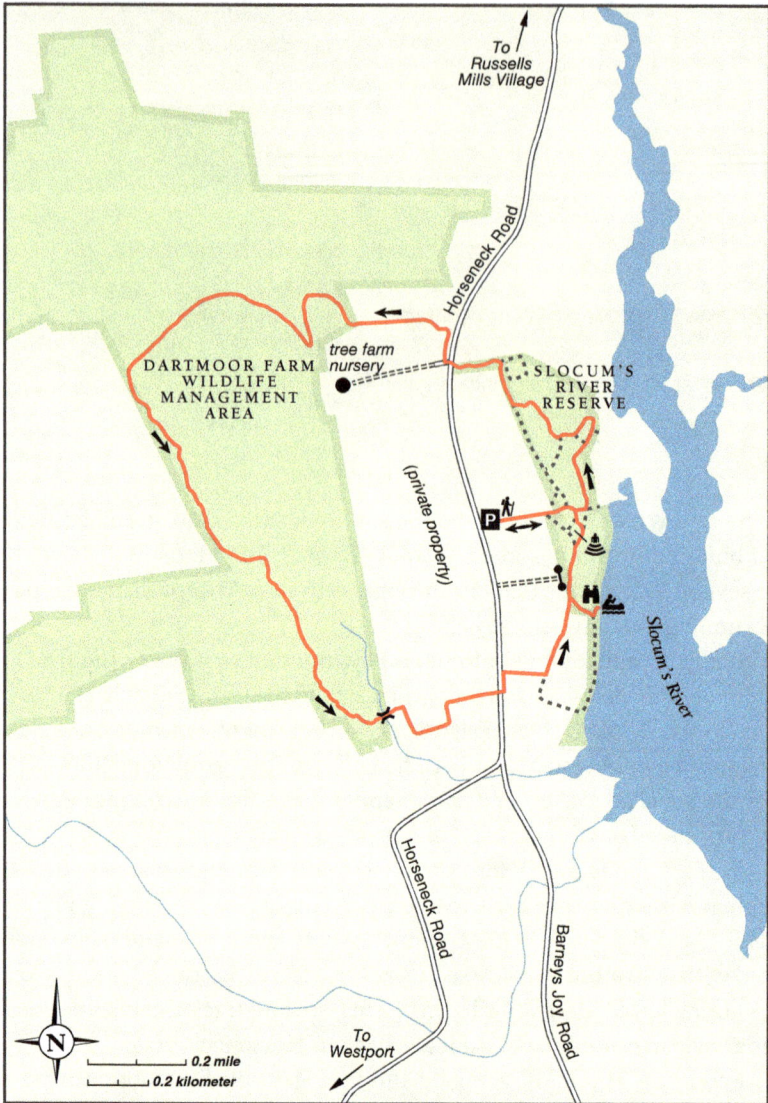

fairly grown over in spots. Have a map, preferably a compass, and the skills to use them both. You can't get too lost in here, but it's the difference between emerging from the woods near your car or on the other side of the reservation.

The Dartmoor trail threads through tree cover, staying close to the wire fence. After a run south, the trail reaches the end of the nursery and splits to the right as it nears a maintenance yard. Covering relatively level ground, it continues northwest to eventually meet a stone wall built along a property line, whereupon it begins a gentle arc south. Embossed with moss and fringed with ferns, the trail is neither well marked nor well defined as it disappears beneath puddles and streams. Stay the course by hiking straight whenever faintly etched paths divert left or (most often) right.

At 0.86 mile from Horseneck Road, the trail intersects with a broad cart road running west to east. Shake off the mud; bear left onto this dry, even plane; and enjoy easy walking through woods of oak and pine for the next 0.3 miles, passing an abandoned camper on the right a few hundred yards along.

Reaching a junction where the trail splits off to a clearing on the right, continue straight once again on a narrow footpath. Fortunately, just as the trail becomes impossibly vague, a gap in a stone wall confirms the path's direction. Once through this passage, keep the stone wall to the left, and continue hiking east.

Winding onward, the trail travels through another section of stone wall and momentarily aims north, passing a tremendous knotted holly tree on the left just before it reaches a cellar hole containing great flanks of granite. Hike along the right edge of the cellar hole, and continue 100 or so yards to find another trail dead ahead. Bear right to hike southeast on this new trail through older woods of maple and holly. Stone walls shadow to the left and right, indicating pasture laboriously cleared centuries ago and now once more glutted with trees.

Bending directly east, the trail loses breadth as it slopes back to wetland. Then it steers straight beyond a stream bridged by slabs of stone to an enormous commercial hayfield. Hike right to trace the farmland's border around this field, then head east along a mowed strip outside an electric fence to return to Horseneck Road.

Cross over to a burly stone wall framing the pasture. Continuing from a sign marking another easement, hike east along a field of grazing cattle to arrive at a point where four walls meet. Standing on this hill that rises above Slocum's River, you can see for miles. Continue left, following the arrow on the Trustees of Reservations sign posted beside the stone wall, and cross the top of the agricultural fields.

Ahead, where the trail splits, bear right to hike downhill. This path leads directly to a canoe landing on the riverbank; follow it to its end, or bear left at the fork midway. From the left turn, the trail undulates upward through a grassy meadow dotted with wildflowers to arrive at a stone seat set back from a grassy lookout. Veer right again to cross a meadow gone feral and right once more before swinging left to meet the path that leads to the parking lot.

## NEARBY ATTRACTIONS

Horseneck Beach State Reservation (follow Horseneck Road south until you see a sign for the beach) is well worth a visit if you have some spare time while visiting the Dartmouth area. Wine lovers may also want to plan a visit to the Westport Rivers Winery, also down the road from the beach at 417 Hixbridge Road, Westport (800-993-9695, westportrivers.com).

**GPS TRAILHEAD COORDINATES:** N41° 33.117'  W71° 00.550'

**DIRECTIONS**  From Boston take I-93/US 1 S 12.5 miles. At Exit 4 merge left onto MA 24 S toward Brockton. Exit onto MA 140 S and turn right onto MA 6 W. At the fourth set of traffic lights, turn left onto Old Westport Road and follow it 0.4 mile. Bear left onto Chase Road and follow it 3.6 miles to the end. Take a right onto Russells Mills Road and follow it 1 mile through historic Russells Mills Village. Continue straight onto Horseneck Road and follow it 1.4 miles to the entrance; there is parking for about 10 cars on the left.

An old stone wall punctuates the land at the reserve.

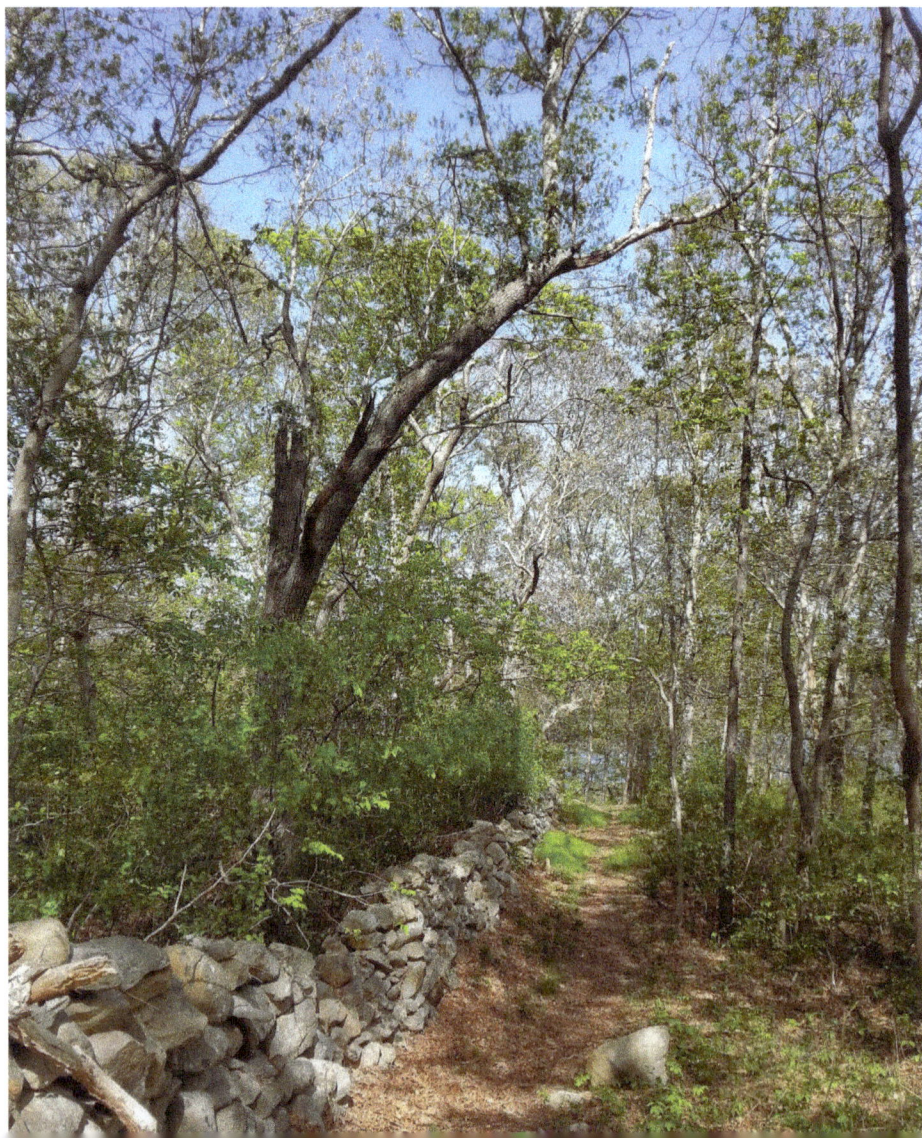

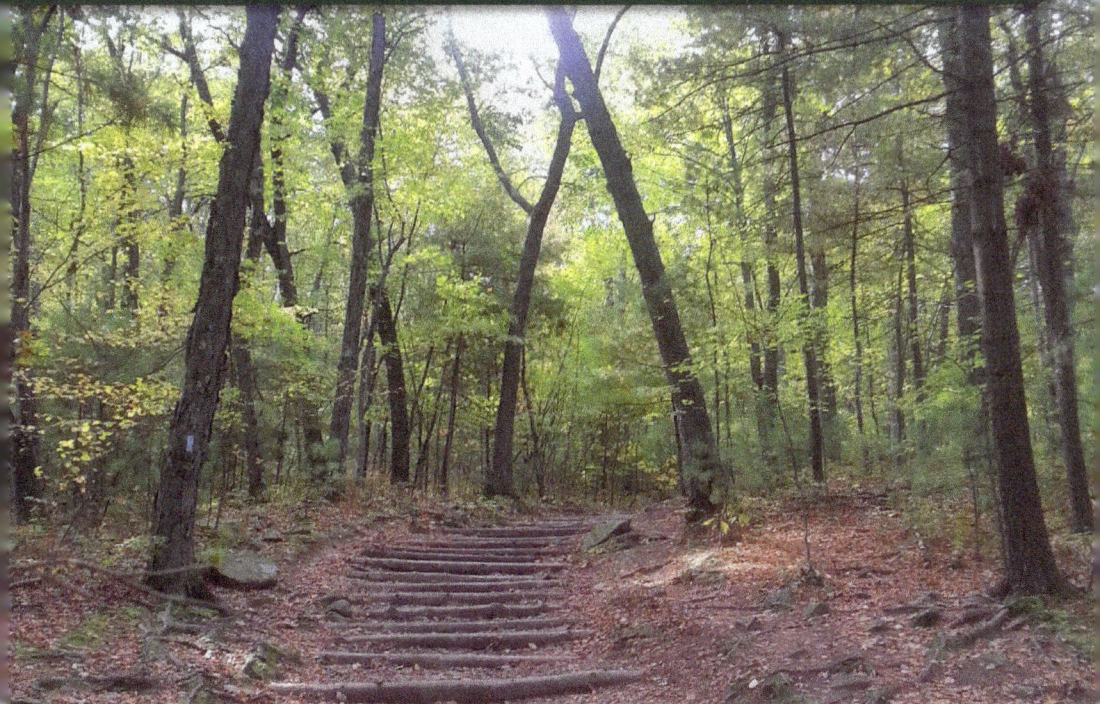

There's a nice mix of trails suitable for anyone at Wilson Mountain Reservation.

**TALL ENOUGH TO** befit its name yet accessible to hikers of all abilities, the 295-foot Wilson Mountain is minutes away from the center of Boston's neighbor, Dedham. Following a trail that loops around the mountain's base then climbs to its rocky peak, you will enjoy peaceful woods, gurgling streams, and a meadow that at the height of summer is resplendent with wildflowers and butterflies.

## DESCRIPTION

To get to the network of trails that traverse the 207 acres of the Wilson Mountain Reservation, head uphill from the parking lot, following the wide, gravel-topped path into woods. Keep right, passing another path bearing left. Within a few hundred yards, this path, identified by blue blazes, forms a V with the red-and-blue trail. The intersection is marked with the number 21.

Follow the narrow red-and-blue trail. Traveling southwest over exposed roots and angular rocks spit up by the hill, and what looks like the forehead of an earth-enshrined granite giant, the trail reaches a high point.

From here, hiking becomes less strenuous. The trail itself is less rocky, with more firmly packed dirt mottled with patches of sand, the remains of pulverized boulders. After passing through a stone wall, the trail rounds a bend and climbs to intersection

**DISTANCE & CONFIGURATION:** 3.5-mile loop

**DIFFICULTY:** Easy–moderate

**SCENERY:** Woods, spring-fed wetlands, meadow of wildflowers

**EXPOSURE:** Mostly shaded

**TRAFFIC:** Moderate–heavy

**TRAIL SURFACE:** Packed dirt topped by loose gravel, some open rock faces

**HIKING TIME:** 1–2 hours

**DRIVING DISTANCE FROM BOSTON COMMON:** 19 miles

**ELEVATION:** 108' at trailhead, 280' at highest point

**SEASON:** Year-round

**ACCESS:** Sunrise–sunset; free

**MAPS:** Posted at entrance or at mass.gov /eea/docs/dcr/parks/trails/wilson.pdf

**WHEELCHAIR ACCESS:** No

**FACILITIES:** None

**CONTACT:** Massachusetts Dept. of Conservation and Resources, mass.gov/locations /wilson-mountain-reservation, 617-626-1250

**LOCATION:** Dedham, MA

**COMMENTS:** This is a good family hike.

24. Here the red trail hikes up and right, and the green trail goes left, easing downhill. This slope is cooled by shade cast by pine, hemlock, ash, and basswood trees.

The next trail intersection is marked 18. Bear left to stay on the blue trail. For a pleasant, virtually rock-free stretch, the trail travels south up a slight grade. Then, closing in on the reservation's boundary, it narrows and doubles back to head northeast, descending past knotted swamp oak and spry sassafras. This sheltered eastern side of the hill harbors mountain laurel and woodland wildflowers, including lady's slippers (*Cypripedium acaule*). Easy to miss, this endangered member of the orchid family can live for 100 years but may flower only 10–20 times in its lifetime.

Several unmarked paths split off from the blue trail as it sweeps uphill again over pine needles and moss. Stay on course with the green trail at intersections 16 and 17; at a split beyond, cross planks bridging a modest stream. In summer, the leaves of linden and basswood trees fan the air above the trickling water. A fractured stone wall rests nearby, left over from when this was farm and pasture land.

Heading north past abutting residential property, the trail crosses more wetland. Rough slabs of wood provide dry footing over pooled, tea-colored water. Granite-hewn upland casts a shadow from the right. Pitching downhill, the blue trail passes junction 15, veering away to cross a stream. In the heat of a summer day, dragonflies and butterflies stir the vaporous atmosphere. Weaving north then west, up then down between hill and mire, the trail expands and flattens as it nears a road.

The trail winds alongside it to a rock formation that looks like the spine of a monster arching out of the earth. The trail then aims southwest, eases downhill, and frees itself from the road. Leveling at wetland once more, the trail meets an enormous boulder at the center of a clearing. Carried here by creeping ice thousands of years ago, the granite monolith is pinned in place by sassafras trees deeply rooted on opposing sides.

Wetland, perhaps born of glacial meltwater, picks up again beyond the boulder. An inviting pool to the left tempts passersby and dares jaded city slickers to give up

# Wilson Mountain Reservation

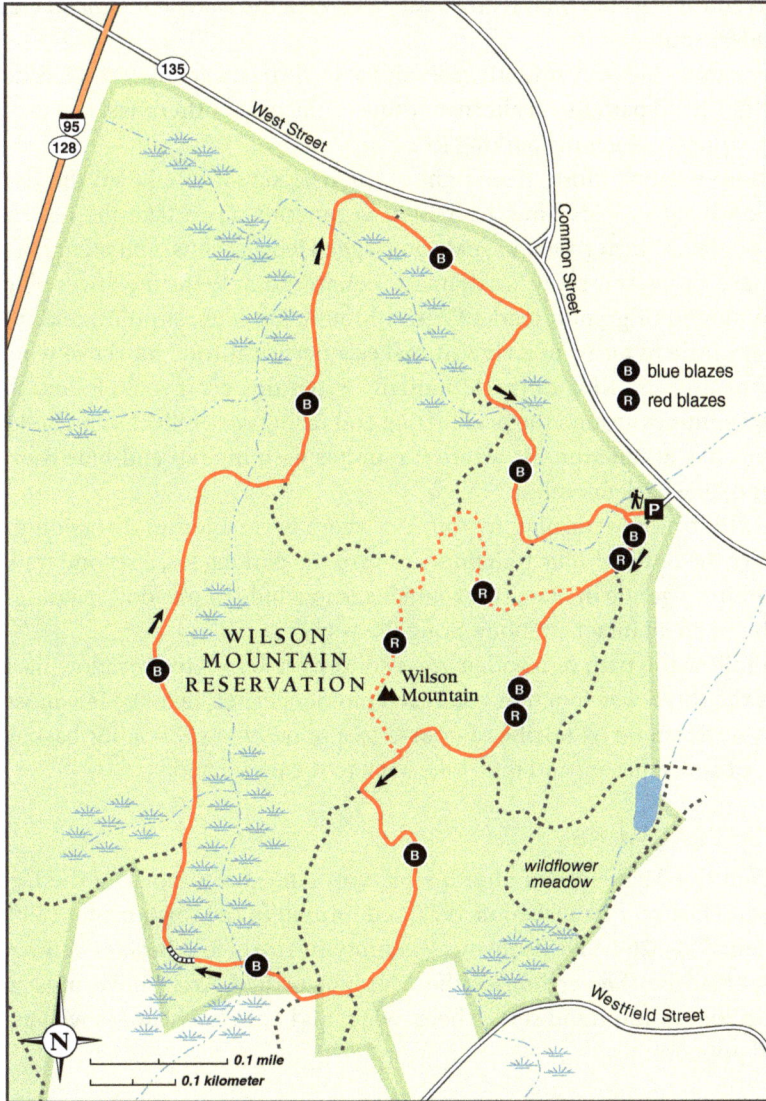

95
128

135

West Street

Common Street

B blue blazes
R red blazes

P

B
R

R

B

B
R

WILSON
MOUNTAIN
RESERVATION

R

▲ Wilson
Mountain

B

B

*wildflower
meadow*

B

Westfield Street

N

0.1 mile
0.1 kilometer

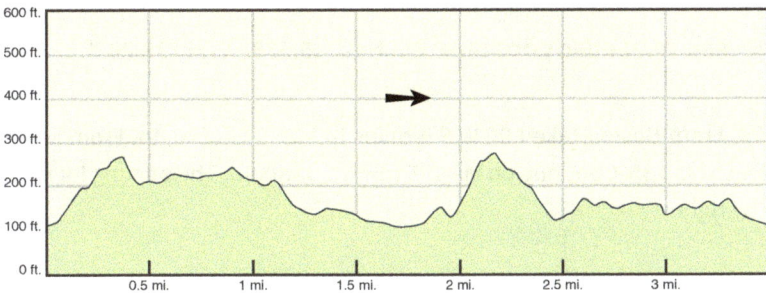

600 ft.
500 ft.
400 ft.
300 ft.
200 ft.
100 ft.
0 ft.

0.5 mi.   1 mi.   1.5 mi.   2 mi.   2.5 mi.   3 mi.

inhibitions and at least dip their feet. Passing between the water and upland crag, the trail meanders southeast.

Dipping downhill over smooth ground, the trail arrives at junction 11. Sidetrack onto the right-hand path for an alternate route to the peak; otherwise, stick with the blue trail to quickly reach the parking lot.

For those wanting more, steer right of the parking lot to take up the red-and-blue trail once again. This time, bear right at junction 21 to take the red trail up Wilson Mountain's western slope. Featuring jagged ledges, cliffs, and plenty of mammoth glacial erratics, this route is a dramatic counterpoint to the mellower blue trail. A massive mound of granite marks Wilson Mountain's highest point, and, though it offers very little in terms of a view, it makes a perfect throne for those who want to crown themselves "King of the Mountain." From this great rock, follow the red trail as it serpentines around the peak, rising and falling with hillocks and hollows to eventually arrive at junction 24, where it reunites with the red-and-blue trail. Bear left here and hike back downhill.

If you still balk at returning to your car, there is yet another diversion to consider. Where the red-and-blue trail filters toward the parking lot, a second trail veers right. Climbing a gentle incline, this route leads to a hidden meadow, passing a collapsed cabin with an intact chimney along the way.

Then follow the path of trodden grass southwest across the meadow back into woods. At the three-way junction you reach moments later, take the left-most trail, and follow a stream on its northeast course to a pond below. Look for basking turtles, frogs, or a blue heron, and then hike back to the parking lot.

## NEARBY ATTRACTIONS

To round out the day before or after hiking, you can catch a movie at the Dedham Community Theatre, established in 1927 and located in the town center (580 High St., Dedham; 781-326-0409; dedhamcommunitytheatre.com). Besides showing the best in cinema, the theater houses the Museum of Bad Art. Unlike most movie houses, the concession stand serves beer, wine, and hot chocolate, as well as soda, candy, and popcorn.

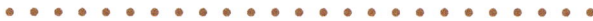

• • • • • • • • • • • • • • • • • • • • • • • • • • •

**GPS TRAILHEAD COORDINATES**  N42° 15.533' W71° 11.867'

**DIRECTIONS**  From Boston take I-90 W 9.4 miles to I-95 S via Exit 15. From I-95 S take Exit 17 to reach MA 135. Continue on MA 135 toward Dedham. The parking lot is 0.5 mile ahead on the right.

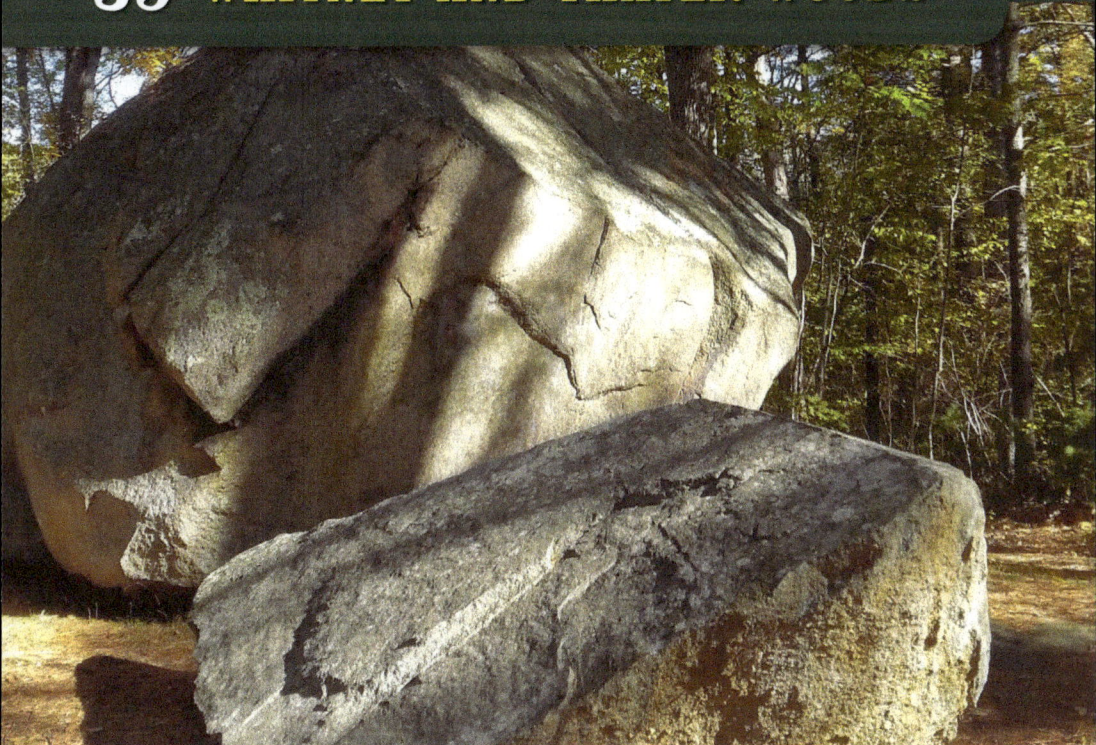

The entrance to Boulder Land is well guarded.

**HIKING THROUGH MILES** of groomed carriage roads and rugged footpaths through hemlock and holly groves, you'll see such spectacles as a magnificent woodland garden and spectacular granite gardens left by the glaciers.

## DESCRIPTION

Set out hiking southwest on Howes Road, the carriage path located at the head of the lot. Winding down a gentle grade, this road cuts a wide path through woods. After a few strides, the world outside fades as another replaces it—a place first settled by the Wampanoag Indians.

An unmarked trail or two diverts left and right, but stay with Howes Road until it reaches junction 2. Turn right to leave the manicured carriage road for a narrower, more rugged trail leading west over roots and granite rubble between two stone walls, one edging wetland, the other tracing a line across upland.

Ahead you'll see an enormous boulder that looks somewhat out of place. Bigelow Boulder is named for Reverend E. Victor Bigelow, the author of the first volume of *A Narrative History of Cohasset.* Bigelow Boulder sits at junction 3, where the footpath crosses Boulder Lane. To continue, pass to the left of the granite monolith, and stay on the narrow, rocky trail as it travels northwest back into the woods. Small

**DISTANCE & CONFIGURATION:** 6.25-mile loop

**DIFFICULTY:** Easy–moderate

**SCENERY:** Woods, ponds, vernal pools, enormous glacial erratics

**EXPOSURE:** Mostly shaded

**TRAFFIC:** Light–moderate

**TRAIL SURFACE:** Packed earth

**HIKING TIME:** 2.5–3 hours

**DRIVING DISTANCE FROM BOSTON COMMON:** 13 miles

**ELEVATION:** 82' at trailhead, no significant gain

**SEASON:** Year-round

**ACCESS:** Sunrise–sunset. Admission is free, but the Trustees welcome donations.

**MAPS:** Available at kiosk near trailhead or at tinyurl.com/whitneythayerwoodsmap

**WHEELCHAIR ACCESS:** Some of the wider carriage roads may be traversable by wheelchair, but the trails included in this hiking route are not.

**FACILITIES:** None

**CONTACT:** The Trustees of Reservations, thetrustees.org/places-to-visit, 617-542-7696

**LOCATION:** Cohasset, MA

**COMMENTS:** The Whitney and Thayer Woods property, combined with Trustees of Reservations–owned Turkey Hill and Weir River Farm, covers 824 acres. Wompatuck State Park, another neighbor of the Whitney and Thayer Woods, adds another 3,500 acres and 262 campsites (140 with electricity).

white squares mark the way. The trail leads downhill at first, winding through young beeches and pines. A couple of times, you'll cross one of the many stone walls, built when this was farmland. After crossing wetland via a sturdy 20- to 30-foot-long boardwalk, the trail bows south at a stream and rambles back uphill.

Emerging from the dense forest at junction 6, the trail continues across Boulder Lane. For the sake of variation, bear right and hike west on the carriage road.

Leading down to a swampy brook, the trail then winds its way back uphill to meet Whitney Road. For a shortened loop, hike left. Otherwise, continue northwest on this road packed hard by clopping hooves and colored orange by a veritable carpet of pine needles.

At junction 8, leave the predictable footing of the carriage road for the root, rock, and water hazards of the narrower trail through the dense woods to the right. Starting off with a steep but brief climb, the trail reaches a pinnacle then zigzags erratically on a northeastern course, mostly downhill, to a well sitting in a clearing.

At marker 12, the trail crosses Adelade Road, which stretches east toward Scituate Hill. Beyond this intersection the trail arcs west, shedding hardwoods and hollies for hemlocks as it touches the outer reaches of Great Swamp.

Arriving at the footpath's end at marker 13, hikers happy to be back on flat ground can continue right, on the wider flat trail of Turkey Hill Lane. But for a more adventurous trek, cross the carriage road and resume the footpath that leads back uphill into woods. Climbing the heap of glacial debris, the trail shimmies past a boulder crumbling like a last piece of layer cake sitting among crumbs to reach an overlook at junction 14. After surveying the view and maybe settling in for a picnic, continue west on the path to the right.

## Whitney and Thayer Woods

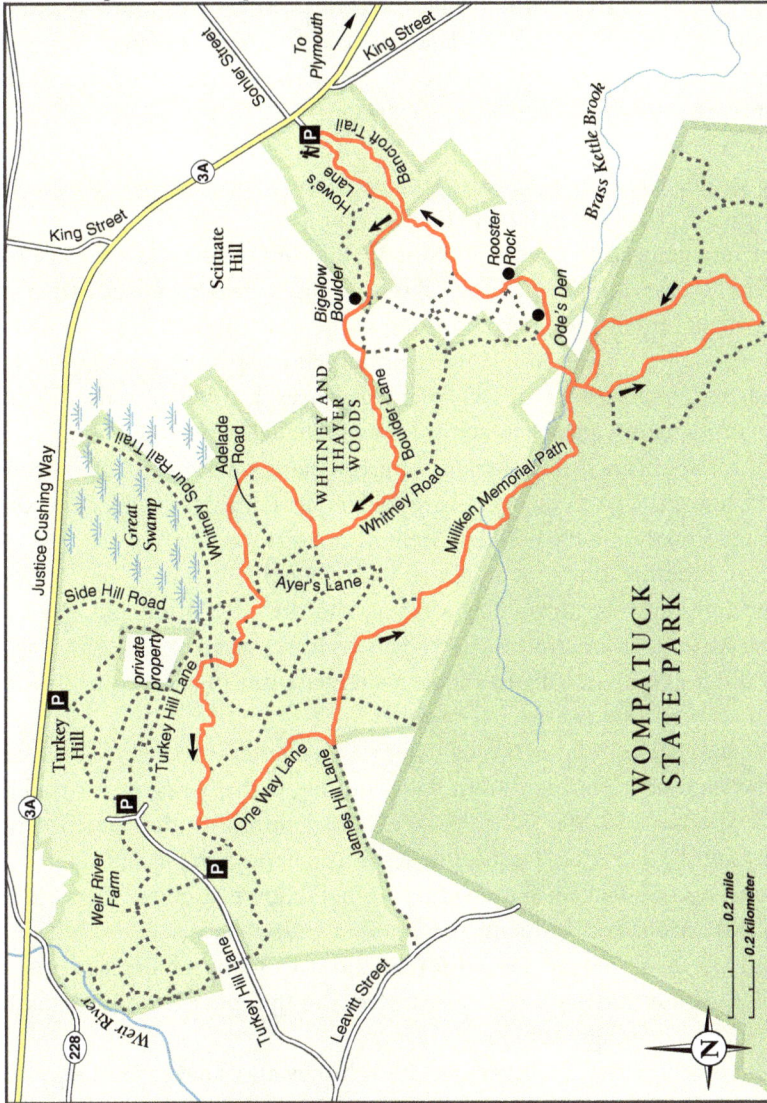

Map labels: To Plymouth, King Street, Sohier Street, Bancroft Trail, Howe's Lane, 3A, King Street, Scituate Hill, Bigelow Boulder, Rooster Rock, Ode's Den, Brass Kettle Brook, WHITNEY AND THAYER WOODS, Boulder Lane, Milliken Memorial Path, Justice Cushing Way, Great Swamp, Adelade Road, Whitney Spur Rail Trail, Whitney Road, Side Hill Road, Ayer's Lane, private property, Turkey Hill Lane, WOMPATUCK STATE PARK, Turkey Hill, 3A, Weir River Farm, One Way Lane, James Hill Lane, Turkey Hill Lane, Leavitt Street, Weir River, 228, 0.2 mile, 0.2 kilometer

Follow white markers as the trail slopes back down to level ground and bears right at a broad, vaguely marked junction. Around a bend, the trail crosses a glade walled in by a great wedge of rock greened by ferns and moss.

Twisting its way north, the trail soon crosses paths with an abandoned railroad track that has been converted into a hiking trail called the Whitney Spur Rail Trail. Stay on the narrower trail footpath as it bisects the former rail line.

205

Aiming west toward Turkey Hill, the trail continues to follow white markers. After winding through muddy lowland, the trail gradually steepens as it gains traction beneath red pines on the eastern slope of Turkey Hill. Ahead, where the plane levels and the trees thin out, the trail meets One Way Lane.

At junction 16, bear left and follow the wider smooth cart road southeast down a gentle grade. The gangly woods, made up of early successional species, hints that this hilltop offered an open vista in the last century.

Reaching James Hill Lane at junction 17, hike left to descend to a glacier-scoured valley cradling the defunct rail line. Follow the lane across the valley and up and over the lofty drumlin beyond. At junction 18, at the base of the hill, steer right to leave the carriage lanes for the Milliken Memorial Path, a path Arthur Milliken cleared and made magnificent with densely planted azaleas, rhododendrons, mountain laurels, and other showy shrubs to honor his wife, Mabel Minott Milliken.

You'll hike through this corridor of green, surrounded by dense shrubs, trees, and wildflowers. The path eventually widens as it bridges wetland and ascends to another funky-looking boulder. Behind it are more glacial erratics, clustered together in a picturesque spot equipped with a bench.

Traveling between Brass Kettle Brook and the edge of upland, the path soon arrives at its end, at junction 19. Here Howes Road, bearing left, offers a neat link back to the parking lot. To add a longer circular jaunt to and through Wompatuck State Park's nature study area, bear right.

Here the trail leads up a gravelly slope, past a marker that reads N7 to a map kiosk inside the state park's border. From this post, follow the hardscrabble trail to placid hemlock woods above. Stay left at marker N6 to continue south to junction N5. Here, the path to the right leads to Doane Street, the former property line of Whitney Woods.

Turn left and left again at each junction that follows, to complete the loop begun at the kiosk. Mounded and soft, the wooded landscape resembles a hastily made bed. Though disturbed by natural forces and axes many times, it is now remarkably quiet. About midway along this stretch, the trail passes the Burbank Boulder, another glacier-age vagrant biding its time.

Upon reaching the kiosk, reenter the Whitney and Thayer Reservation and follow Howes Road, taking a right at junction 19. Elevated to evade seasonal flooding, the carriage road crosses Brass Kettle Brook then, taking a northeast tack, meets Bancroft Trail at junction 20. To visit two more points of interest, switch tracks and bear right. A handful of twists and turns away, the path reaches a castlelike rock cave.

As the trail swings northwest on the edge of a valley, it passes a massive rock configuration painted with the letter *R* to identify it as Rooster Rock. Catch it at the right angle in the right light, and it is the spitting image of a rooster sporting a fancy comb.

A few yards farther, the trail reconvenes with Howes Road at junction 21. Bear right to proceed northeast. Arriving at an orange chain gateway just after junction 22, the route continues past a private home. Continue down the wider path to junction 2. Leave the carriage road once more, and hike the Bancroft Trail back to the parking lot.

When Henry M. Whitney owned much of these 824 acres in the first half of the 20th century, he reshaped the stagnating farmland into a grand estate. As president of the West End Street Railway, Whitney presided over the development of the Boston rail system, now known as the MBTA.

## NEARBY ATTRACTIONS

The 75-acre Weir River Farm, owned and managed by The Trustees of Reservations, boasts hayfields, managed woodlands, a stable and barn, and, best of all, friendly livestock. Access the farm via MA 228 in Hingham. From MA 228, turn right onto Levitt Street, continue 0.6 mile, and bear left onto Turkey Hill Lane. Follow it to the end.

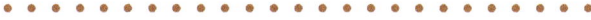

• • • • • • • • • • • • • • • • • • • • • • • • • • •

**GPS TRAILHEAD COORDINATES** N42° 14.067' W70° 49.450'

**DIRECTIONS** From Boston, take I-93 to MA 3 (Cape Cod). From MA 3, take Exit 14 to MA 228 north. Continue 6.5 miles through Hingham. Turn right onto MA 3A east and follow it 2 miles to the entrance and the parking lot on the right.

There are miles and miles of winding trails at Whitney and Thayer Woods.

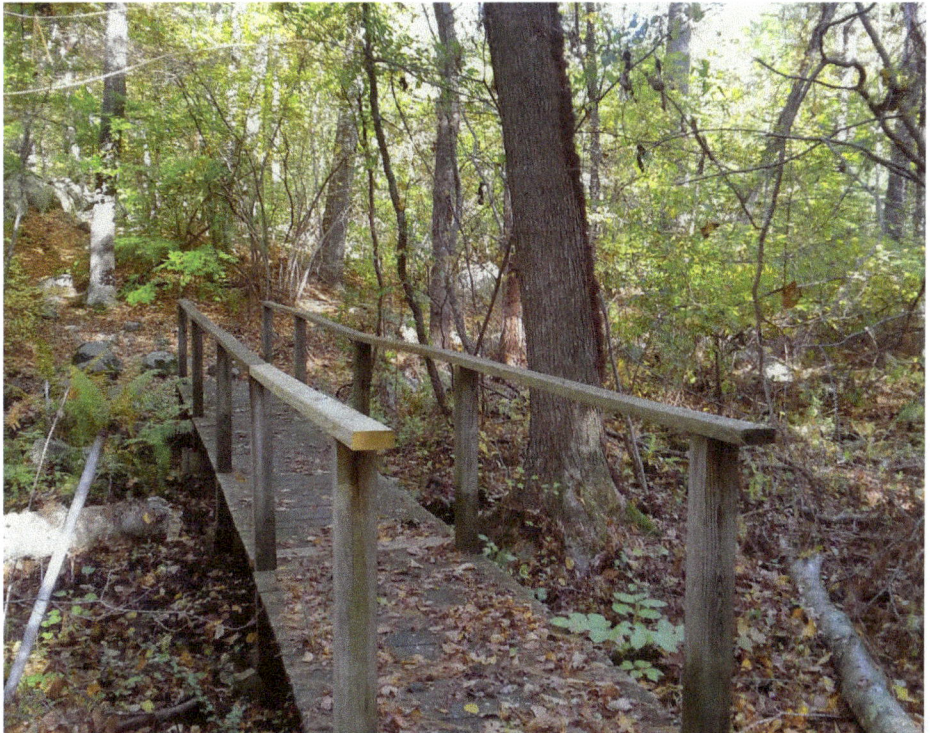

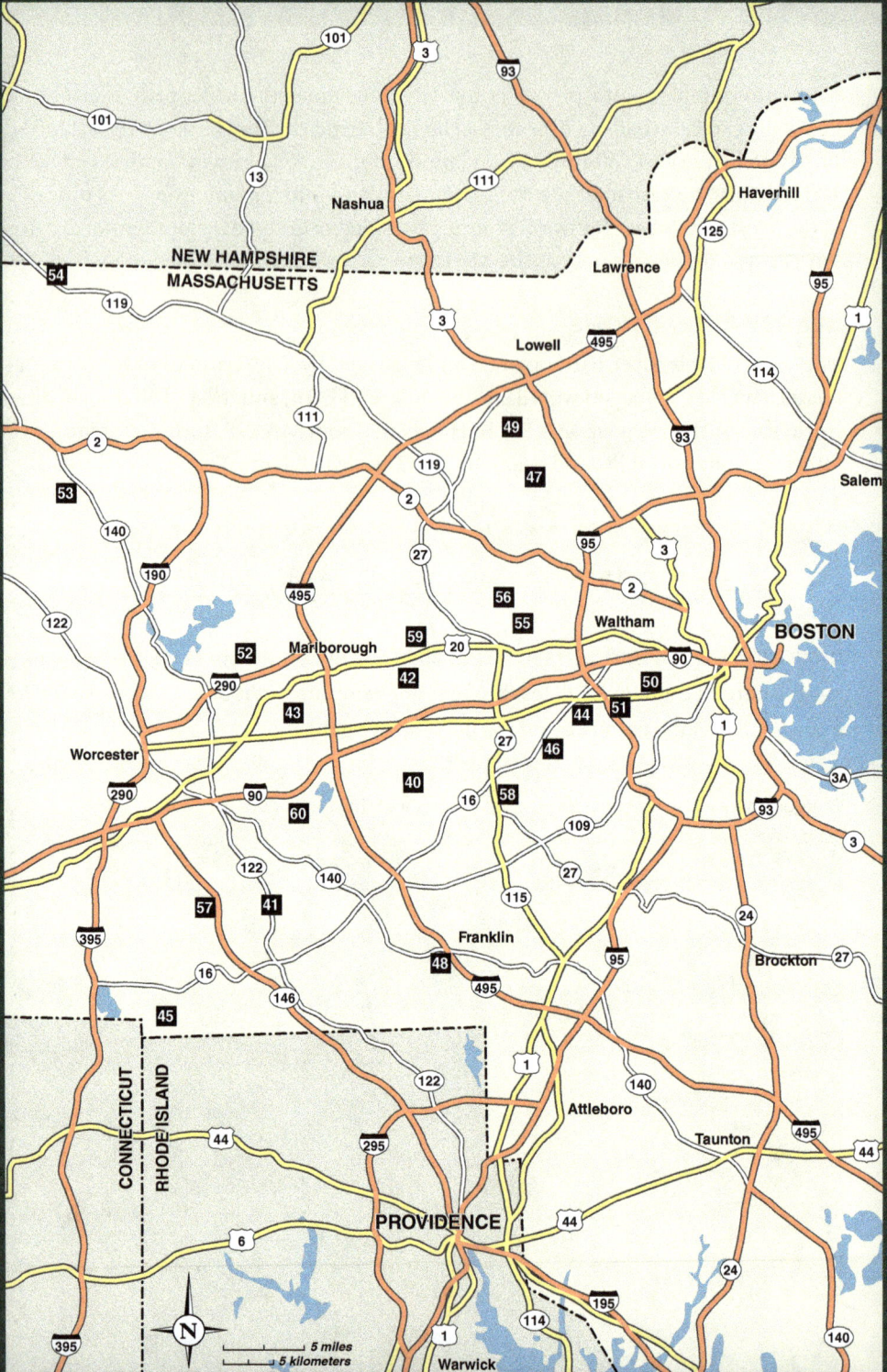

# WEST OF BOSTON

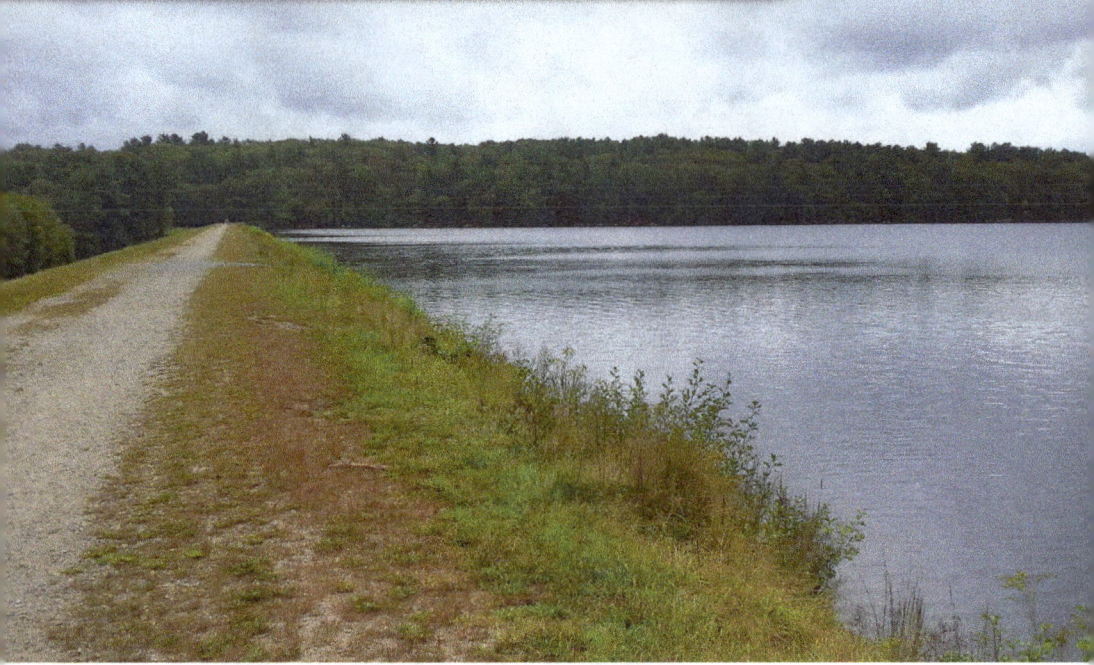

The straight shot down along the reservoir

**THIS TRAIL WINDS** around the 157-acre Ashland Reservoir, taking you on a rugged journey through the forest and rewarding you with spectacular views of the water.

## DESCRIPTION

Tucked away in the suburban town of Ashland, you'll find Ashland State Park located right off MA 135, down past the Ashland Community Center, playground, and soccer field. For a hike that feels wild and remote in spots, Ashland State Park is remarkably accessible. During the off-season, you'll need to park up here. During the summer, there is plenty of parking down near the beach and picnic area.

To start your circumnavigation of the Ashland Reservoir, head down toward the beach and picnic areas. Continue around to the left, past the restroom building, to find the yellow-blazed trail that will lead you around the reservoir—the 3.5-mile Ashland State Park trail. From the picnic area, the trail starts off wide, flat, and firm, like a dirt and gravel road. That will certainly change once you enter the forest past the dam.

Ashland State Park is a heavily used park, especially the beach and picnic area during the summer on a clear day. As such, the trail and all the facilities are well maintained. And you will most likely have a fair amount of company on the trail. Follow the early parts of the Ashland State Park trail through the picnic area. You

**DISTANCE & CONFIGURATION:** 3.5-mile loop

**DIFFICULTY:** Moderate

**SCENERY:** Views of Ashland Reservoir and a small island

**EXPOSURE:** Mostly shaded

**TRAFFIC:** Fairly light along the trail

**TRAIL SURFACE:** Rough, with rocks and roots; muddy in some spots

**HIKING TIME:** 1 hour, 45 minutes

**DRIVING DISTANCE FROM BOSTON COMMON:** 28 miles

**ELEVATION:** 261' at trailhead; considerable rise and fall along the trail, but no significant gain

**SEASON:** Year-round

**ACCESS:** Sunrise–sunset; free

**MAPS:** Available at the visitor center or at mass.gov/eea/docs/dcr/parks/trails/ashland.pdf

**WHEELCHAIR ACCESS:** No

**FACILITIES:** Restrooms, picnic tables

**CONTACT:** Massachusetts Dept. of Conservation and Resources, mass.gov/locations/ashland-state-park, 617-626-1250

**LOCATION:** Ashland, MA

can clearly see the water to the right through the trees. Follow the yellow blazes around to the right after passing the turnoff for the pavilion. There the trail descends slightly. Continue, bearing slightly right toward the water.

When you come out of the woods, you'll see a straight shot across the top of the Ashland Reservoir Dam. Follow this and enjoy the sweeping views of the reservoir. At the far end of the dam, you'll pass over a fascinating stone aqueduct and reenter the woods. Bear right to continue on the Ashland State Park loop trail.

As you reenter the forest here on the far side of the dam, the trail becomes much more narrow and rough. It's a true hiking trail surfaced with rocks and roots. There's not too much elevation gain, as you're essentially circling the reservoir, but it can be tough going in spots, so watch your footing. The trail is quite well defined and well marked. As mentioned before, it's also a fairly heavily used trail, so the course of the trail is clear. There are open views to the water to your right all the way around as you hike around the reservoir.

Don't get too caught up admiring the views of the water. You'll want to watch your step as you hop over roots and rocks as the trail twists and winds its way through the forest. In spots, the trail dives right down to the water's edge and becomes muddy and swampy. In one spot, perched right at the water's edge and shaded with loose-leafed deciduous trees, there's almost a Japanese Zen garden feel—very peaceful and relaxing. There are plenty of places like this along the trail to stop and ponder for a moment or just to take a break from the root- and rock-hopping this trail demands.

You'll eventually come to another, smaller beach on the far side of the reservoir, almost right across from the larger primary beach. After passing through this other beach, you'll see some houses through the loosely spaced forest on the left. Be respectful and stay on the trail. Toward the end of this residential border, you'll pass over a couple of funky footbridges. These bridges are cleverly crafted to work with the placement of the granite boulders. Shortly after this crossing, you'll come out

## Ashland State Park

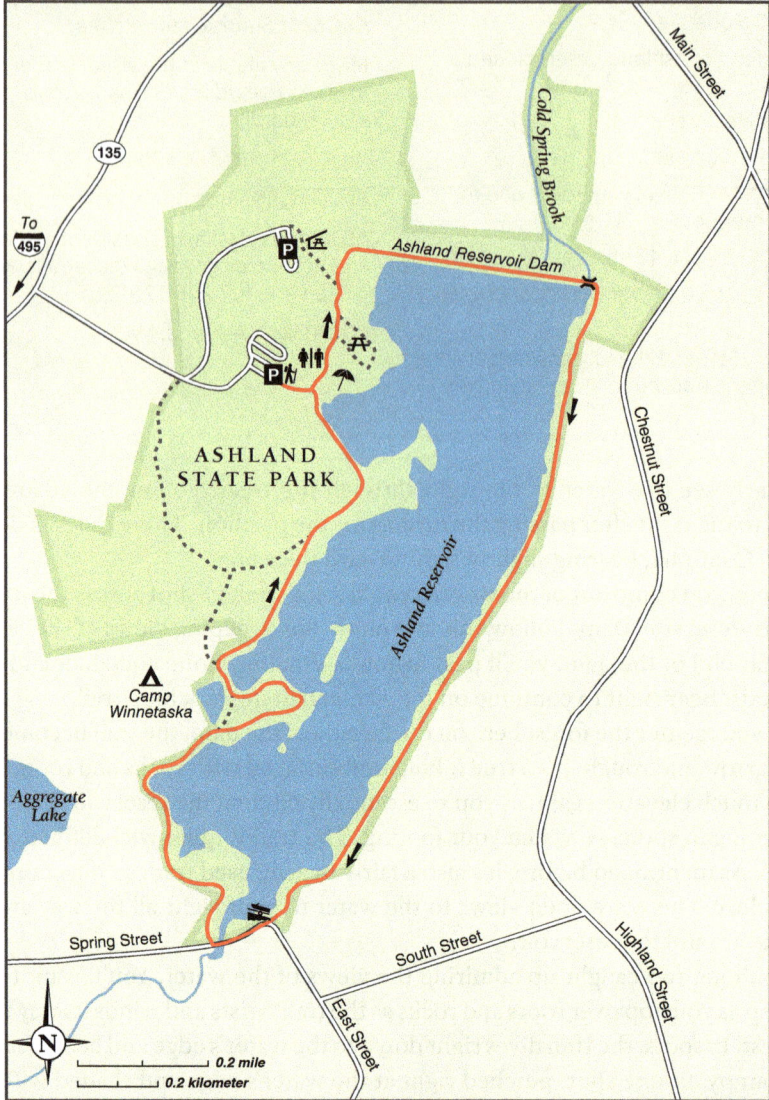

Ashland State Park

135

To 495

Cold Spring Brook

Main Street

Ashland Reservoir Dam

Chestnut Street

**ASHLAND
STATE PARK**

Ashland Reservoir

Camp
Winnetaska

Aggregate
Lake

Spring Street

South Street

East Street

Highland Street

N

0.2 mile
0.2 kilometer

into another parking area located at the far end of the reservoir. A lot of fishing boats launch from here. Cut straight across this smaller lot, and get back on the Ashland State Park trail.

The trail leads you through a loose grove of conifers, then out onto the road leading into the parking area you just traversed. After 50 feet or so on the road, you dive back into the woods with a dramatically steep climb up a side hill. Watch your step here if it has recently rained, as it could be quite slick. The water is still to your right as you continue around the reservoir.

The trail here is just as rocky and rooty as before, but it does take you up and over a series of small hills, especially right after you reenter the woods from that brief passage on the road. After a few ups and downs and twisting and winding, the trail settles down and flattens out briefly. You're still following the yellow blazes here, and the trail is still fairly well marked and well defined. Plus, you're following the contour of the reservoir, so there's little chance of taking a seriously wrong turn.

As the trail gets closer to the shoreline, the surface gets rougher, with more roots and rocks to traverse. Eventually, the trail takes you out and around a small peninsula. At the outer end, you pass over a soft bed of pine needles and can look out to the water and see a small island. Here it feels as if you're hiking along the coast of Maine. Continue looping around the peninsula and enjoying the pristine views. The trail continues, rising and falling through the forest and eventually coming out at the beach where you started.

## NEARBY ATTRACTIONS

Ashland is a fairly suburban spot, but if you need someplace to grab a bite after this energetic hike, check out Stone's Public House in downtown Ashland (508-881-1778, stonespublichouse.com). If it's a slow night and you suddenly feel something, it may be because the inn is apparently home to several restless spirits. Read the fascinating full story on their website.

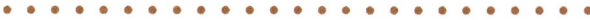

• • • • • • • • • • • • • • • • • • • • • • • • •

**GPS TRAILHEAD COORDINATES** N42° 14.661' W71° 28.074'

**DIRECTIONS** From Boston, take I-90 W to Exit 12 (Worcester Road/Boston Worcester Turnpike) in Framingham. Follow this east to Country Club Lane and turn right. Take a slight left onto Gates Street, then turn right onto Salem End Road. Turn left onto Badger Road. This turns into Myrtle Street, then Main Street. Turn right onto Summer Street, and then right again onto MA 135/W. Union Street. Ashland State Park is behind the Ashland Community Center.

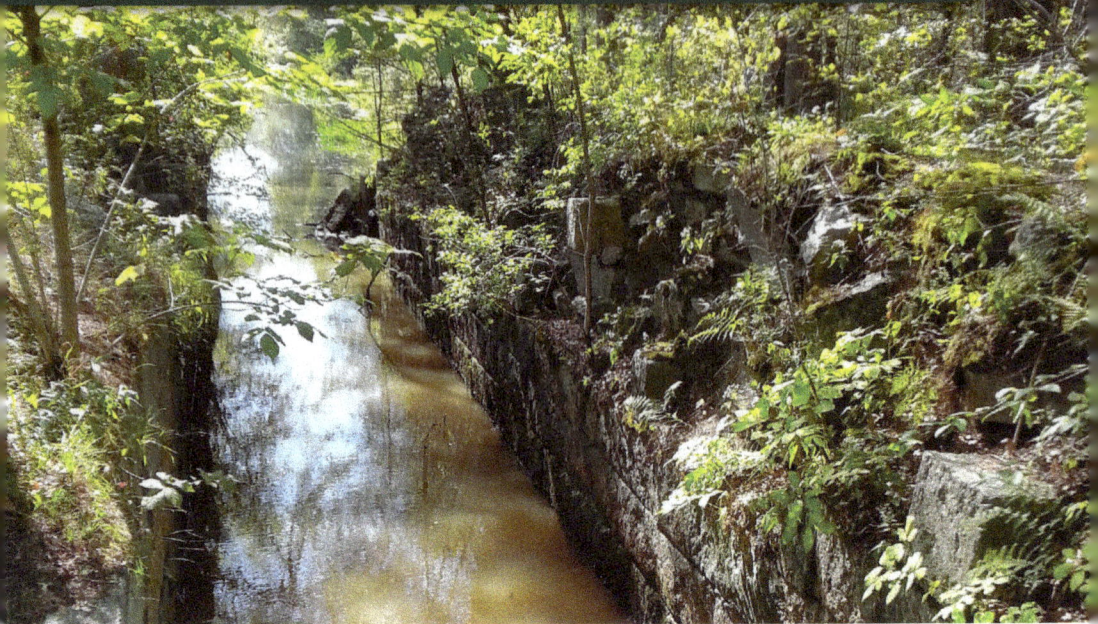

The Blackstone River hike takes you past the historic canal.

**ON THIS HIKE,** you will explore the Blackstone Canal, following it lock by lock through tangled woods, feral meadows, and preserved farmland to the site of the recently reclaimed Stanley Woolen Mill.

## DESCRIPTION

Like many hikes around Boston, the Blackstone Canal hike is rich with history. Late in the 1700s, John Brown, an industrious businessman of the family for whom Brown University is named, endeavored to build a canal along the Blackstone River. It was finally built 30 years later by General Edward Carrington. Then, in 1793, Samuel Slater established the first hydro-powered cotton mill in the United States along the canal.

The trail begins just beyond the parking lot to the left of the Blackstone Heritage Park sign. Follow the wide, firmly packed trail as it heads southeast along the canal. Trees have filled in between the canal and the Towline Trail. Seen through tangled branches, the slow-moving, sometimes stagnant canal waters are the color of strong tea. The rushing water you hear is the freer-flowing Blackstone River that parallels the canal's northern bank.

Though flooding or a fallen tree may temporarily alter the Canal Towpath, there's little risk of getting lost, as the trail parallels the canal. As you continue, the woods to the right give way to wetland. The trail surface is mostly firmly packed dirt.

**DISTANCE & CONFIGURATION:** 7.5-mile out-and-back

**DIFFICULTY:** Easy

**SCENERY:** Historic Blackstone Canal, with views of River Bend Farm and Stanley Woolen Mill

**EXPOSURE:** Mostly shaded

**TRAFFIC:** Light

**TRAIL SURFACE:** Packed dirt and grass

**HIKING TIME:** 3–3.5 hours

**DRIVING DISTANCE FROM BOSTON COMMON:** 49 miles

**ELEVATION:** 249' at trailhead, 463' at highest point

**SEASON:** Year-round

**ACCESS:** 8 a.m.–sunset; free

**MAPS:** Posted at the entrance, also available at visitor center at River Bend Farm or at mass.gov /eea/docs/dcr/parks/trails/blackstone.pdf

**WHEELCHAIR ACCESS:** A 0.6-mile portion of the trail from River Bend Farm to the Stanley Woolen Mill is wheelchair accessible. Then the trail simply becomes too rugged.

**FACILITIES:** Visitor center, restrooms, and picnic tables with grills at River Bend Farm

**CONTACT:** Massachusetts Dept. of Conservation and Resources, tinyurl.com/blackstoneriver, 617-626-1250

**LOCATION:** Uxbridge, MA

**COMMENTS:** Hiking is allowed in hunting season, except on Sundays. If you hike during hunting season, wear an orange reflective vest.

Here and farther along, the trail functions as a causeway, elevating you above water on either side. The waterway's ecosystem is a breeding ground for an array of insects, amphibians, and a wonderful variety of birds. Along with throngs of robins and catbirds, you may see a muscular kingfisher dash by. In June, dragonflies and damselflies dart about like winged jewels.

After running tight with the river for a stretch, the trail swings right to pass through a small meadow. A remnant of farming days, this shrinking patch of grassland now gives way to wildflowers and shrubs. Before rejoining the river, the trail crosses a tributary by way of a short, elevated boardwalk. Farther down, the trail turns east to cross a small dam. From here the causeway between the river and the canal becomes more pronounced as it straightens again on a southeasterly course.

The trail is quite well maintained. The trail surface varies from packed soil to gravel brought in to add reinforcement after washouts. Once past this section, where the Blackstone runs particularly fast and strong, the Canal Towpath splits from the river to follow the canal instead. You'll be shaded by a forest of mixed hickory, beech, and pine. Ferns, bamboo, and other wetland plant species conceal toads and baby snapping turtles at ground level.

Soon the trail bends left to meet the river's edge. Here you will notice big pieces of carved-out granite blocks. These are remnants of stone quarried to construct the canal's lock system. A few yards on, where the trail dead-ends upon reaching Rice City Pond, you encounter lock 25 at Goat Hill.

On the other side of the lock, the trail ascends to an intersection. Take the trail left and continue hiking along the bank of the river, gaining elevation as you go. Soon you arrive at an imposing granite boulder to the right of the path. Stopping to look,

# Blackstone River and Canal Heritage State Park

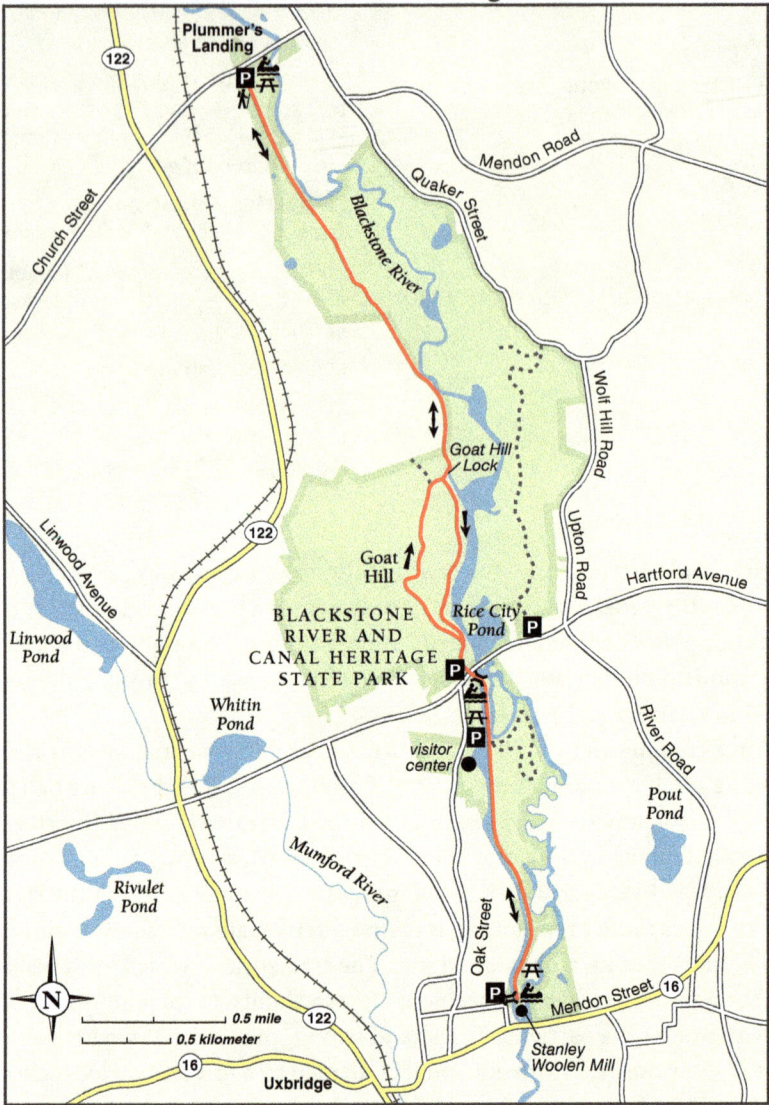

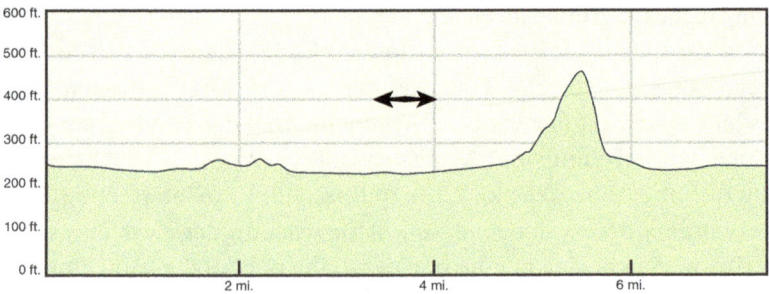

you will notice stonecutters' tools stuck in a long crack at eye level. Apparently the rock refused to break, and the wedges remain where they were driven.

Continuing southeast, the trail undulates along in a cleft between the Blackstone wetlands and Goat Hill under a spectacular canopy of beech, oak, hickory, and pine. Looking down the banking to the left, you will see what used to be a storage pond for the Taft Central Mill, which later became the Stanley Woolen Mill. Dammed after the Blackstone Canal Company shut down, the waters covered the towline until a hurricane came through in 1955.

Ahead, the Canal Towpath Trail meets another route coming down the hill to the right. On the left, a stone wall forms a clean 90-degree angle, enclosing a meadow of bygone days, now grown in. Just beyond here, the trail leaves the woods and crosses a field to arrive at Hartford Avenue. Across to the right is a visitor center. As you make your way over this quiet road, you can hear the water rushing through the remains of the mill owner's dam-control gate.

At the canoe landing on the eastern side of Hartford Avenue, pick up the Canal Towpath Trail again, and follow it as the river is diverted slightly northward. From here the towpath causeway is particularly pronounced as it approaches the bridge at River Bend Farm. Across the pond to the right sits an enormous red barn that once housed one of the largest dairy herds in the region.

Continuing south from River Bend Farm to the trail's end at the Stanley Woolen Mill, there is an unmistakable change in the canal. After the Blackstone Canal Company shut down, the owner of the Stanley Mill, Moses Taft, obtained water rights so that he might increase water flow to his machines. To accommodate the greater volume of water, the trench was deepened and its banks reinforced with rock.

After taking in the picturesque mill, you read the informational plaque posted at the trail's end. Return to the Canal Towpath Trail, and retrace the trail back to Goat Hill. To vary your return trip, you can split from the Canal Towpath Trail at Goat Hill and follow the trail northwest as it climbs left, away from the canal and up and over Goat Hill. Follow blue markers, continuing northwest to the top of the hill. Soon the trail turns due north and descends steeply, flush with a stone wall. Soon after reaching the stone wall's great end-stone, the trail arrives at a junction. Continue right and walk a short distance to find Goat Hill Lock. From here, follow the Canal Towpath Trail 1.7 miles back to Plummer's Landing.

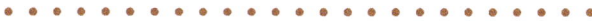

• • • • • • • • • • • • • • • • • • • • • • • • • •

**GPS TRAILHEAD COORDINATES** N42° 07.667'  W71° 38.333'

**DIRECTIONS**  From Boston, take I-90 W to Exit 11. Turn right (south) onto MA 122 toward Grafton. Drive 10.3 miles on MA 122 S to a light. Turn left onto Church Street. Continue 0.4 mile to the parking lot at Plummer's Landing.

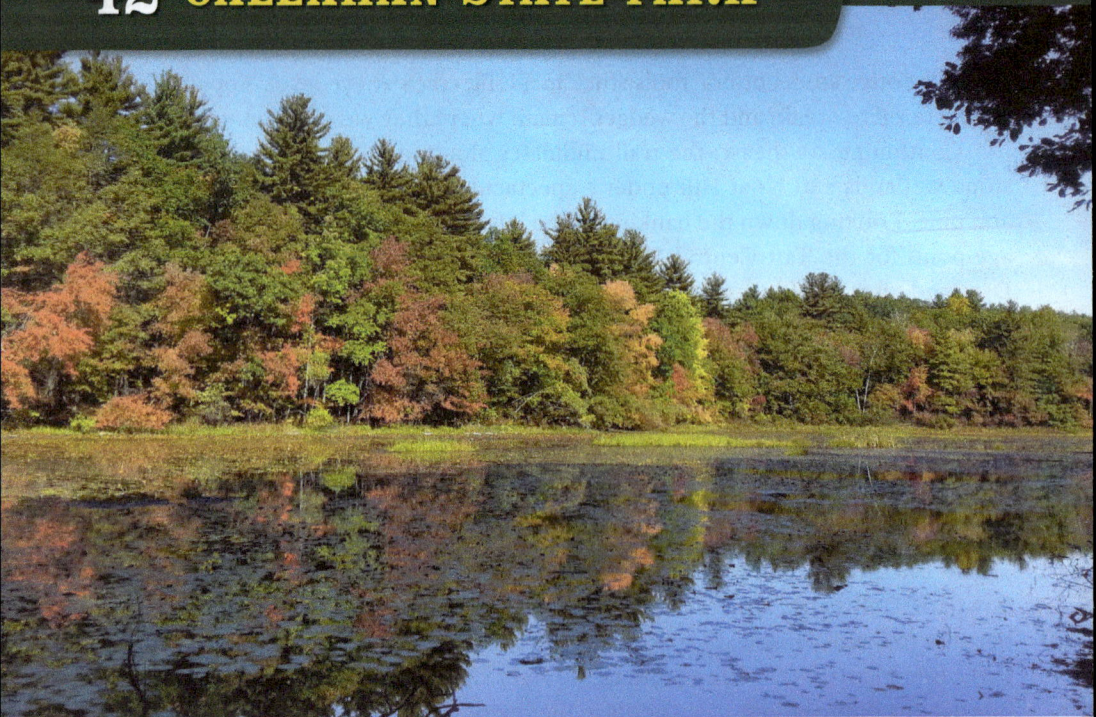

Callahan State Park is a varied mix of easily accessible wilderness.

**OF THE TWO** portions of this hike, the northern half is the more rugged and less popular. The southern side has woods, wetlands, and tracts of meadowland.

## DESCRIPTION

From the parking area at Stearns Farm off Edmands Road, you're right between the north and south sections of the park. Starting off toward the southern section first, locate the trailhead by hiking northeast to the Pipeline Trail, which travels directly south from Edmands Road along a centuries-old cart road. Follow this route past aged oaks and other hardwoods. The first junction comes beyond a footbridge. Here the trail comes to a T intersection. Bear left to continue south.

Cutting a wide swath through hemlocks, the trail rises on an even grade above a sunken floodplain to the east. Various paths divert left or right from this main trail, but you continue south to Packard Pond. At the three-way intersection ahead, bear left away from the hill. Crossing a brook via a small footbridge, the trail bears left at another split and passes a farmhouse. The trail gains definition upon reaching a great undulating meadow tamed by regular mowing.

Follow the trail as it scales the hillside next to woods to arrive at a four-way intersection just off the park's south entrance and parking lot. The dense forest gives way to

**DISTANCE & CONFIGURATION:** 7.37-mile double loop

**DIFFICULTY:** Easy–moderate

**SCENERY:** Woods, reforested farmland, working farm, kettle pond, earthen dam

**EXPOSURE:** Mostly shade

**TRAFFIC:** Moderate

**TRAIL SURFACE:** Packed dirt with some rocky areas and mud in wet seasons

**HIKING TIME:** 2.5–3 hours

**DRIVING DISTANCE FROM BOSTON COMMON:** 25 miles

**ELEVATION:** 285' at trailhead, 438' at highest point

**SEASON:** Year-round

**ACCESS:** Sunrise–sunset; free

**MAPS:** Available at trailheads or at mass.gov /eea/docs/dcr/parks/trails/callahan.pdf

**WHEELCHAIR ACCESS:** No

**FACILITIES:** None

**CONTACT:** Massachusetts Dept. of Conservation and Resources, mass.gov/locations/callahan -state-park, 617-626-1250

**LOCATION:** Framingham, MA

**COMMENTS:** The park is a favorite destination for mountain bikers, horseback riders, and cross-country skiers.

open field here, as you follow the Dam Trail along the edge of the open space. Bear right away from the earthen dam, and follow Moore Road downhill into a verdant basin.

Dipping to its lowest point, this gravel road meets Baiting Brook then cuts a straight line past Eagle Pond and open meadow to reenter the forest. Immediately after a boardwalk across a muddy zone, the trail splits at a V. Bear right and hike north beneath tree cover along the edge of the adjacent meadow on the Juniper Trail. This trail also takes you up and over a small hill. If you went left at that intersection, you'd be on the Deer Run Trail, marked with blue and red blazes that indicate that both hikers and equestrians are welcome.

Traveling over level ground, the Deer Run Trail passes through reforested farmland. Now and again a strand of stone wall materializes amid the maze of standing and fallen trunks.

Shortly after encountering the Fox Hunt Trail running east to west, the Deer Run Trail briefly departs state-owned land and crosses another parcel owned by the Sudbury Valley Trustees. The trail is occasionally rerouted, so pay attention to trail markings and be mindful of trail erosion.

Both the Deer Run Trail and the Juniper Trail eventually rejoin the Rocky Road, a path that appears to split left and right. To shorten the hike by half, hike to the right on the true Rocky Road Trail, which travels 0.3 mile back to Stearns Farm. Otherwise, stay left, heading northwest on what becomes the Red Tail Trail.

Traveling across a drumlin's gritty slope, the Red Tail Trail descends, swings west on a hairpin turn, then converges with the Bay Circuit Trail, which enters from the east. Continuing straight, the Red Tail Trail passes private property on upland to the west as it crosses level ground to reach a gate at Edmands Road.

From this understated entrance, equipped with little more than a sign asserting the park's rules and regulations, stride across the two lanes of pavement to a scenic,

# Callahan State Park

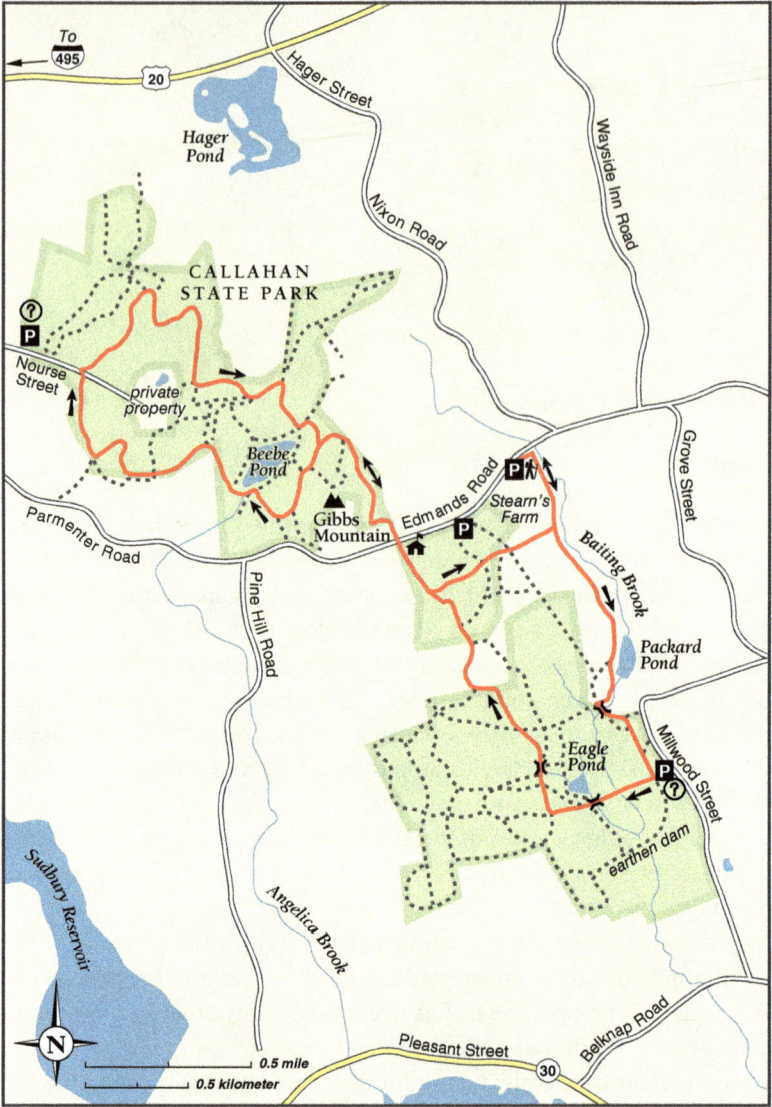

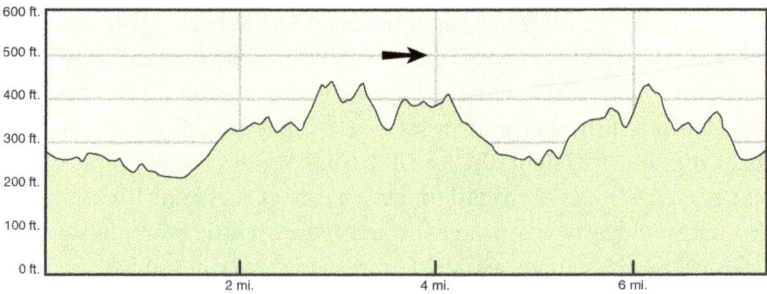

To 495

20

Hager Street

Hager Pond

Nixon Road

Wayside Inn Road

CALLAHAN STATE PARK

Nourse Street

private property

Beebe Pond

Parmenter Road

Gibbs Mountain

Edmands Road

Stearn's Farm

Grove Street

Baiting Brook

Packard Pond

Pine Hill Road

Eagle Pond

Millwood Street

earthen dam

Sudbury Reservoir

Angelica Brook

N

0.5 mile

0.5 kilometer

Pleasant Street

30

Belknap Road

600 ft.
500 ft.
400 ft.
300 ft.
200 ft.
100 ft.
0 ft.

2 mi.

4 mi.

6 mi.

weed-filled field. Look for the white blazes of the Bay Circuit Trail and a small sign bearing the silhouette of a backpacker. Follow this lightly etched trail as it ascends and curves west to the foot of Gibbs Mountain. The trail here is narrow and slightly strewn with roots and rocks.

A state park sign marks the start of Backpacker Trail and reassures you you're on the right track. Taking the mountain straight on, the trail ascends steeply at first and then eases as it winds northeast on a horizontal plane, allowing hikers to take in the setting and its natural history.

Making its way downhill, the trail passes first a path to the left and then one to the right. Take note of these, but stay on course with the Bay Circuit Trail, At the second junction, the trail bears left to round the mountain's northern face. At the next intersection, which is not all that well-marked, the Bay Circuit Trail bears right to descend farther off the mountain. The seemingly more pronounced trail continues straight. Choose either route—they meet again farther on. To continue the hike as mapped, leave Bay Circuit Trail temporarily, and bear left to travel south.

Just beyond a path cascading down a slope to the left, the trail arrives at a field. Climb along the narrow, lightly trod route as it circumnavigates this grassland, first climbing to its high point and then easing off to its western wooded border.

When the path loops back north, meeting the Bay Circuit Trail at a T, bear left to continue west. At the foot of a gravel embankment, the trail meets Beebe Pond. This is a picturesque glacial kettle hole pond neatly hidden among the dense maple forest. Cross a causeway lined with hemlocks to reach a junction on the northwest side of the pond. Here both the Bay Circuit Trail's white blazes and the park's blue markers lead uphill to the left.

Leveling off in a pine stand above the pond, the trail splits through one stone wall and then tracks another out of the woods to a meadow. Hike left and travel west along the meadow's fringe. When the sunny grassland meets woods once more, follow along as the trail leads down a gentle grade and corrects its course at a hairpin turn.

Spilling into a stone-wall avenue, the trail soon meets the stark path of a power line. The route then exits north through another stone wall at the next immediate right. Until this junction, Bear Paw Trail (blue) and the Bay Circuit Trail travel as one, but here they part ways. Follow the path heading north, marked with a blue bear claw.

Easing down a slope riddled with stones and roots, the trail soon ends at an unpaved service road. Continue across on a diagonal aiming west to pick up Acorn Trail.

Turning uphill to skirt the swamp, the Acorn Trail rejoins the Backpacker Trail. Bear right at this precarious junction, and retreat downhill and across a stream. After some loopy turns, the trail straightens and travels south beside a stone wall. Tacking east, Backpacker Trail then passes through a lumber tract. Encountering an old north–south cart road on this hill of packed sand and gravel, the trail accompanies it south briefly then departs east. After gently rising and falling over the landscape, the trail brings you to another junction at the base of Gibbs Mountain.

Having completed this significant loop, hike left and you will backtrack over Gibbs Mountain and Edmands Road to the park's south side. Cross the road again, then follow the Red Tail Trail to the first junction, and bear left onto Wren Trail (which serves as a section of the Bay Circuit Trail).

Two more junctions break the rhythm, but stay on course with the Bay Circuit Trail to head east. At the second junction, where the route is splintered by the Pipeline Trail, hike uphill several feet to find the way marked by a white triangle. The last stretch is sketchy but short. At the final junction, bear left and follow white blazes back to the parking area on Edmands Road.

## NEARBY ATTRACTIONS

Along MA 9 in Framingham, you have myriad dining options, from fancy to casual and everything in between.

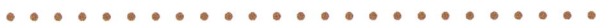

• • • • • • • • • • • • • • • • • • • • • • • • • •

**GPS TRAILHEAD COORDINATES** N42° 20.033'  W71° 28.333'

**DIRECTIONS** From Boston, take I-90 W 11.9 miles, then merge onto Worcester Road via Exit 12 toward Marlborough. After 1.7 miles bear left onto the Pleasant Street Connector, which becomes Firmin Avenue. Continue 0.1 mile, then turn right onto MA 30. At 0.7 mile turn left onto Pinehill Road. Turn right onto Parmenter Road, which shortly becomes Edmands Road. Continue 0.1 mile and turn right to stay on Edmands Road. Parking is on the right.

Dramatic foliage on display atop Cedar Hill.

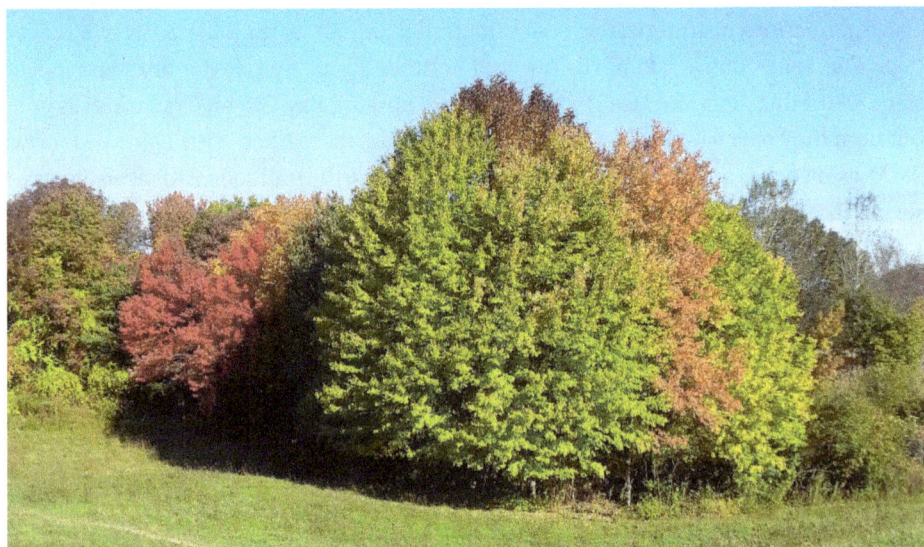

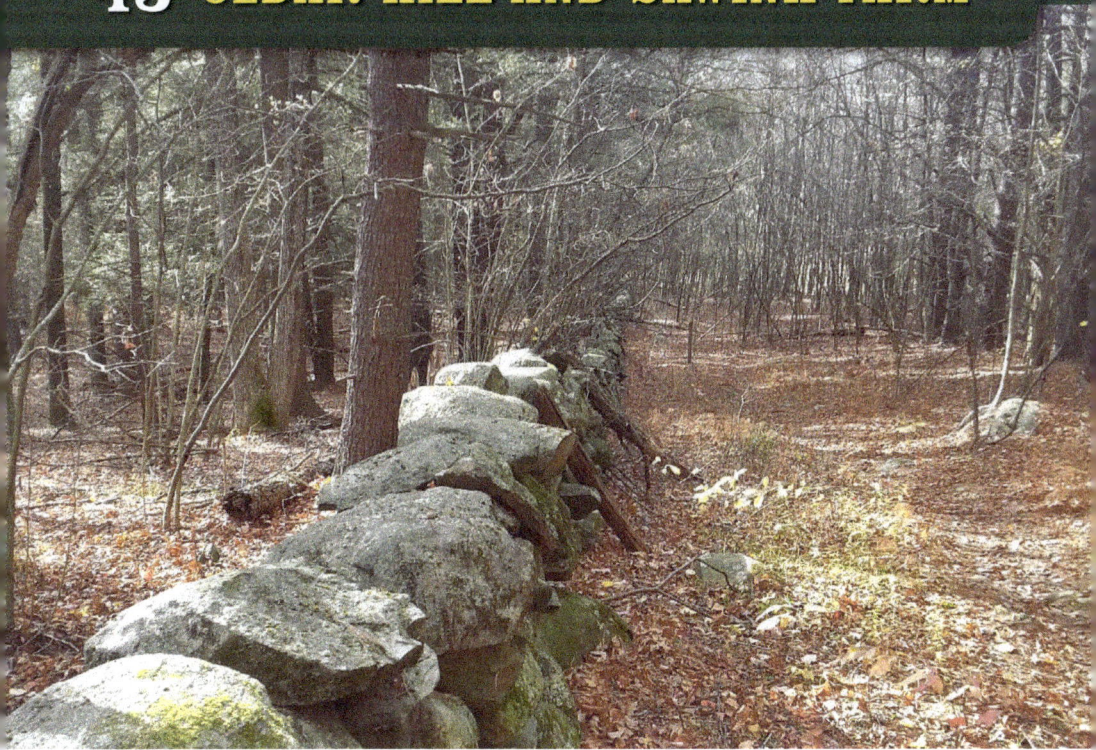

The Cedar Hill and Sawink Farm hike traverses a varied landscape.

**THIS HIKE TRAVELS** within the borders of three towns—Northborough, Marlborough, and Westborough—crossing abandoned farms, several drumlins, numerous streams, diverse forests, and magnificent swamplands rich with wildlife.

## DESCRIPTION

From the parking area, walk toward Lyman Street to find the Little Chauncy Trail trailhead on the left. Crossing through an abandoned farm, the flat, grassy path skirts a convex meadow on the last high ground above Little Chauncy Pond.

Volunteer members of Northborough and Westborough trails organizations installed a boardwalk here to provide passage for hikers and mountain bikers. The marshy field has been usurped by milkweed, goldenrod, Queen Anne's lace, burdock, and thistle. The wildflowers feed a great diversity of vibrant birds, such as goldfinches and bobolinks.

Three quarters of the way along the pond, the trail climbs from the meadow into pinewoods. Follow the plentiful trail markers as they weave through enormous creaking trees, jackknife around a boulder, and head east. In spots, the abundance of markers causes confusion. For clarity, keep your sights on the triangular red tags

**DISTANCE & CONFIGURATION:** 8-mile out-and-back with 2 loops

**DIFFICULTY:** Easy–moderate

**SCENERY:** The reserve's nearly 2,000 acres include abandoned farmland, deciduous woodland, and a drumlin next to a magnificent swamp. As many as 38 species of birds, including ruffed grouse, willow flycatcher, and a variety of warblers, nest within this reservation.

**EXPOSURE:** Mostly shaded

**TRAFFIC:** Light

**TRAIL SURFACE:** Packed dirt, grasslands, boardwalks through wetland

**HIKING TIME:** 3 hours

**DRIVING DISTANCE FROM BOSTON COMMON:** 35 miles

**ELEVATION:** 278' at trailhead, 430' at highest point

**SEASON:** Year-round

**ACCESS:** Sunrise–sunset; free

**MAPS:** Available at trailhead, at the Northborough town hall, and at tinyurl.com/cedarsawinkmap

**WHEELCHAIR ACCESS:** No

**FACILITIES:** None

**CONTACT:** Sudbury Valley Trustees, tinyurl.com /sudburyvalleytrustees, 978-443-5588

**LOCATION:** Northborough, MA

initialed *N* for Northborough, and continue east, staying left at a junction at the crown of the wood. Easing downhill, the trail leads southeast 200 yards or so past an aspen grove to Lyman Street.

Emerging into a thicket of maples rooted in a seasonal floodplain, the trail crosses a field over a low-slung boardwalk. In the heat of a late summer day, the altitude at waist level is dense with zooming dragonflies.

Leaving the field, the trail (now called Talbot Trail) ascends into woods. The trail here is a more traditional hiking trail—a narrow winding trail over hard-packed dirt, punctuated with some roots and rocks. The surrounding forest is composed of white pine, oak, and a good number of birches. The trail shortly comes to a two-way junction. Bear right to continue on Talbot Trail, and when the trail splits again a short distance on, bear left. Skirting the peak of the hill, the trail cuts a narrow route through pasture consumed primarily by Norway maples.

As Talbot Trail continues across the slope, it passes a steep trail shooting straight to a water tower on the hilltop. Changing its trajectory, the trail then bends to meet Cole Trail, which ascends from the west. At this junction, bear right to stay with Talbot Trail, now aimed toward a hemlock-shaded brook at the base of the drumlin called Cedar Hill. Once across the sturdy bridge built by local Eagle Scouts, follow the trail up a sandy pitch to a three-way split. Here the Plantation Trail and Chestnut Trail bow off to the right. The Cedar Hill Trail branches left. Choose the latter, and hike north onto land protected by the Sudbury Valley Trustees (SVT).

The scruffy hillside is jumbled with weeds, unpruned fruit trees, and assorted shrubs. The pastoral setting is punctuated with several huge pine and cedar trees. Stay alert and you might see golden-winged warblers, eastern meadowlarks, brown thrashers, or American kestrels. Coyotes and red fox also prowl the hillside's thickets.

From the summit of Cedar Hill, follow the mowed path north among the goldenrod, traveling downhill to reenter the woods. Pine and cedar trees frame the way,

# Cedar Hill and Sawink Farm

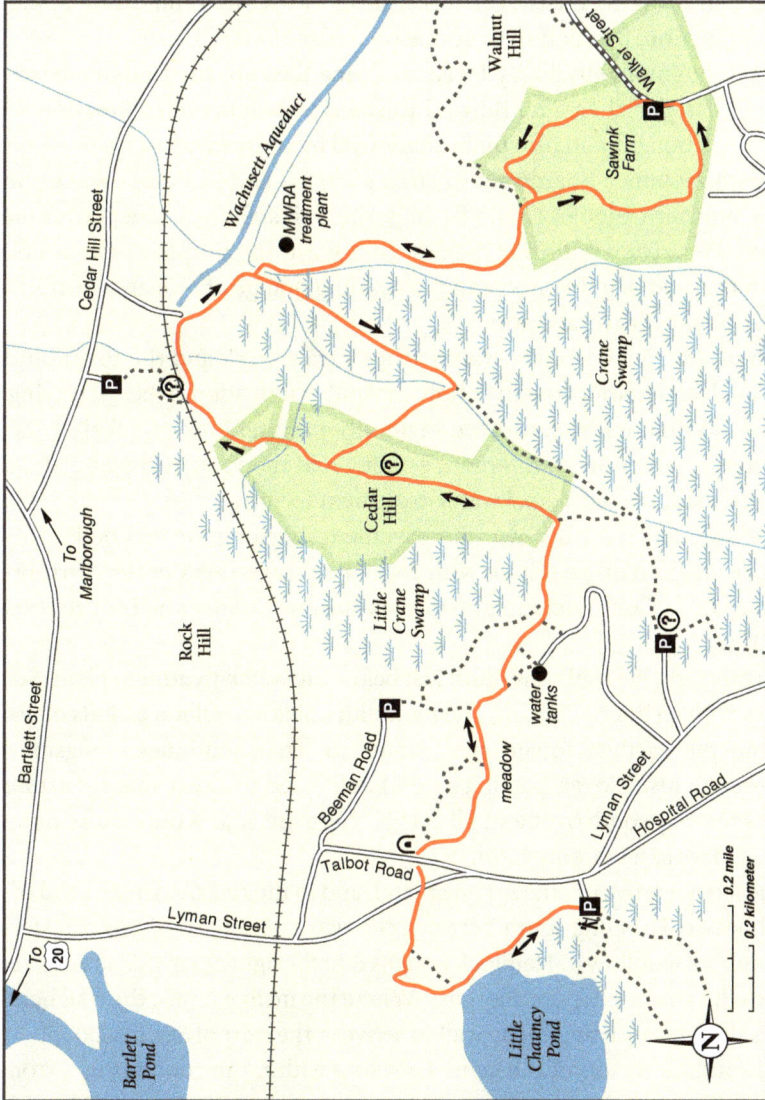

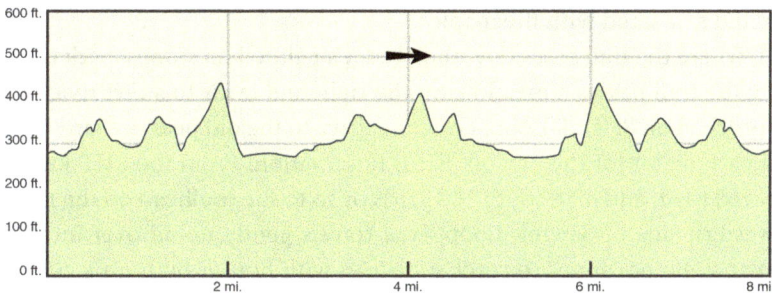

Walnut Hill

Walker Street

Sawink Farm

*Wachusett Aqueduct*

MWRA treatment plant

Crane Swamp

Cedar Hill Street

To Marlborough

Bartlett Street

Rock Hill

Cedar Hill

Little Crane Swamp

Beeman Road

meadow

water tanks

Lyman Street

Hospital Road

Talbot Road

Lyman Street

To 20

Bartlett Pond

Little Chauncy Pond

0.2 mile
0.2 kilometer

and as the trail turns northeast, the forest fills in with birch, pine, and apple trees. Ahead, at a junction, bear left to continue on Cedar Hill Trail.

As the topography gradually levels to Crane Swamp, the trail bends around a massive and flat glacial erratic. Beyond this, a sign points right, directing the trail under hemlock boughs and into pines shadowed by sugar maples.

The path mounts a boardwalk to cross a stream and its overflow. Leaving this part of the northern edge of Crane Swamp, the trail spills into a generous meadow sowed with 25 native wildflower species. In August, the purple of the asters juxtaposed with the gold of goldenrod and the dazzling orange of monarch butterflies is a spectacular blend of natural colors.

North of this rich oasis, the trail reaches a train track and the town borders of Northborough and Marlborough. Follow the trail as it bends northeast, staying south of the track. Within a few yards, the idyllically pastoral look and feel of the place is supplanted by an entirely different aesthetic and mood. Directly ahead, across a paved utility road, is a municipal water-treatment facility.

Crane Swamp Trail runs over the pavement, hugging the wooded edge of the wetland to a junction marked both with an SVT sign and the *N* of the Northborough Trail Association. Continue straight to pick up the Connector Trail that leads to Sawink Farm.

From this fork, the trail runs south just below the water-treatment plant. Solid like a mountain with an internal spring, the monolith holds 3.6 million gallons of water.

Beyond the earthen tower, the Connector Trail continues alongside Crane Swamp through lush clover, passing a pond bulldozed to a tear shape. Farther on, a sign points the way south over a small bridge. Here the land is once more untouched since its last days as a working farm.

To the left is a grove of pine set on upland, and to the right, a dense wood of young birch and beech. Traveling south between the two, the trail soon meets a stone wall and bends uphill to follow it. Hemlock boughs dim the light along this stretch, scenting the air with the essence of pure antiquity. Where the incline levels, the trail bears right and passes through a parting in the wall to arrive at the start of Sawink Loop.

Head south here, left of the sign. Traveling within the confines of a stone-wall grid, the trail jogs northeast between epic sugar maples. Giant pines that somehow escaped ax and saw stand with the maples.

Ahead, where the trail eases downhill, red X's painted on stones mark the way.

Shortly the trail passes a meadow on the right and leads to a dirt road straight ahead. To proceed on Sawink Loop, cross the drive to the old pear orchard that now serves as a parking lot for the Sawink Farm Reservation. From the SVT kiosk, exit onto the paved road, and hike south 100 yards or so to the trailhead on the right.

The western side of Sawink Loop Trail travels gently uphill over interwoven roots and flat stepping-stones to reach a plateau with houses built on a cul-de-sac.

From here it turns north and descends steeply to hemlock-sheltered wetlands. After navigating the wetland rather erratically through a convergence of stone walls, the trail climbs back onto dry ground. Passing sisters of the sugar maples seen earlier, the trail soon returns to the start of Sawink Loop.

From this spot, follow the Connector Trail to its end at the water-treatment plant. At the trail junction, turn left to pick up Crane Swamp Trail heading south. Forming a straight causeway across the dense swamp, the trail leads back to the eastern side of Cedar Hill. Where the hillside meets the swamp, divert onto Plantation Trail heading northwest. After crossing a small bridge, the narrow path makes a crooked run up the side of the hill to rejoin a section of Cedar Hill Trail, hiked earlier. Bear left at this fork and retrace your footsteps back to the parking lot on Lyman Street.

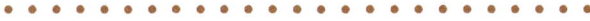

• • • • • • • • • • • • • • • • • • • • • • • • •

**GPS TRAILHEAD COORDINATES** N42° 18.309'  W71° 36.668'

**DIRECTIONS**  From Boston, take I-90 W (parts of which are toll roads). Drive 27.5 miles, then merge onto I-495 north via Exit 11A toward Marlborough. Continue 2.7 miles before merging onto MA 9 west via Exit 23B toward Worcester. After 2.5 miles turn right onto Lyman Street. The parking area is on the left. There are other parking areas and trailheads for this trail network near the end of Walker Street in Westborough, at the end of Beeman Road in Northborough, and on Cedar Hill Street in Northborough.

The trail up and over Cedar Hill is the most dramatically scenic.

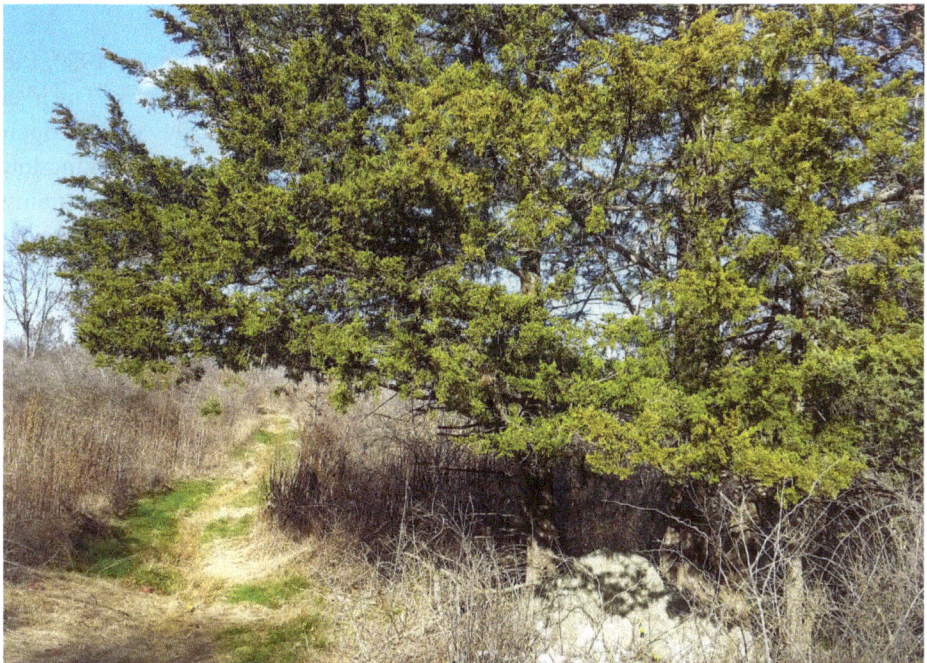

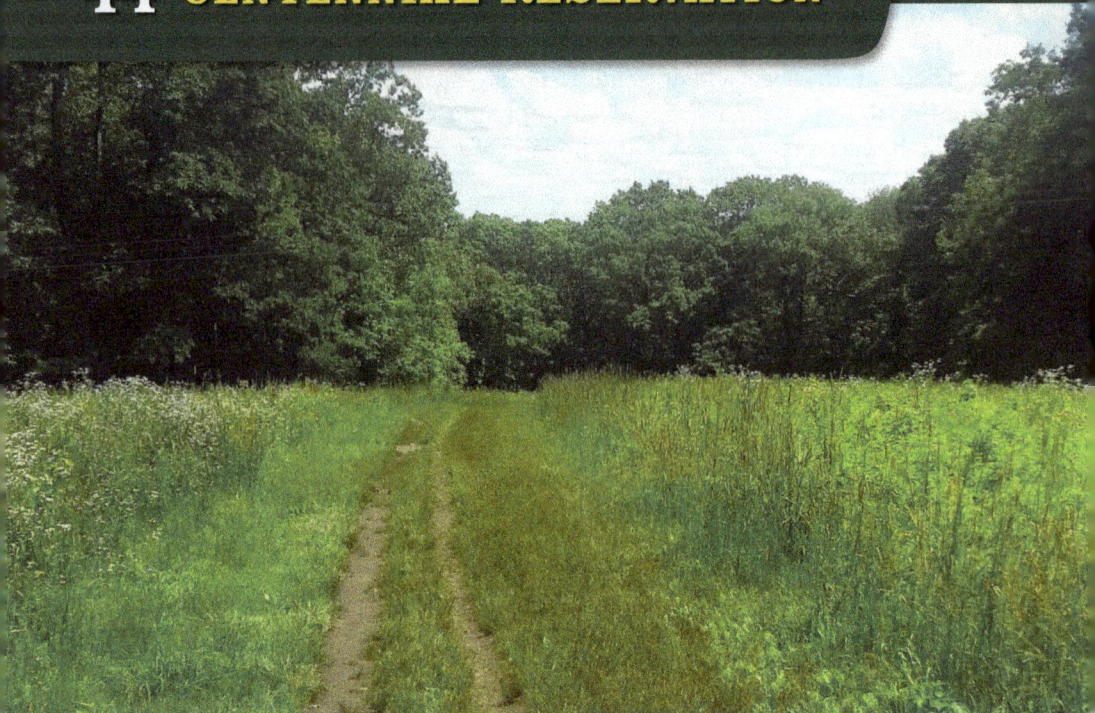

Centennial Reservation is a quick and easy walk through the woods.

**JUST ONE OF** the many hikes possible on Wellesley's extensive trail system, Centennial Reservation is a place where the entire family can enjoy the pristine forest, kettle pond, and rolling meadows.

## DESCRIPTION

In an inspired look to the future, on town-meeting day in the spring of 1980, the citizens of Wellesley voted to purchase the 42 acres that make up this park. The idea was to celebrate the township's first 100 years by preserving this lovely tract of open space for future generations. The trailhead is scarcely a foot from the parking lot, behind a notice board greeting visitors with maps, news, and a calendar of upcoming events. This is truly a wilderness gem amid the dense band of suburban neighborhoods surrounding the Boston area.

Head west on the sprawling trail marked with purple. Within several yards, a sign points both left and straight to two ends of the same trail. Continue west down an incline surfaced with wood chips to a small kettle pond. Stay on this path as it curves left, rimming the water. On the far side of the pond, the trail, now reduced to a thin track, climbs up the face of a cascading meadow and then shoots into woods.

Proceeding uphill gently through a dark tunnel of trees, the path quickly emerges at the bottom of another, larger, steeper expanse of grass and wildflowers.

**DISTANCE & CONFIGURATION:** 1.58-mile loop

**DIFFICULTY:** Easy

**SCENERY:** Views from Maugus Hill and woods surrounding acres of wildflower-rich meadowland maintained to provide sanctuary for breeding songbirds and other wildlife

**EXPOSURE:** Mixed sun and shade

**TRAFFIC:** Moderate

**TRAIL SURFACE:** Packed dirt, gravel, wood chips

**HIKING TIME:** 1 hour

**DRIVING DISTANCE FROM BOSTON COMMON:** 14 miles

**ELEVATION:** 163' at trailhead, 317' at highest point

**SEASON:** Year-round

**ACCESS:** Sunrise–sunset; free

**MAPS:** Available at kiosk by parking lot and at wellesleyma.gov/documentcenter/view/6903

**WHEELCHAIR ACCESS:** No

**FACILITIES:** None

**CONTACT:** Wellesley Natural Resources Commission, wellesleyma.gov/documentcenter/view/6904; 781-431-1019, ext. 2294

**LOCATION:** Wellesley, MA

**COMMENTS:** Landscaped by glacial action and generations of farming, the reservation includes the drumlin called Maugus Hill, an esker, and a scenic kettle pond.

Tall blossoms of black-eyed Susan (*Rudbeckia hirta*), Canada goldenrod (*Solidago canadensis*), Queen Anne's lace (*Daucus carota*), and lady's thumb (*Persicaria persiacria*) sway in the breeze above cow vetch (*Vicia cracca*) and purple clover. Poison ivy also shows its three-leaved fronds among the grass.

Once at the top of this rise on Maugus Hill, you will find a bench facing southeast, inviting you to sit for a spell and take in the sweeping pastoral view miraculously free of blight. This is a great spot to rest, enjoy the view, take some pictures, or have a bite of lunch in the middle of your hike. From the bench, continue right, following the purple blazes. A rich, diverse forest of sassafras, maple, pine, and oak quickly envelops the trail as it slopes around the back of the hill.

Entering a grove of beech where the trunks of the trees glint with a metallic shine, the trail levels off. There's a quiet neighborhood close by to the right, the houses slightly concealed by a tangle of leafy twigs and branches. A path from this neighborhood feeds into the purple-marked trail. The proximity to these houses, and even the sight of this neighborhood, does little to disturb the deep woodland feel of Centennial Reservation.

Bearing west now, the trail rises again from the edge of wetland back toward the top of the meadow, passing a trail to the grassy peak of Maugus Hill to the right. Continue left, hiking southeast on the purple trail. Ahead, where the route splits, veer right, easing downhill again over a smooth expanse of packed dirt.

Arriving at a broad intersection, hike straight through, following the purple trail to descend a slightly steeper slope. Bristled swamp oak, hickories, and hemlocks grow along this stretch. You'll also see ferns and mushrooms soon after the trail makes a sweeping turn southeast.

Stay on the purple-blazed trail through the next junction, and continue south, tapering off the wooded hill. Gradually bending east, the trail curves back toward

**229**

## Centennial Reservation

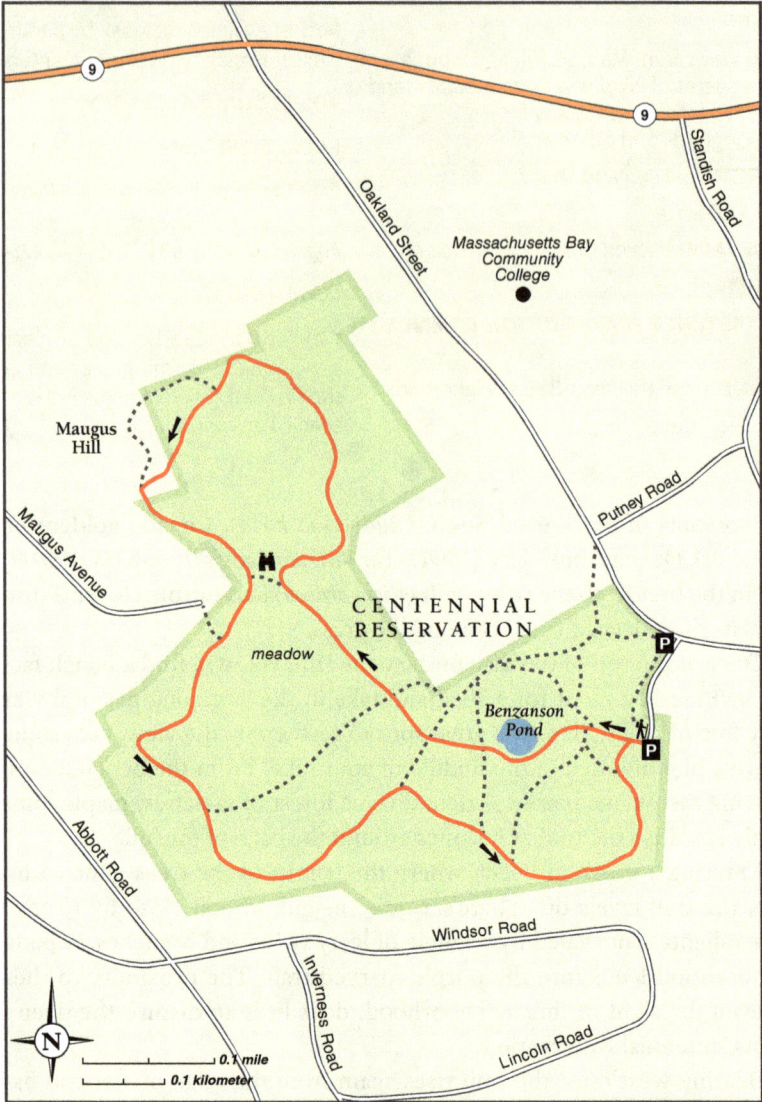

**Centennial Reservation**

9

Oakland Street

Standish Road

Massachusetts Bay
Community
College

Maugus
Hill

Putney Road

Maugus Avenue

CENTENNIAL
RESERVATION

meadow

P

Benzanson
Pond

P

Abbott Road

Windsor Road

Inverness Road

Lincoln Road

N

0.1 mile
0.1 kilometer

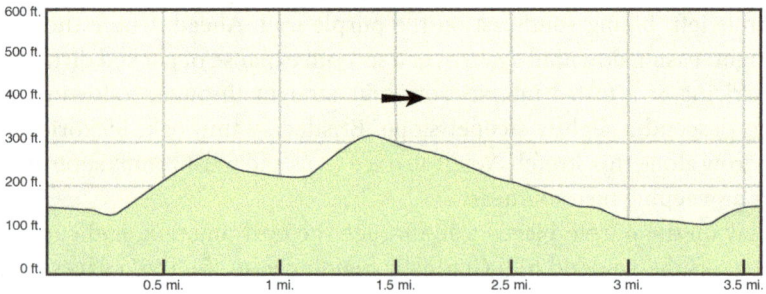

600 ft.
500 ft.
400 ft.
300 ft.
200 ft.
100 ft.
0 ft.

0.5 mi.    1 mi.    1.5 mi.    2.5 mi.    3 mi.    3.5 mi.

the meadow. Bear right along a sliver of trail through lilting grass stalks to a small wooden bridge that leads through a brief bushy corridor to another small field bordered by houses.

At the end of this field, where the trail diverts left to run up a slope into woods, stay right. Here the trail proceeds along sandy ground on the edge of an esker to a row of birdhouses erected among a cultivated patch of purple coneflowers. The path drops beside a brook flowing from the left and follows beside woods festooned with wild grapes and vinca.

Reaching a split, turn left and aim north toward ground flush with lady's thumb and ghostly moonflowers. Climbing a brief but steep pitch, the trail passes a magnificent old oak tree. A few hundred yards farther along, the purple trail loops back to its beginning at the head of the parking lot.

## NEARBY ATTRACTIONS

Wellesley has numerous well-maintained trails linking greenspace throughout the town. For more information and maps, visit the Wellesley Trails Committee website at wellesleyma.virtualtownhall.net/pages/wellesleyma_trails.

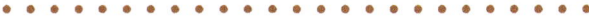

• • • • • • • • • • • • • • • • • • • • • • • • • • •

**GPS TRAILHEAD COORDINATES** N42° 18.417'  W71° 15.683'

**DIRECTIONS** From Boston take MA 9 westbound to the Cedar Street ramp. Go through lights and continue on Cedar Street 0.25 mile. Bear right on Hunnewell Street and proceed 0.25 mile. Turn right onto Oakland Street and continue about 0.8 mile down the hill. The park is on the left, marked by a wooden sign.

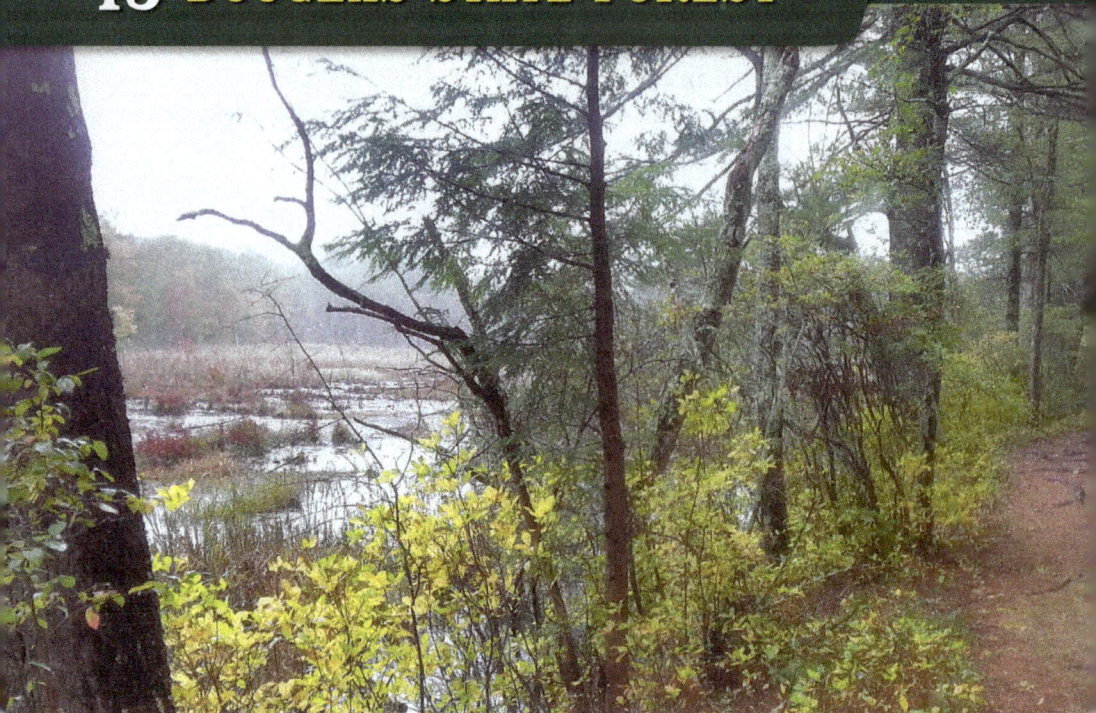

Douglas State Forest isn't hard to reach but feels wonderfully remote.

**THE COFFEEHOUSE LOOP** at Douglas State Forest takes you through a diverse forest and traverses a large scenic marshland.

## DESCRIPTION

Douglas State Forest is perched near the borders of Massachusetts, Connecticut, and Rhode Island. It isn't that far away but feels wonderfully remote. Once you enter the park, follow the long road down to the first ranger booth. The road to the left leads to the boat ramp. The road to the right leads down to the ample parking lots for Douglas State Forest.

Down on the shores of Wallum Lake, there is a large picnic area with numerous picnic tables and restroom facilities. From the large map and information kiosk, walk to the right toward one of the restroom buildings. You'll see a sign leading you to the 2.2-mile Coffeehouse Loop. Turn up the long, sloping dirt road toward the nature center and the Coffeehouse Loop trailhead. At the top of the hill, bear left across a small field, and follow the trail into the woods. You are now on the Coffeehouse Loop.

For the most part, this trail is remarkably consistent in character. It does pass through a couple of small ravines and alongside a dam later in the hike, but for the first chunk, the trail is moderately wide and fairly smooth, although rocky in spots. The

**DISTANCE & CONFIGURATION:** 2.2-mile loop

**DIFFICULTY:** Easy–moderate

**SCENERY:** Dense forest, pristine marsh

**EXPOSURE:** Mostly shaded

**TRAFFIC:** Light–moderate

**TRAIL SURFACE:** Firmly packed dirt, some rocky and muddy areas

**HIKING TIME:** 60–70 minutes

**DRIVING DISTANCE FROM BOSTON COMMON:** 58 miles

**ELEVATION:** 595' at trailhead, no significant gain

**SEASON:** Year-round

**ACCESS:** Sunrise–sunset; free

**MAPS:** Available at nature center

**WHEELCHAIR ACCESS:** No

**FACILITIES:** Restrooms, picnic tables, grills

**CONTACT:** Massachusetts Dept. of Conservation and Resources, mass.gov/locations/douglas -state-forest, 617-626-1250

**LOCATION:** Douglas, MA

trail takes you through a fairly dense and quite diverse forest with several species of conifers and deciduous trees. In spots, there is also a lot of scrubby ground cover.

A few minutes into your hike, you'll come to an intersection with a red-blazed trail. Continue straight to stay on the Coffeehouse Loop. Shortly after that intersection, the trail is almost as wide as a fire road, with the edges clearly defined by low scrub brush. You'll come to a few gentle rolling hills, but for the most part there will be very little elevation gain or loss. And the character of the trail surface remains remarkably consistent throughout this loop—fairly smooth packed dirt with the occasional rocks and roots. Continuing a bit farther, you'll encounter another intersection where the Coffeehouse Loop heads right. Here it also overlaps the yellow-blazed Midstate Trail.

If you are interested in exploring the entire Midstate Trail (which bisects the state of Massachusetts) or even part of the trail, Douglas State Forest is a good starting point. You could have someone drop you off there and pick you up wherever you finish. The Midstate Trail and the Bay Circuit Trail farther east are both excellent multiday excursions.

Continuing on the Coffeehouse Loop and Midstate Trail, you're still following a fairly even course. You may encounter a few muddy spots, but for the most part, the trail is still mostly smooth, firm-packed dirt. The trail bends and weaves a bit but follows a fairly straight tack. You'll pass down through a couple of small ravines and a fairly dense forest with lots of undergrowth. Off to your left, you may start seeing swampy areas through the trees.

You'll come to another intersection where the Midstate Trail continues straight and the Coffeehouse Loop breaks off to the right. Turn right to continue following the blue-blazed Coffeehouse Loop. Shortly after this turn, you'll see a large marsh to the left. You'll also traverse a short footbridge at the base of a rocky culvert. Here the trail gets a bit rockier as it climbs over and through this culvert.

After coming out of the dense woods, you'll see a faded sign that directs you to the right to stay on the Coffeehouse Loop. Here the trail is wide, flat, and firm like

**Douglas State Forest**

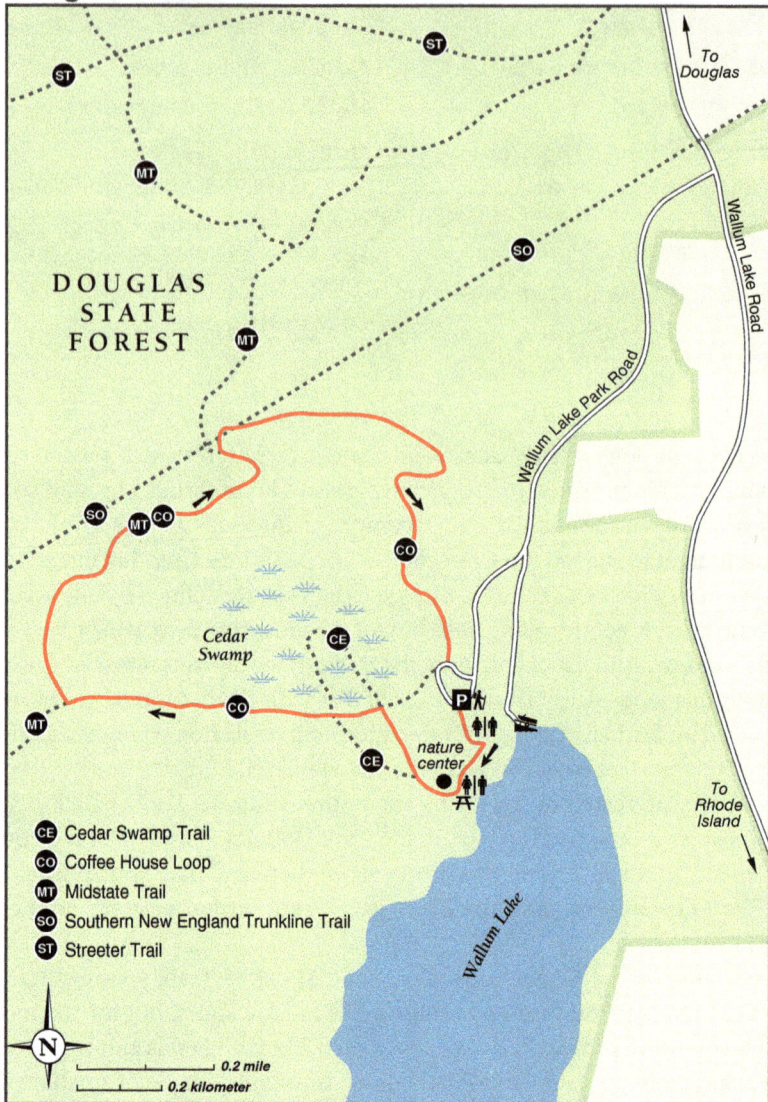

**DOUGLAS
STATE
FOREST**

*Cedar
Swamp*

nature
center

*Wallum Lake*

To
Douglas

*Wallum Lake Road*

*Wallum Lake Park Road*

To
Rhode
Island

**CE** Cedar Swamp Trail
**CO** Coffee House Loop
**MT** Midstate Trail
**SO** Southern New England Trunkline Trail
**ST** Streeter Trail

N

0.2 mile
0.2 kilometer

an old fire road. There are spectacular views of the marshland to the left as you continue along this long, straight trail.

Not long after, you'll come to another intersection where the Coffeehouse Loop dives to the right back into the forest. If you continued straight here, you'd come out on the paved road leading to the parking lots and beach area. It's also posted as the Spur Trail if you came in from that road.

Turning left and continuing on the Coffeehouse Loop, the trail here is firmly packed dirt, with a few rocks here and there. There's minimal elevation gain as you pass through the moderately dense forest. The trail is fairly well marked with blue blazes and quite well defined, especially as it winds through the dense undergrowth.

The moderately wide trail takes you through a forest of tall, slender pines, red oaks, and maples. After a relatively straight passage, it veers left and climbs slightly. The trail surface is still relatively smooth, punctuated with the occasional rock or root outcropping. In spots, the trail edges are particularly well defined by the scrubby undergrowth of the forest.

After winding through the woods at a leisurely pace, you'll come out to the dirt overflow parking area. The trail skirts the edge of this parking area then cuts back into the woods, eventually returning you to the larger paved parking lots and the beach and picnic area where you first picked up the Coffeehouse Loop. If you get an early start, plan ahead and bring a picnic or something to grill after your hike.

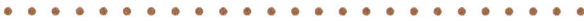

• • • • • • • • • • • • • • • • • • • • • • • • • •

**GPS TRAILHEAD COORDINATES** N42° 01.291'  W71° 46.120'

**DIRECTIONS**  From Boston, take I-90 to Exit 10A toward MA 146/US 20 (Worcester/Providence). Turn right to merge onto MA 146 S toward Millbury and Providence. Take Exit 4 for Lackey Dam Road toward Douglas/Northbridge. Turn left onto North Street then right on Main Street. Continue on Main Street about 3.4 miles. Turn left onto Wallum Lake Road and then right on Wallum Lake Park Road.

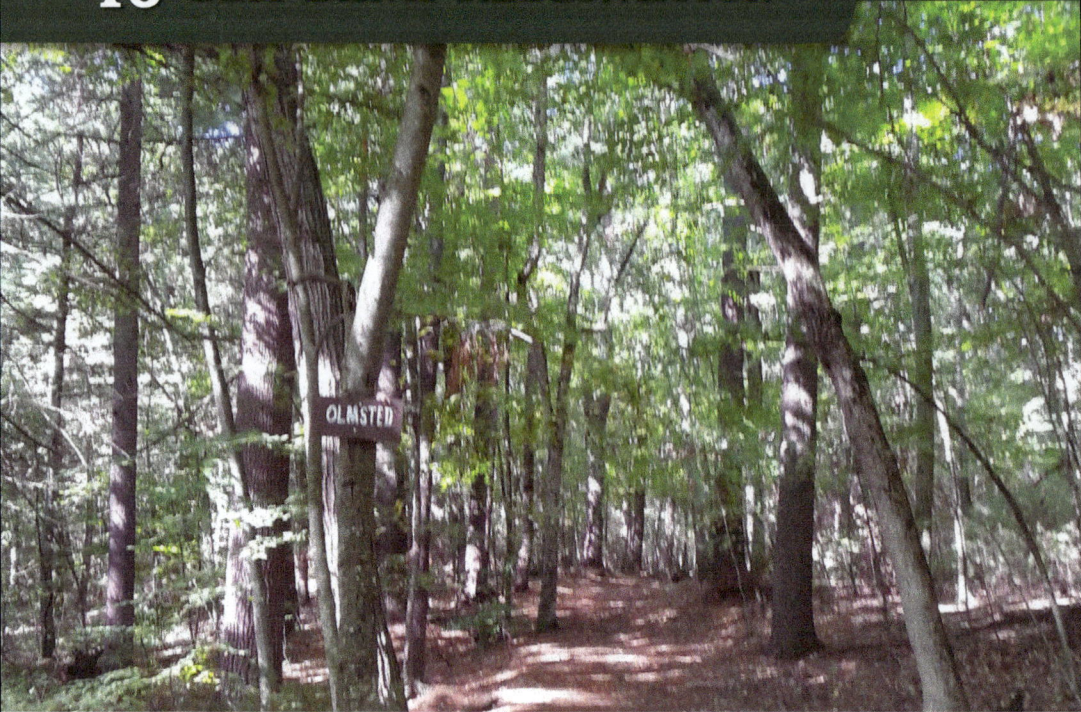

Elm Bank Reservation is an easy-to-reach walk for families and younger hikers.

**LOCATED IN AN AREA** that has maintained a charmingly rural character despite its proximity to Boston, Elm Bank's well-tended 182 acres offer miles of hiking both along the wooded banks of the Charles River and over landscaped grounds.

## DESCRIPTION

Originally a private estate from the 17th century until the dawn of World War II, Elm Bank was given its name by one of its earliest owners, Colonel John Jones, who planted elm trees along the banks of the Charles River. In 1999, the Massachusetts Horticultural Society arranged to lease the buildings and gardens and made Elm Bank its new headquarters.

This is more of a walk than a hike. The trail follows a gentle path through stately forest and along the banks of the Charles River. Starting at the parking lot located beside the Massachusetts Horticultural Society, follow the paved road northwest. As the road curves gently downhill, you will pass the Horticultural Society's demonstration gardens on the left and the redbrick Hunnewell Building on your right. A short distance farther, the road makes a T. Cross here to find the trailhead marked by a posted map.

The trail sets off immediately into magnificent woods made all the more impressive by a row of enormous white pines. The Charles River lies to the left, just a few feet

**DISTANCE & CONFIGURATION:** 1.9-mile loop

**DIFFICULTY:** Easy

**SCENERY:** Charles River, stately forest

**EXPOSURE:** Mostly shaded

**TRAFFIC:** Moderate

**TRAIL SURFACE:** Packed dirt

**HIKING TIME:** 45 minutes–1 hour

**DRIVING DISTANCE FROM BOSTON COMMON:** 15 miles

**ELEVATION:** 111' at trailhead, no significant gain

**SEASON:** Year-round

**ACCESS:** Sunrise–sunset; free

**MAPS:** Posted at the entrance or at tinyurl.com/elmbankmap

**WHEELCHAIR ACCESS:** Much of the grounds of the Elm Bank estate are wheelchair traversable; however, depending on condition, several sections of the hike described are not.

**FACILITIES:** Restrooms at the Metropolitan District Commission (MDC) ranger headquarters; soccer fields; canoe/kayak launch

**CONTACT:** Massachusetts Dept. of Conservation and Resources, mass.gov/locations/elm-bank-reservation, 617-626-1250

**LOCATION:** Wellesley, MA

**COMMENTS:** The Massachusetts Horticultural Society is headquartered here. Visitors can tour the society's demonstration gardens and the Elm Bank Estate.

from the edge of the trail and down a steep slope, flowing northeast 21 miles from the headwaters in Hopkinton. According to the Charles River Watershed Association, the river's rich tea color is normal, no matter the month or recent weather. Leaves, wetland grasses, and debris from other natural sources tint the water with their tannins. Years of concerted efforts to stop dumping and other contamination have borne exciting results. Today 74% of the 80-mile river is clean enough for swimming.

The broad trail, cushioned with a layer of pine needles, continues along the river's right bank. Before long, the trail descends to just a few feet above water level. You'll come to a narrower path splitting off to the right. Stay with the river route to the left at this break and at each of the next few intersections.

Just ahead, the trail arrives at a broad opening suitable for a canoe or kayak landing. On the opposite side of the trail, a few feet farther on, there is a large vernal pool that is well fed from overflow of the Charles River. Here beech and birch add lightness to the woods that earlier had been dominated by more-somber hemlocks and pines. The character of the woods is cool and relaxing.

The river bends abruptly southeast at this point, creating a deep oxbow as it changes course to flow first south and then southwest. The bend is so sudden and tight that it is no wonder that, after the winter thaw and healthy rains, the engorged river redraws the map. Looking across it, you can spot private houses through the budding trees in May. During the summer months when the trees are full, the houses will be hidden. Having experienced limited cutting since the 1700s, the woods along the river are remarkably diverse. Along with species of oaks and pines, there are some tulip trees, hackberries, silver maples, and ashes, and even one towering lilac.

Once the trail has veered decidedly southwest, you will encounter a fork. Both routes lead back to the playing fields at the Elm Bank mansion. For this hike, follow

237

## Elm Bank Reservation

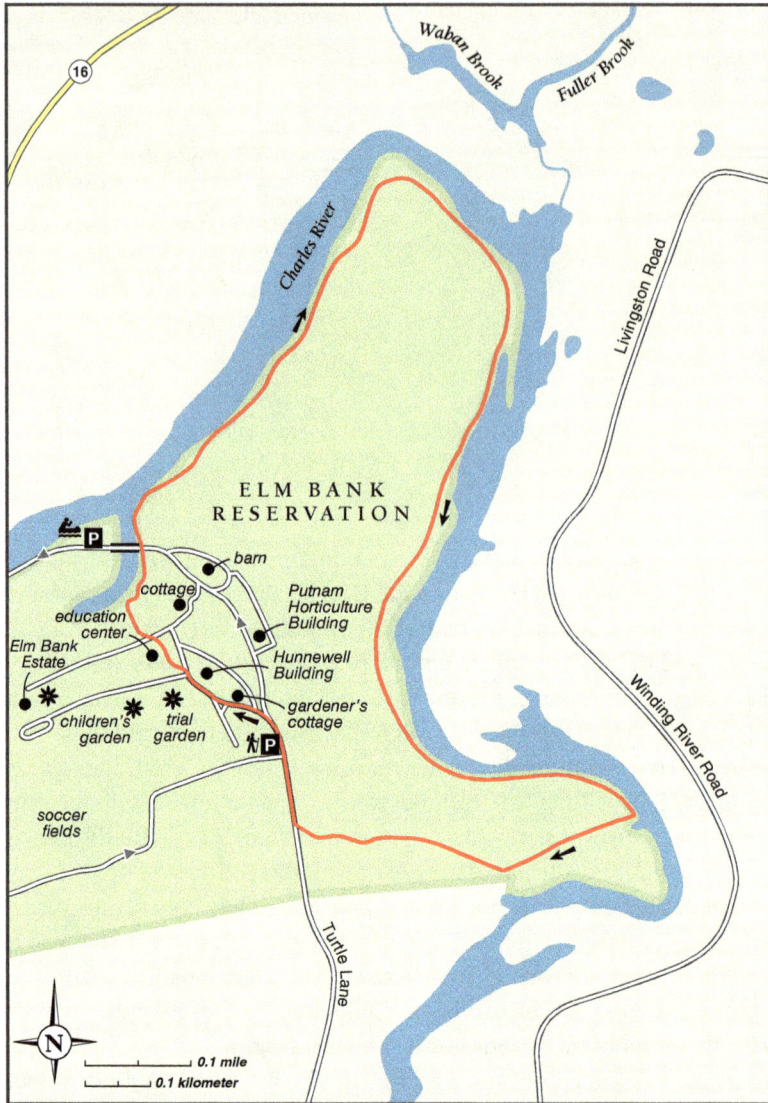

the right-hand route. This path makes a hairpin turn back to the river, heading north before turning west at another split. On this last stretch, the trail is recessed below the level of the dense woods. Mature trees cast shadows from far overhead.

Shortly the trail meets another packed-earth trail coming in from the left; stay to the right. Not much farther beyond this, the trail reaches a paved road. On the other side, you will see the playing fields. Cross here and walk right to arrive back at the Horticultural Society's parking lot.

Today, Elm Bank Reservation's acres, although somewhat reduced in number over the years, are owned by the Commonwealth of Massachusetts, which originally declined them as a gift.

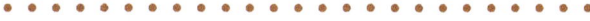

• • • • • • • • • • • • • • • • • • • • • • • • • •

**GPS TRAILHEAD COORDINATES** N42° 16.500'  W71° 18.200'

**DIRECTIONS**  From Boston, take I-90 W to Exit 15A. Follow I-95/MA 128 S to Exit 21B (MA 16 W). Follow MA 16 W 2.9 miles. On MA 16 W you will come to a stoplight (at a five-way intersection) in Wellesley; bear left to continue 1.7 miles on MA 16. The Elm Bank Horticultural Center will be on your left, marked by a small green sign. The street address is 900 Washington St. (MA 16).

The views of the placid Charles River add to the Elm Bank hike.

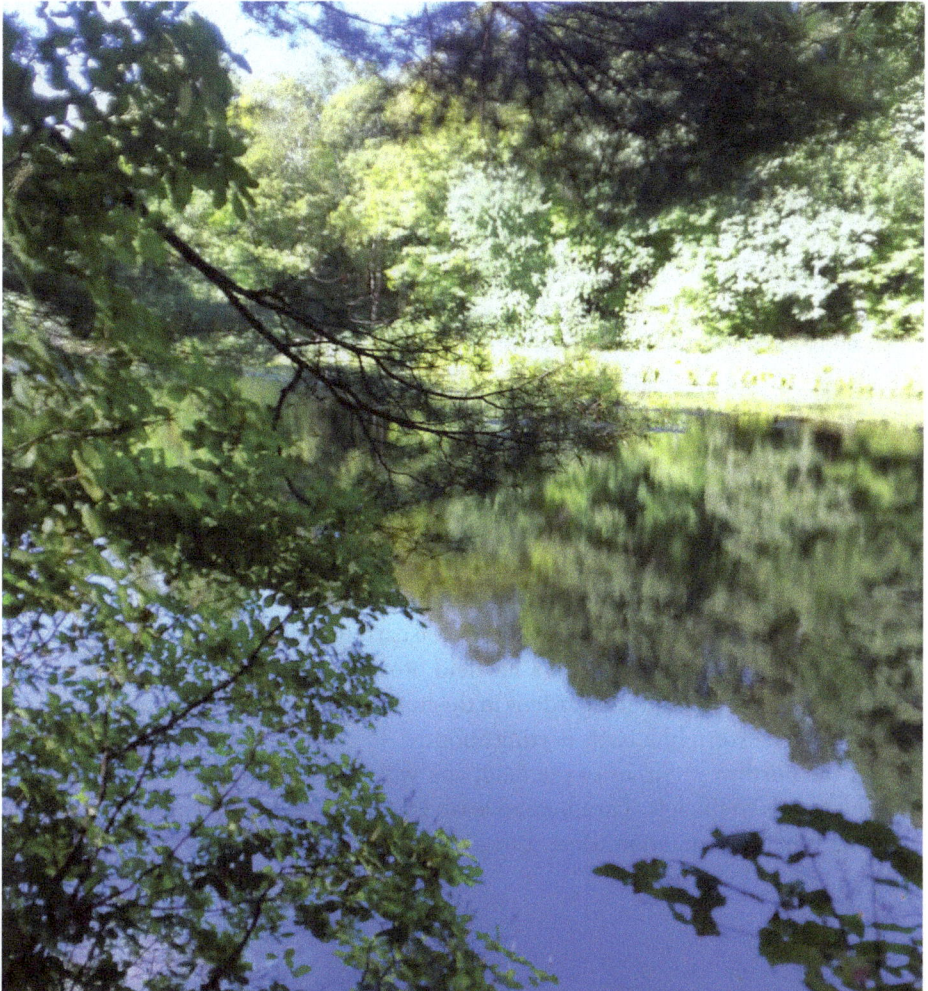

# 47 FOSS FARM

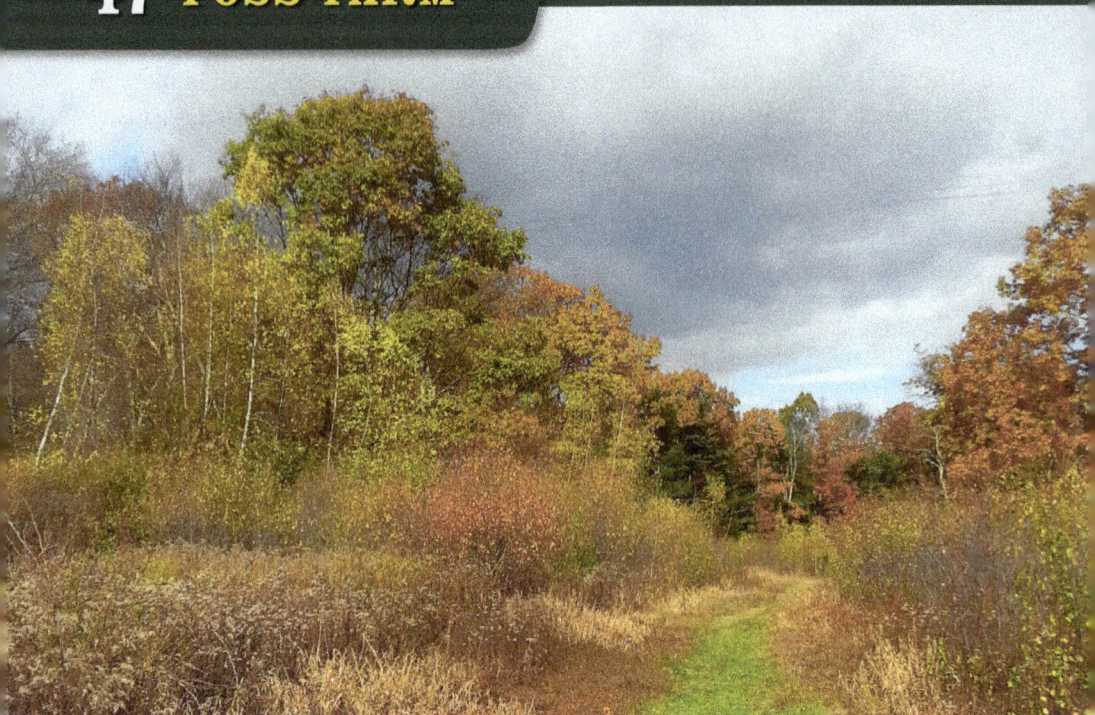

Foss Farm takes you through dramatic woodlands and swamps.

**ON THIS HIKE,** you will shadow the Concord River, crossing through conserved farmland and a magnificent tract called The Great Meadows owned by the National Wildlife Federation. The trail passes through woods and picturesque farmsteads before rounding a large pond teeming with lily pads and then doubling back to Foss Farm.

## DESCRIPTION

Find the trailhead at the edge of the parking lot, and head northeast across an open field. Rising and falling with the curve of the land, the path soon leads to two horseback-riding rings, one straight ahead and another around a corner to the left. Foss Farm is a popular destination for local equestrians who come to school their horses and to compete in shows held in summer and autumn.

Follow the path, which is more like a wide carriage road at this point, north past the riding rings along the edge of a hayfield. Reaching woods, the path turns right and heads toward community gardens in the northwest corner of the field. Watch for swallows and eastern bluebirds darting about.

At the northwest corner of the field, you will find a sign marking a trail leading into the woods to the left. Turn here to leave Foss Farm and enter land owned by the National Wildlife Federation. Here it begins to feel like you're really hiking. The trail

**DISTANCE & CONFIGURATION:** 6.7-mile out-and-back

**DIFFICULTY:** Moderate

**SCENERY:** Fields, woods, wetlands

**EXPOSURE:** Mostly shaded

**TRAFFIC:** Light

**TRAIL SURFACE:** Grass, packed dirt, boardwalks

**HIKING TIME:** 3 hours

**DRIVING DISTANCE FROM BOSTON COMMON:** 25 miles

**ELEVATION:** 132' at trailhead, no significant gain

**SEASON:** Year-round

**ACCESS:** Sunrise–sunset; free

**MAPS:** Posted at the entrance or online at carlisletrails.pbworks.com/f/greatmeadows.pdf

**WHEELCHAIR ACCESS:** No

**FACILITIES:** None

**CONTACT:** Town of Carlisle, www.carlislema.gov /pages/carlislema_steward/foss; 978-369-6136

**LOCATION:** Carlisle, MA

**COMMENTS:** Waterproof shoes are recommended in wet months.

narrows and traverses through dense forest. A few feet beyond a gap in a stone wall, it reaches an intersection. The River Trail lies to the right, and the Redtail Trail, to the left.

Heading north on the Redtail Trail over level ground ever so slightly out of reach of floodwater, you pass through a grove of red pines dense enough to suppress growth of any underbrush except ferns that thrive in wet, dimly lit conditions. The trail winds through the forest and makes for a peaceful, relaxing hike. Woodcocks also favor these parts, both for the cover they provide and for the earthworms that multiply voluminously in the forest detritus.

Weaving throughout the loosely spaced forest, the trail eventually leads to a particularly scenic marshland, linked to a small pond formed with the help of a dam put in place by farmers in days gone by. A sturdy wooden boardwalk and footbridge help you get across.

After crossing the bridge, bear right (northeast), making your way along a path that skirts the expansive Great Meadows Wildlife area. Because mowing is frequently inhibited by wet conditions, lush grasses are inclined to overwhelm the trail here. In June the humid air is filled with the ecstatic pulsing chirps of bullfrogs. Farther along, the tended side of the field transitions to grassland left to revert to its natural state. Though the area is open and dominated by grasses and wildflowers, aspen, birch, and pine saplings are beginning to assert themselves. The trail is quite well marked and well defined here.

Leaving the Great Meadows area, continue west along a mowed pathway through another field. Near a sign simply marked TRAIL, the path splits in two. Take the left trail to promptly arrive at another intersection. Here, signs point back to Foss Farm and to the Pine Loop. Leave the meadows behind and continue left (west) under the cover of pencil-straight pines. Traveling through this cultivated evergreen grove, the path curves northeast. Shortly you come upon a sign pointing to Maple Street, a pond, and the river to the right. Turn off here to continue north. Still surrounded by lofty pines, you may hear a car pass on the street barely visible to the left.

## Foss Farm

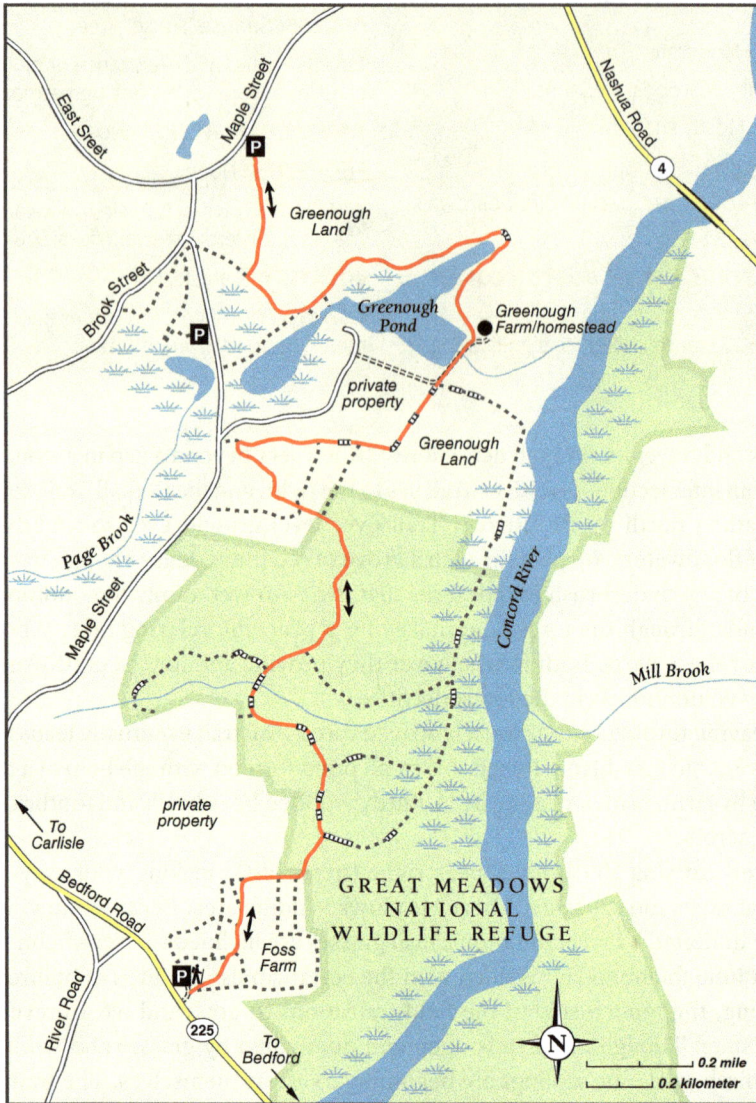

Rounding the knoll, you can catch a glimpse of the river edging into a field on the left. Just ahead, the trail dips to another fork. Continuing straight, the Pine Loop trail leads back to Foss Farm, while the path to the left leaves the woods and heads toward Maple Street. Choosing the latter route, head east across the field toward the river. A picturesque house and barn sit on private property to the left.

After crossing the field, the path reenters a wooded corridor dense with oaks and pines. Several yards away, hidden by a tangled thicket, the Concord River flows southwest, meandering seaward. A sign ahead directs hikers right, away from private property. Behind that, the River Trail emerges from the bog.

Hiking a few hundred yards more on what becomes a dirt road, you arrive at the eastern end of Greenough Pond. A dam and ruler-straight causeway bridge the water, allowing passage from the fields of Greenough Farm to the homestead just within sight. Greenough Farm is now idle conservation land, its handsome white barn and clapboard home ghostly vacant. Follow the road to the barnyard and search to the left to find a weathered post marking where the trail continues along the pond's bank.

Though overcome by weeds at the start, the trail becomes easy to follow as it circles the pond. On the western side of the pond, the trail bends south and crosses a tributary by way of a wooden footbridge. Beyond the bridge, follow the trail now marked with red dots, as it climbs up a banking and bends away from the pond back into woods. After crossing another stream, the trail splits at an unmarked intersection made distinct by a telephone pole at its center. Choose the trail to the right, which widens as it climbs. Beyond a break in a stone wall, a sign points right, to parking. Undulating through woods, this broad, well-traveled path leads to a bold-yellow arrow painted on a rock soon after the trail's end at Maple Street. From this terminus, turn and retrace your steps to hike back to Foss Farm.

Foss Farm doesn't have a lot of elevation gain, but it does take you through some varied woodlands, across lush meadows and some spectacularly scenic swamps. It would be a good hike with smaller kids as it's fairly easy, and you could always turn around whenever you determine they have used up almost half of their energy.

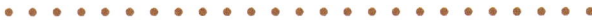

• • • • • • • • • • • • • • • • • • • • • • • • • • • •

**GPS TRAILHEAD COORDINATES** N42° 30.783' W71° 19.117'

**DIRECTIONS** From Boston, take I-90 W 9.4 miles to I-95 N. Continue 9.4 miles to Exit 31B/ MA 4 N toward Bedford. Travel 2.8 miles; turn left onto MA 225 and continue 4.1 miles. Shortly after crossing the Concord River, look for a dirt road on the right leading to a dirt parking lot. There's a sign reading FOSS FARM on the roadside, but it is not easy to see.

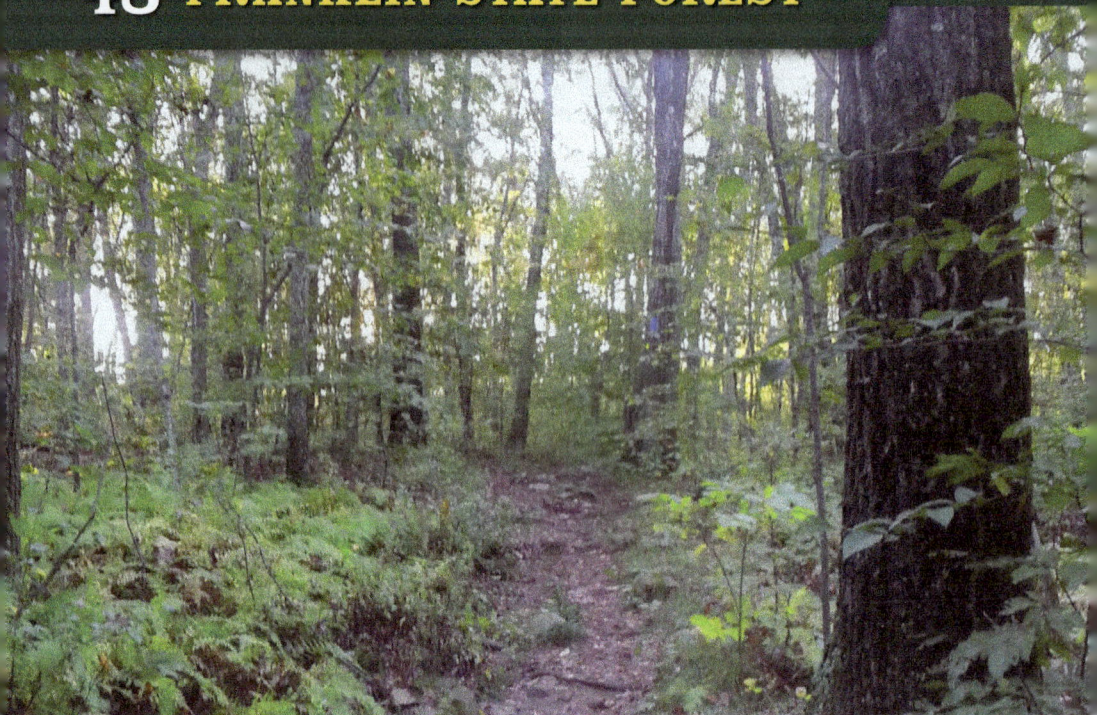

The loop at Franklin State Forest is just long enough for a brief retreat to the woods.

**THIS IS AN EASY TRAIL** when you just need a quick jaunt through the woods. And while this is the hiking-only side of Franklin State Forest, there are many more trails on the multiuse side.

## DESCRIPTION

Far enough from Boston, but not too far, Franklin State Forest provides a respite from the suburban traffic, shopping plazas, and pavement. Find the small parking area near the intersection of Beaver Street and Grove Street. There's room for four or five cars. If you find a spot on Grove Street, start at the metal gate intended to keep motorized vehicles out of this side of the forest. Dirt bikes are allowed in the other side of Franklin State Forest, on the other side of the power lines, but not on this loop.

After passing the metal gate, you start off following the blue-blazed Healthy Heart Trail, one of more than 70 Healthy Heart Trails spread throughout Massachusetts. Shortly into the hike, the trail takes a 45-degree turn right and begins a straight rocky climb of about 30 yards. At this point, the trail roughly parallels Grove Street. At the top of this climb, the trail flattens out and turns left. You'll pass a bench positioned there if you'd like to stop and simply look around the forest.

After passing this bench, the trail takes you through a few sweeping S turns, then up a short, slightly steep climb to the left, and then around a corner to the right.

**DISTANCE & CONFIGURATION:** 1.5-mile loop

**DIFFICULTY:** Easy

**SCENERY:** Open mixed forest

**EXPOSURE:** Shaded

**TRAFFIC:** Light

**TRAIL SURFACE:** Firmly packed dirt, with some rocks and roots

**HIKING TIME:** 45 minutes

**DRIVING DISTANCE FROM BOSTON COMMON:** 44 miles

**ELEVATION:** 255' at trailhead, 404' at highest point

**SEASON:** Year-round

**ACCESS:** Sunrise–sunset; free

**MAPS:** Available at kiosk or at tinyurl.com /franklinstateforestmap

**WHEELCHAIR ACCESS:** No

**FACILITIES:** None

**CONTACT:** Massachusetts Dept. of Conservation and Resources, mass.gov/locations/franklin -state-forest, 617-626-1250

**LOCATION:** Franklin, MA

The trail surface here is quite rocky, so watch your step. After these steeper, rocky S turns, the trail flattens out slightly. The forest here has fairly dense undergrowth but is loose enough and comprises mostly deciduous trees, which let in a lot of light on a sunny day. Up ahead, you'll see the backs of some condo buildings through the trees.

Still following the blue blazes that mark Massachusetts DCR trails, you'll pass over what's left of an old stone wall, staying on what is marked as the Healthy Heart Trail. The path bends right and follows a long straight course. Here you will still see the backs of those condo buildings on the right. It must be nice to have a state forest right in your backyard. Be respectful and stay on the trail here.

Farther down on this long straightaway, you'll pass over another old stone wall. Here the trail begins to veer away from the condos. Pass a second stone wall and then the trail takes a sharp left. The character of the forest changes almost immediately as well. It goes from a mixed, mostly deciduous forest to a grove of impressively tall conifers. After a couple more zigs and zags, the trail follows along another straight- away, this one roughly paralleling that last stone wall you crossed over. You'll pass another bench on the right, if you'd like to take a quick break. Otherwise, hike to the next intersection, where the Healthy Heart Trail takes a 90-degree turn left through the old stone wall.

If you went straight here, you'd come to the power lines. So it's unlikely you'll miss this turn, and even if you do, you'll know right away. If you would like to explore the rest of Franklin State Forest, head out to the power lines, and bear right and then left on the paved road to find more trailheads. At this intersection, you may also hear the sounds of kids playing, as the Forge Park YMCA is nearby through the woods.

Take this left and enter a dark, sylvan grove of mostly coniferous trees. The ground underfoot is padded with a dense carpet of pine needles, so your footfall will be muffled. The trail winds down and around to the left, away from the power lines and the sounds of the YMCA. And once again, the forest is silent.

# Franklin State Forest

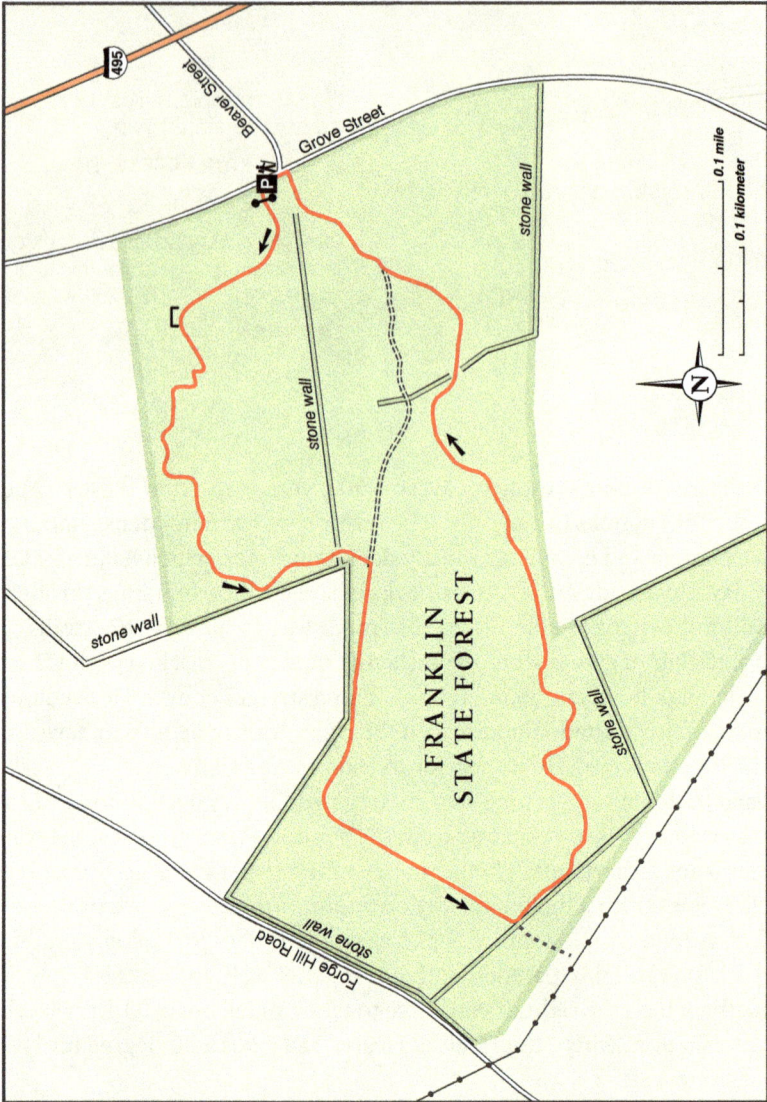

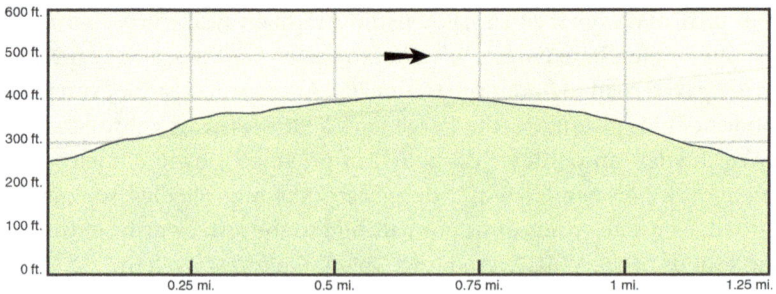

The trail winds left and climbs slightly, then continues winding through the moderately dense forest down to the right. On this side of the forest, you can see blackened trees and stumps, evidence of controlled burns in this well-maintained DCR forest. As the trail descends gently right, you'll pass yet another old stone wall; cross over the wall. The trail takes you on a few racetrack-like S turns, climbing and falling gently, and then bears right again. Shortly after this turn, the Healthy Heart Trail cuts off to the left. Continue straight to stay on the slightly longer loop.

Follow the trail down toward another stone wall. This time the trail wraps around the corner of the wall, which is in better shape than some of the others you've crossed. After you pass this old stone farmland border, the character of the forest loosens and lightens up. This is especially noticeable on a bright sunny day.

This winding trail then takes you on a few more S turns, and the trail surface gets a bit rougher and rockier. Watch your step as you pass through. The trail descends ever so slightly then takes you on a short, straight shot through a column of young deciduous trees. After this brief straightaway, the trail climbs a bit and veers left and then right. The forest is quite open here as well.

Now you're getting closer to the trailhead where you began, so you may start hearing traffic on Grove Street or even I-495. Follow the trail through a few more shallow S turns and over another stone wall. Shortly after this, the Healthy Heart Trail rejoins this loop, coming in from the left. Then the trail drops dramatically over a considerably rocky surface. Going down this section will likely involve rock-hopping. The trail follows the contour of the hillside back down toward Grove Street. Near the bottom, there is one final zig to the left, which brings you back to where you started.

## NEARBY ATTRACTIONS

There are plenty of places to refuel after your hike. If you're in the mood for sushi, try Ichigo Ichie (508-541-8882, ichigoichieus.com). The British Beer Company (508-440-5190, britishbeer.com/location/franklin) is in the Stop and Shop plaza across I-495 from the trailhead. And a bit farther down MA 140 W and well worth checking out is the upscale restaurant 3 (461 W. Central St., 508-528-6333, 3-restaurant.com), which features classic and contemporary bistro fare.

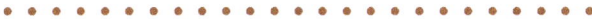

• • • • • • • • • • • • • • • • • • • • • • • •

**GPS TRAILHEAD COORDINATES** N42° 04.802'  W71° 25.388'

**DIRECTIONS**  From Boston, take I-93 S to I-95 S toward Providence. Follow this to I-495 N toward Worcester. From I-495 N, take Exit 17. Bear left off the exit and cross over I-495. Take a sharp left onto Grove Street and continue about two-thirds of a mile to small parking area on the right (across from Beaver Street).

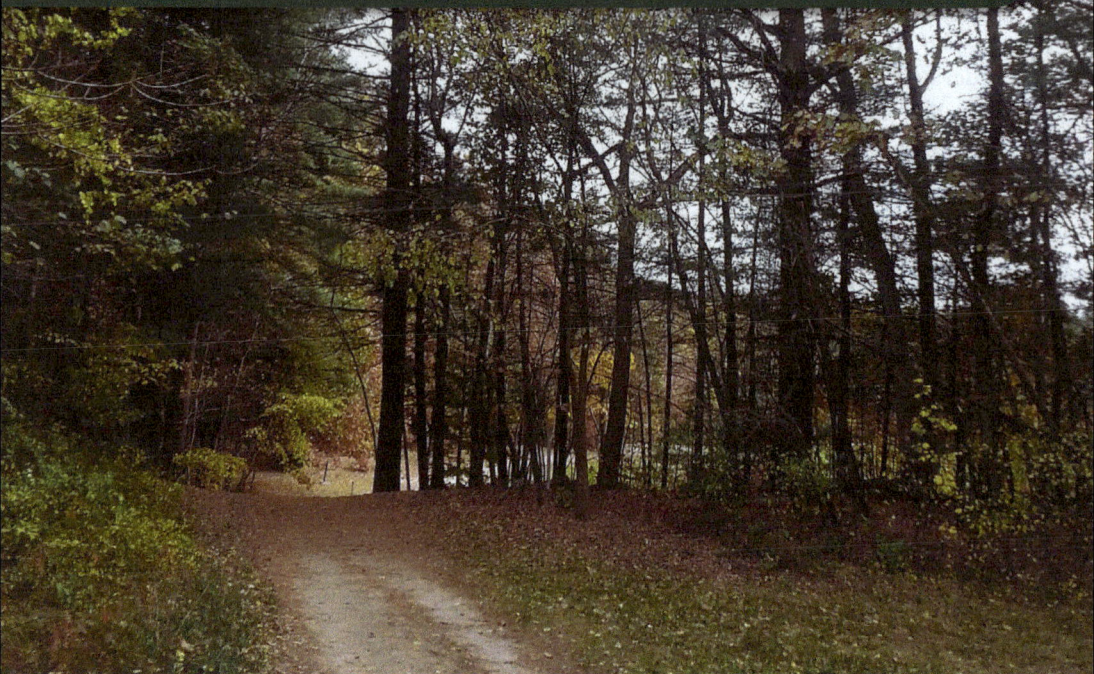

Great Brook State Farm has miles of overlapping trails inviting hours of exploration.

**THIS HIKE PROVIDES** a full tour of the nearly 1,000-acre Great Brook Farm State Park, passing over terrain that varies from rugged, rocky slopes to boardwalks stretched across swampland.

## DESCRIPTION

Like many of the state parks and reservations near Boston, you could spend days hiking here. Get a map, and then either follow the hiking route described here or take off exploring on your own.

From the parking lot, head north on the trail to the left of the interpretive center, passing a butterfly garden planted with bee balm and other perennials. Ahead at junction 4, two loop trails converge. Continue straight, crossing the gravel road to hike north on Litchfield Loop Trail. Stretching across a meadow, the trail bears right and enters woods.

Winding along over glacial mounds, the Litchfield Loop Trail leads to a sliver of meadow bordered by wildflowers. The trail here is fairly flat with a firmly packed surface. Beyond this corridor, the trail broadens to another field. Ahead, at the three-way junction (6), proceed on the blue-marked Indian Hill Trail. When you take the Indian Hill trail into the woods, this feels more like a hiking trail. It's narrow, winding, and occasionally filled with roots and rocks.

**DISTANCE & CONFIGURATION:** 6.82-mile loop

**DIFFICULTY:** Easy–moderate

**SCENERY:** Glacial landscape with vernal pools, eskers, woods, swamp, and a large pond

**EXPOSURE:** Mostly shaded

**TRAFFIC:** Moderate

**TRAIL SURFACE:** Packed dirt with loose gravel in some places

**HIKING TIME:** 3–3.5 hours

**DRIVING DISTANCE FROM BOSTON COMMON:** 28 miles

**ELEVATION:** 174' at trailhead, no significant gain

**SEASON:** Year-round

**ACCESS:** Sunrise–sunset. Parking is $2 per car.

**MAPS:** Maps are available at the park and at mass.gov/eea/docs/dcr/parks/trails/greatbrook -summer.pdf

**WHEELCHAIR ACCESS:** No

**FACILITIES:** Great Brook Farm's dairy concession sells freshly made ice cream and lunch mid-April–mid-October, 11 a.m.–dark. Other facilities include restrooms and a cross-country ski center at the Hart Barn.

**CONTACT:** Massachusetts Dept. of Conservation and Resources, mass.gov/locations/great-brook -farm-state-park, 617-626-1250

**LOCATION:** Carlisle, MA

After winding through the forest, the Indian Hill Trail makes a hairpin turn to head northeast under a canopy of pines. Reaching the top of the hill at junction 33, the trail continues straight on its northeast trajectory, gradually easing downhill.

The foot of Indian Hill marks the border between the towns of Carlisle and Chelmsford. Great Brook Farm is entirely in Carlisle, so the trail ends its north-bearing run and aims southeast, keeping flush to the town line. Several houses abutting the park are visible through the woods on this stretch. Keep left at the next junction, staying on the trail that doubles as a gas line. Then bear right (south) at the split that soon follows.

On encountering a brook, the trail (marked with blue blazes) hugs the bank of the wetland, crossing first a small bridge and then another wide enough to accommodate three horses walking abreast. The Indian Hill Trail runs uphill and to the right at junction 10. Continue straight, heading east on the grand woodland avenue humbly named Woodchuck Trail. This raised trail cuts a dry, curved route south, despite the wetlands on either side. You'll pass a minor path or two to arrive at the end of a massive stone wall at junction 11.

For a shorter hike, stay on the Woodchuck Trail as it veers west. You could also vary the hike with a quick jaunt on a more intimate path, detouring left onto the Deer Run Trail. After adding a loop to the east at junction 30, the Deer Run Trail cuts west across wetland via one of the park's many boardwalks built by members of the New England Mountain Bike Association (NEMBA), then links with the Garrison Loop at junction 31. Just northwest of this crossroads, the trail leads uphill to a historic site called The City.

Past the cellar hole of the garrison house, the trail retreats under pines and hemlocks to reunite with the Woodchuck Trail. Those interested in viewing a log cabin built by Great Brook Farm's original owner, Farnham Smith, will want to bear right at this junction. The cabin is several yards down the trail on the left. After visiting

**Great Brook Farm State Park**

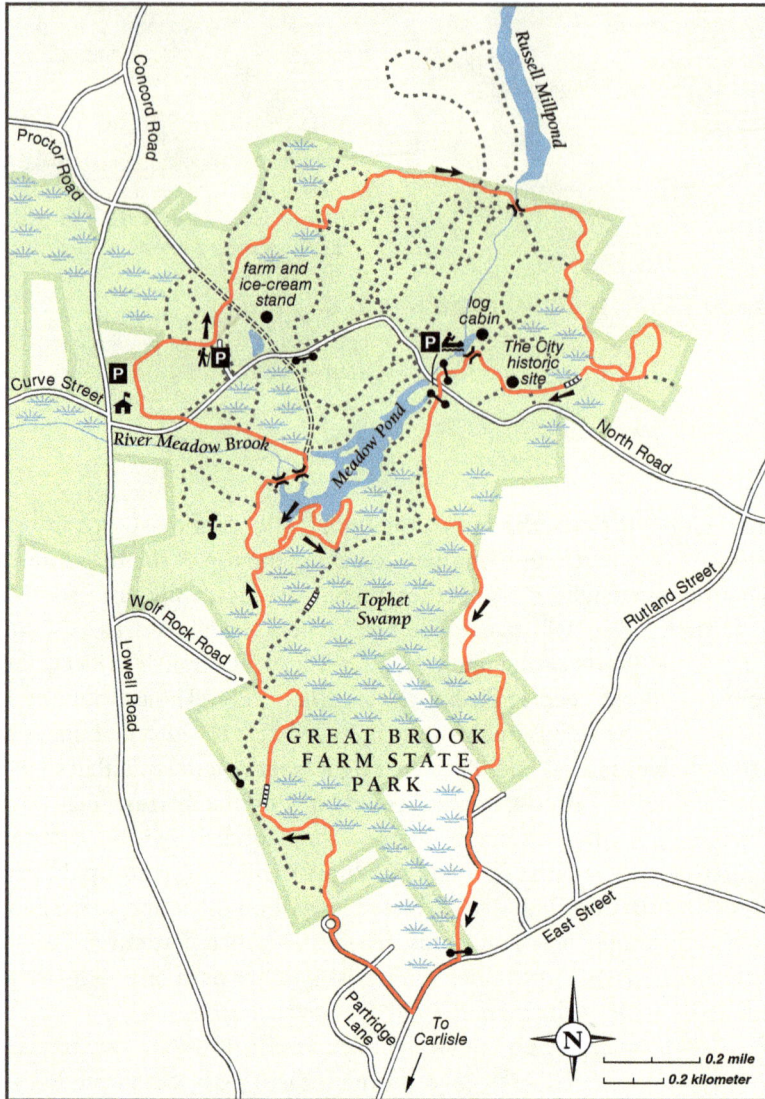

the cabin, follow the Woodchuck Trail southwest to its end at North Road. Navigate the metal gate, then cross the road to reach the canoe launch at Meadow Pond—a kettle pond created when the Wisconsin Glacier retreated.

Pick up the Pine Point Loop Trail to the left of the canoe launch, and follow this wide, firmly packed dirt cart road south along the edge of the wetland surrounding Meadow Pond. Here you can bear right onto the Beaver Loop, a lightly traveled trail that leads to the water's edge. Otherwise continue straight to junction 15—the gateway to Tophet Swamp.

Swinging west, the Pine Point Loop Trail forms a causeway across a glacial outwash plain lying south of Meadow Pond. To shorten the hike by half, stay on this route. Otherwise bear left to set out around Tophet Swamp. The trail begins with a length of boardwalk that NEMBA built over a section that can get particularly sticky during wet months. Beyond this, the trail makes its way through woods along the swamp's outer reaches, following the park's eastern border approximately 1.3 miles.

Emerging from woods, the trail arrives at a cul-de-sac at the end of Aberdeen Drive. Several hundred yards up the drive, the trail reenters woods to the right. Bearing southwest, it travels through a beech grove punctuated with sassafras to reach a gate at East Street. Having left the park, Tophet Loop Trail continues to the right along the street and passes several houses before bearing right at Woodbine Road. Tracking this peaceful road to a turnaround at its end, the trail leaves pavement and forges north.

Next the trail arrives at junction 44. Here the Heartbreak Ridge Trail bears left and the terraced Tophet Loop Trail continues right, mirroring the swamp's irregular edge.

Beyond a short boardwalk the trail winds east then west, bringing you to an enormous glacial erratic sitting in the center of junction 29. To stay on the Tophet Loop Trail, keep right. Follow the Heartbreak Ridge Trail to the left if you'd like to survey the landscape from atop a prominent esker (a ridge of sand, earth, and stone created by a stream running deep beneath a glacier). This trail bears west around the boulder.

Either way, both trails leave Tophet Swamp as they snake north. The Heartbreak Ridge trail passes a pond teeming with fantastic life forms, then tapers to end at junction 18 on the Pine Point Loop Trail. Bear left on the Pine Point Loop Trail if you'd like to shorten your hike. This route leads back to the parking area by way of North Road and the Lantern Loop Trail. Whichever way you choose, you'll once again be on the wide, relatively flat, firmly packed surface of an old carriage road.

To continue your tour of Great Brook Farm, bear right at junction 18, and backtrack east to junction 16. Taking up the Tophet Loop Trail once more, bear left to hike north. The main trail, more deeply etched than the others, follows the pond's outline and then bends south to return to the Pine Point Loop Trail at junction 17. Bear right to follow this convoluted route past the Heartbreak Ridge Trail and then a cornfield encircled by the Erickson Loop.

Past junction 21, the Pine Point Loop Trail swings east, crossing between wetland and Meadow Pond. Continue hiking east over a stone bridge, and the carriage road passes an idyllic picnicking spot.

Bear left (west) at junction 22 to follow the clay-surfaced Maple Ridge Trail. Traveling across a wooded floodplain, this trail passes a path to the right and, after bearing left at junction 23, joins the Lantern Loop Trail at North Road.

Crossing the road on a diagonal, take up the Lantern Trail, and arc north past picturesque cornfields and the ski center at Hart Barn. When the trail meets junction 2, leave the Lantern Loop Trail and follow the dirt road, bearing east toward the top of the parking lot.

## NEARBY ATTRACTIONS

History buffs will want to explore nearby Concord—a town as rich in history and appeal as any other New England town. It's also home to Walden Pond, made famous by Henry David Thoreau and his book of the same name.

• • • • • • • • • • • • • • • • • • • • • • • • • •

**GPS TRAILHEAD COORDINATES** N42° 33.45'  W71° 20.917'

**DIRECTIONS**  From Boston, take I-93 N to I-95 W/MA 128, then take Exit 31B (MA 4 N/MA 225 W). Follow MA 225 W 8 miles to the Carlisle center rotary, then turn right on Lowell Street (following the sign to Chelmsford). Fern's Market is on the corner. The park entrance is 2 miles ahead on the right. The park office is on the right at 984 Lowell St., just beyond the entrance. To park, turn right onto North Road. The parking area is 0.5 mile down on the left.

Great Brook's trails wind around pastures and through the dense forest.

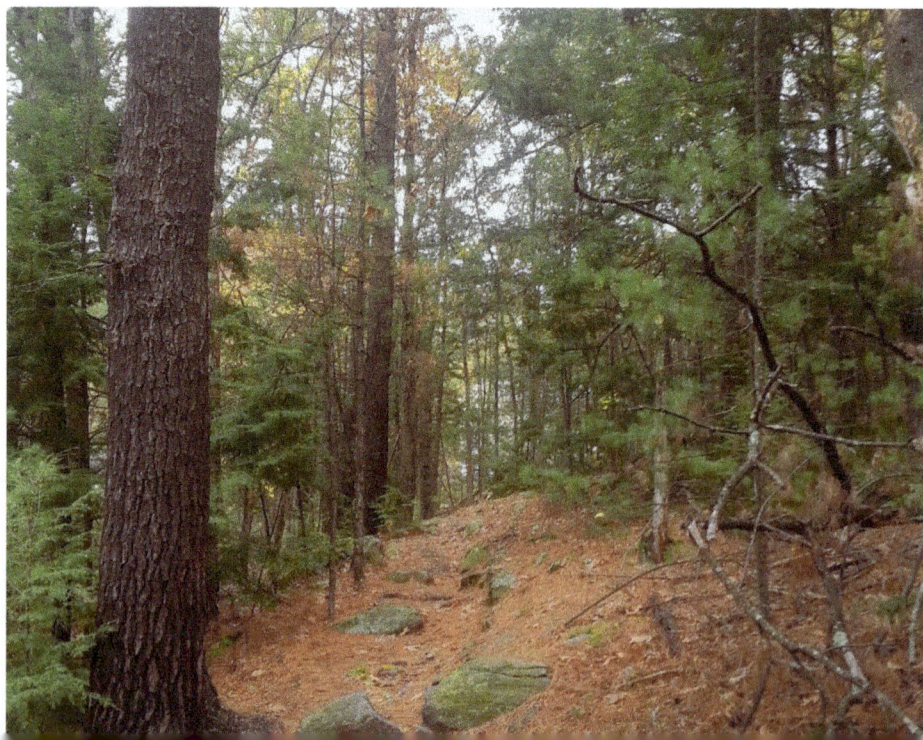

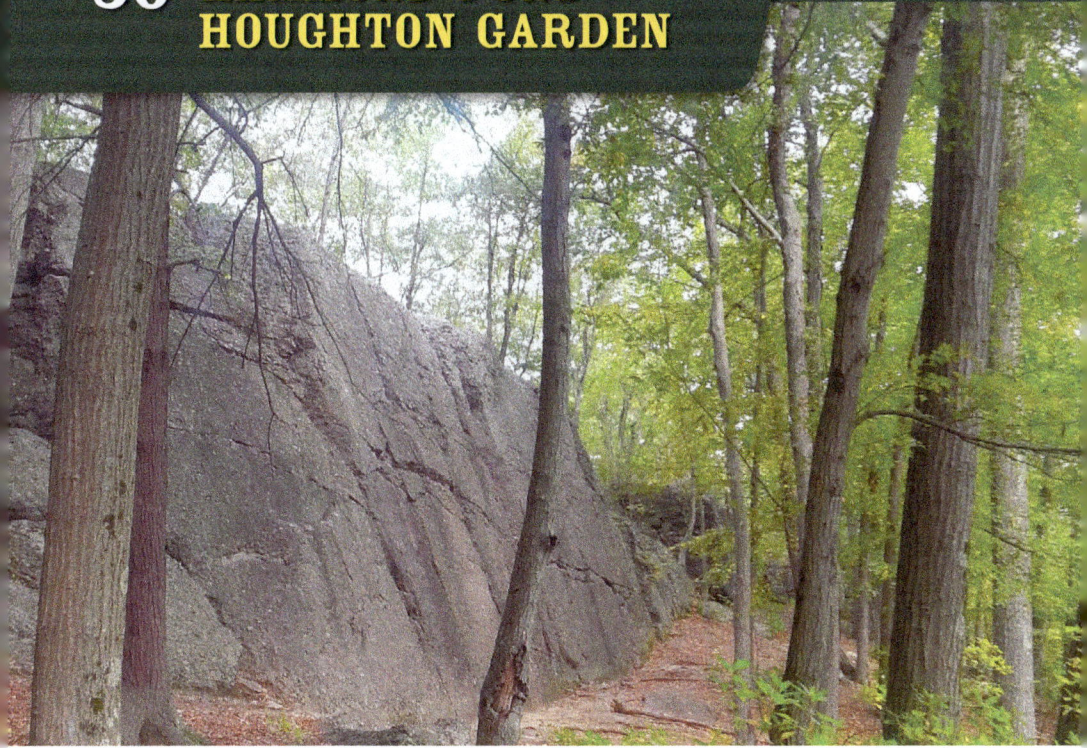

# 50 HAMMOND POND– HOUGHTON GARDEN

Mere feet from the bustle of MA 9, this refuge is indeed a welcome diversion.

**A HIDDEN GEM,** this historic and scenic hike passes a 10-acre pond and crosses the tracks of part of the nation's oldest subway system before touring a 19th-century deer park and a garden listed on the National Register of Historic Places.

## DESCRIPTION

In the mid-1600s, Thomas Hammond and his wife, Elizabeth, relocated from the coastal town of Hingham to Newton, then a part of Cambridge. Over the centuries, the Hammonds' original property passed through the hands of many others, including the Webster and Houghton families. Between 1968 and 1979, the City of Newton purchased parcels totaling 113 acres to ensure they remain open wooded space.

Locate the trailhead at the northwest corner of the Chestnut Hill Mall parking lot next to a kiosk displaying a map of the reservation. Departing from this unlikely spot, set out hiking north on the wide packed-earth trail shaded by an elegant awning of hemlock boughs. Though visible from the paved ground outside, Hammond Pond quickly vanishes behind a thicket of brush once you're in the woods. The trail arcs along the border of the pond, keeping within close range of the water.

**DISTANCE & CONFIGURATION:** 2.2-mile loop

**DIFFICULTY:** Easy

**SCENERY:** Woods, pond, peat bog, 6-acre deer park, 10-acre historic wild garden

**EXPOSURE:** Mostly shaded

**TRAFFIC:** Light

**TRAIL SURFACE:** Packed dirt, crushed stone, rough wooded sections

**HIKING TIME:** 1.5–2 hours

**DRIVING DISTANCE FROM BOSTON COMMON:** 6 miles

**ELEVATION:** 171' at trailhead, no significant gain

**SEASON:** Year-round

**ACCESS:** Sunrise–sunset; free

**MAPS:** Available at newtonconservators.org/map18webster.htm

**WHEELCHAIR ACCESS:** Recent rehabilitation work and upgrading has made parts of the Houghton Garden wheelchair accessible.

**FACILITIES:** None

**CONTACT:** Newton Conservators, newtonconservators.org; Massachusetts Dept. of Conservation and Resources, mass.gov/locations/hammond-pond-reservation, 617-626-1250

**LOCATION:** Newton, MA

**COMMENTS:** Be exceptionally careful, as this hike crosses the tracks of the MBTA D train Green Line. Houghton Garden is popular among birders.

Looking like the steel prow of a grounded ship, a massive wall of granite looms to the left on a still sea of fallen leaves. This ledge is a huge draw for the area's novice rock climbers. The granite wall almost always has a group of climbers, whether newbies taking organized lessons or seasoned climbers stopping in during the workday.

Bending northeast, the trail reaches a clearing where suddenly the tannin-dark pond materializes to the right, reflecting metallic light to the sky. Here the trail forks left and right. Bear right and continue into the thicker woods of oak and maple. The trail here is firm and flat but gets a bit narrower where it enters the woods. Beyond where a minor path connects the main trail to the pond below, the trail passes a boulder so striated by glacial wear that it looks like a worry-creased brow.

The pond disappears behind a dense hedge of leatherleaf, elderberry, chokecherry, pussy willow, and other shrubs growing beside the pond and the peat bog separated from it by a dam jutting east. Staying on upland, the trail winds west along the boundary of the bog. It is lightly worn and therefore vague on this section, but it soon arrives at a sign identifying the land as part of the Webster Conservation Area. From this point, blue blazes mark the trail.

A boardwalk provides dry passage over a wet patch. Just beyond this, the trail splits. Either way will do; however, the trail to the right maintains a view of the bog. Traffic sounds waft from overhead as cars whoosh by on Hammond Pond Parkway. Below that, the woods are remarkably quiet. Track for the Green Line of Boston's commuter rail system runs along the far bank of the wetland, and from time to time a rattling train clatters by. Built around 1852, the downtown parts of the Green Line are the oldest and most heavily traveled in America. This rail is the D train that leads to Riverside station. It also provides T access to the trailhead if you'd like to avoid driving.

## Hammond Pond–Houghton Garden

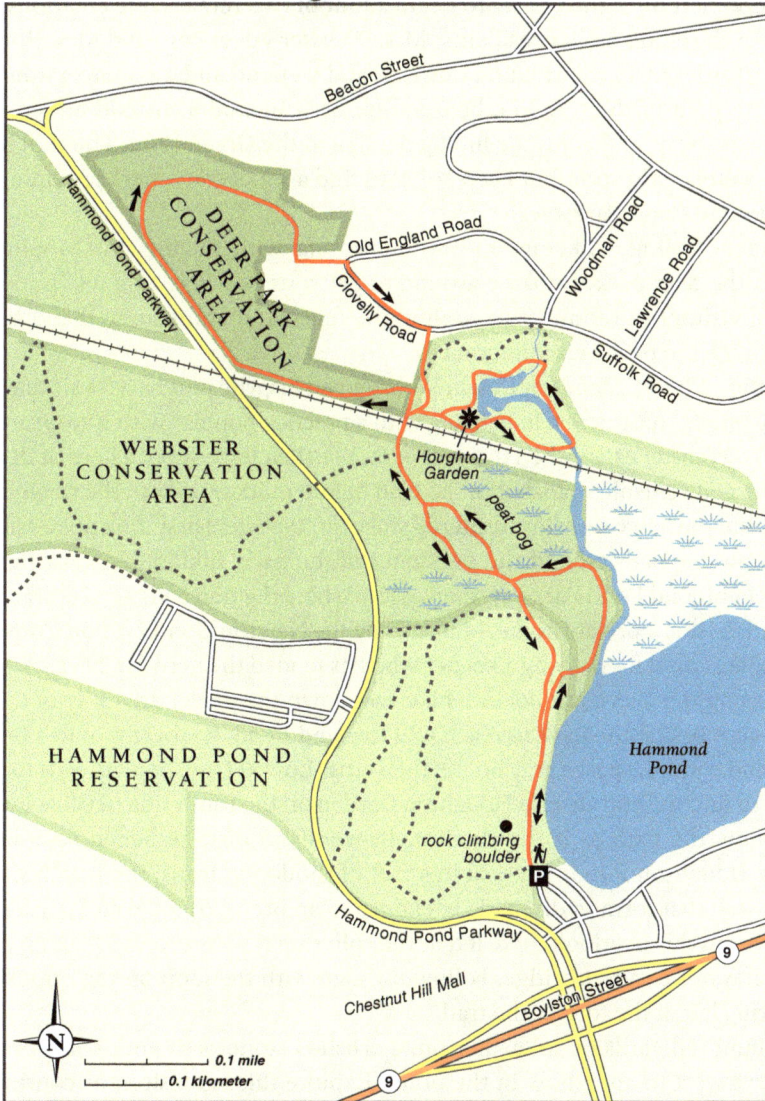

Ahead the trail veers west, away from the peat bog and a moment later meets with its other half joining from the left. Stay with the trail as it passes another path diverting left and arrives at a junction. Here Hammond Pond Parkway and the MBTA tracks cross paths, forming the northern boundary of the reservation. The trail to the left fords the flow of the parkway to connect with additional Webster conservation land. For this hike, continue right and follow blue blazes over the rails of the Green Line.

Set out left on a grassy lane to begin a tour of two remarkable creations that are gifts from the land's earlier residents: Mrs. Webster's deer park and Mrs. Houghton's garden. Bordered by the train on one side and wetland and a private garden on the other, the path leads west to a boarded-up barn behind a forbidding fence. Look left for a gateway, and continue hiking parallel to the Green Line. The trail becomes sketchy in this tight spot, but keep going to find a set of steel stairs providing an exit to Hammond Pond Parkway.

The sprawling, unkempt meadow erupting with granite outcroppings lying ahead is the deer park. Looking around to get your bearings, you will notice a sign advising visitors to refrain from scaling the fence and confirming that a trail does indeed trace the park's circumference.

In the early 19th century, Edwin Webster and his wife purchased a sizable piece of land, including these acres. In keeping with a practice popular with European aristocracy, Mrs. Webster established the deer park. She then introduced a herd of 24 animals. A unique and valuable snapshot of the land before modernization, the rugged grazing land within the fence remains unaltered since the Websters first took possession.

Follow the path around the perimeter of the park, hiking first west then north beside Hammond Pond Parkway, then east to where the trail ends at an entrance to the deer park beside a private home. Managed by the Newton Conservation Commission, the deer are cared for daily by a keeper who has tended the herd for 20 years.

Leaving the deer park behind, hike east down the gravel driveway of the stately brick house beside the park to reach Old England Road. Bear right onto a horseshoe curve, and continue past a gray house, then cross Lowell Lane (which leads to the train tracks) to find the entrance to Houghton Garden on the south side of Clovelly Road.

Follow the path as it travels through woods to a stone bench on a hill overlooking Houghton Pond. Dressed in a ruff of rhododendrons, the bench sits atop a granite wall that forms a dramatic backdrop to an orchestrated water garden 20 feet below. From this overlook, hike left at the split that travels southeast along a slender finger of water to a footbridge. Follow through with the loop on the opposite bank by bearing left at the fork in the trail.

A hundred yards or so farther on, a crushed stone path enters from the street and flows west to an oxbow in the pond. Explore this extension, or continue right to access a wooden bridge that crosses to meet an array of paths woven through an alpine rock garden on a bank beside the pond.

Martha Houghton established the garden in 1919. Today members of the Chestnut Hill Garden Club, in partnership with the friends of Houghton Garden and the City of Newton, strive to maintain it in accordance with Houghton's high standards. Said to be one of the first of its kind, the alpine rock garden includes climbing hydrangea, lily of the valley, wood hyacinth, and exotic evergreens such as the umbrella pine. When you're ready, follow the trail as it curves around a stone bench, climbs the steps, and joins the path to the entrance.

Once back on Clovelly Road, bear left onto Lowell Lane and backtrack across the Green Line to the south side of the reservation. Taking up the blue-blazed trail again, follow it southeast, staying right at each of its splits to return to the parking lot.

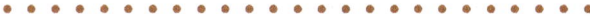

• • • • • • • • • • • • • • • • • • • • • • • • •

**GPS TRAILHEAD COORDINATES** N42° 19.378'  W71° 10.370'

**DIRECTIONS**  From Boston by car: Take MA 9 to the Hammond Pond Parkway exit. Turn right onto Hammond Pond Parkway and then right into the parking lot of the Chestnut Hill Mall. The trailhead is located in the northwest corner of the parking lot.

From Boston by public transportation: Take the D train (outbound to Riverside Station) on the MBTA Green Line to the Chestnut Hill station.

The serene swampland set within the forest at Hammond Pond

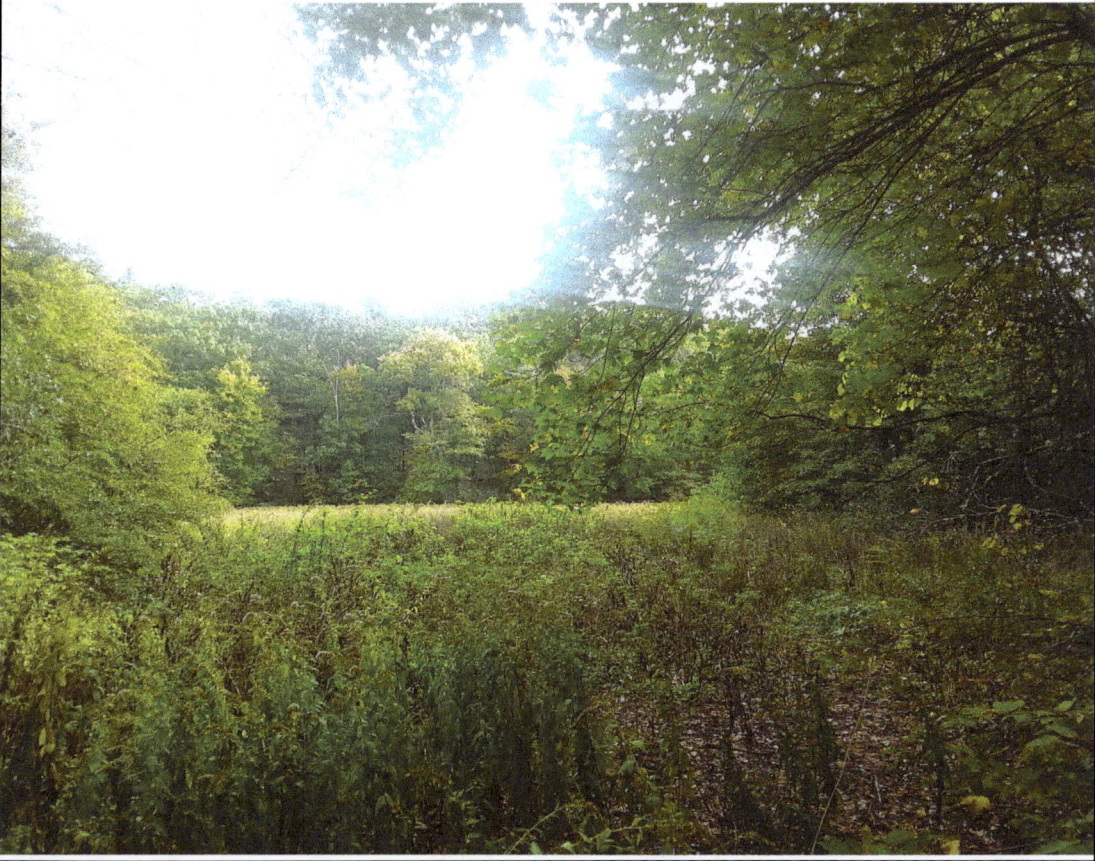

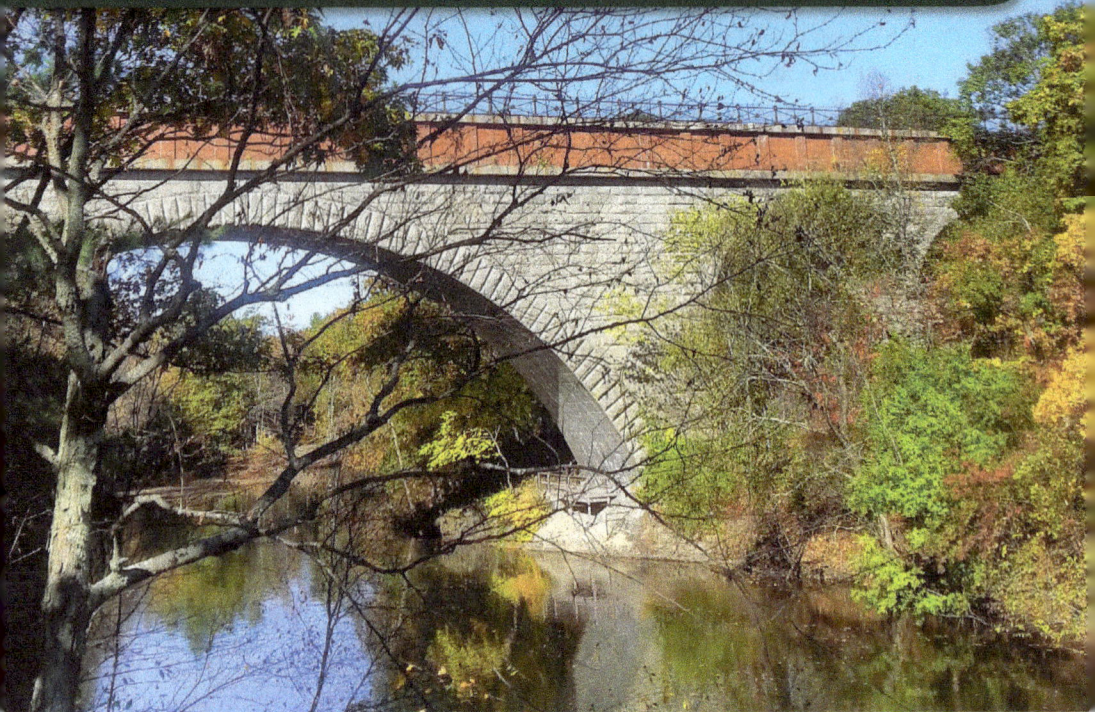

Hemlock Gorge is a great easy hike for your kids' first time out.

**THIS HIKE EXPLORES** the Charles River where it spills through a gorge cut by a glacier 10,000 years ago. After surveying the gorge from within a hemlock forest, the trail circles a small island in the river and then crosses the magnificent Echo Bridge.

## DESCRIPTION

Carved by the force of a retreating glacier 10,000 years ago, the Hemlock Gorge Reservation was once Massachusetts's equivalent of Niagara Falls. The trail that leads to Hemlock Gorge begins at the northern end of the small parking area. Follow the wide dirt road as it heads into woods between a quiet residential neighborhood to the left and the Charles River to the right.

Almost immediately, the road reaches a junction with another path that leads left; pass this and continue straight, even as you meet another trail heading right. A few yards farther on, under the calming canopy of the hemlocks, the whoosh of traffic on nearby MA 9 and I-95 fades and blends with the sound of the river below.

The trail is mostly hard-packed dirt with a few areas of flat rock. There are a couple of short hills, but for the most part this is a gentle hike suitable for anyone. At the next fork, bear left and climb a steep embankment. At the top, look right to

**DISTANCE & CONFIGURATION:** 1.3-mile loop

**DIFFICULTY:** Easy

**SCENERY:** View of the Charles River running through a spectacular gorge with water flowing over 2 dams

**EXPOSURE:** Shaded

**TRAFFIC:** Moderate

**TRAIL SURFACE:** Packed dirt and leaves

**HIKING TIME:** 30 minutes

**DRIVING DISTANCE FROM BOSTON COMMON:** 9 miles

**ELEVATION:** 132' at trailhead, no significant gain

**SEASON:** Year-round

**ACCESS:** Sunrise–sunset; free

**MAPS:** Posted at various locations in the reservation, or at mass.gov/eea/images/dcr /parks/trailmaps/hgorge.gif

**WHEELCHAIR ACCESS:** No

**FACILITIES:** Picnic tables

**CONTACT:** Massachusetts Dept. of Conservation and Resources, mass.gov/locations /hemlock-gorge-reservation, 617-626-1250

**LOCATION:** Newton, MA

**COMMENTS:** Before English colonists settled the area, the gorge was the fishing ground of the Ponkapoag people.

see Echo Bridge reaching across the water. Take a moment to enjoy the view. Then continue following the trail as it descends back into the woods.

The hemlocks of Hemlock Gorge, most well over a century and a half old, have been under attack by an infestation of hemlock woolly adelgid (*Adelges tsugae*) for several years. Though a little haggard, the trees are now showing signs of renewed vigor, thanks to the efforts of the Friends of Hemlock Gorge.

Go left at the next split in the trail, and make your way downhill past beech trees growing among the hemlocks. Follow the trail a short way farther to the northern-most tip of the reservation where the land falls off abruptly, and evergreen boughs block the view of the traffic opposite. The roar of water falling from the lip of a dam in the near distance will lure you to land's end.

Picking up the trail again, turn and follow it southeast against the current. Closer to the water, things are much quieter. Not far along, the trail arrives at a wooden bridge to a small island. Cross over and face south for a spectacular view of Echo Bridge and an old mill. This picturesque scene is nearly the same as it was in the late 1800s.

The trail loops over and around the rugged island. Following it northwest takes you to the circular dam at the end of the gorge. Follow the trail southeast to find the Devil's Den, a natural cave formed in the island's granite face, low on the western side.

Take the footbridge back to the mainland, and pick up the trail to the left, heading up a steep banking to return to where Echo Bridge touches land. Mount the step to this elegant piece of engineering (built in 1877 to bear the Sudbury River Aqueduct), and stroll across to the river's opposite bank.

Once on the other end, take the stairs down to the base of the bridge, cross Ellis Street, and descend one more flight of steps to get to the lookout platform below. Afterward, take the steps back up to the riverbank, and look for a path to the left.

## Hemlock Gorge Reservation

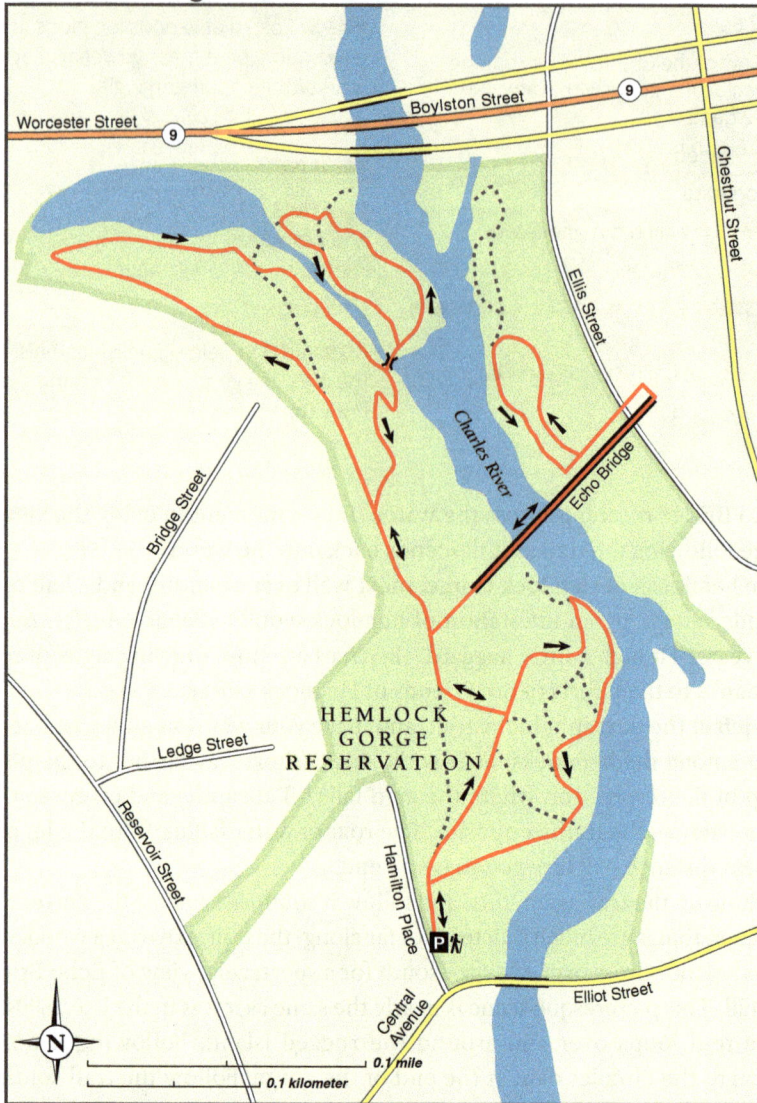

Follow this short route northeast along the river to the edge of a small field, and then loop back to the bridge.

Climb the stairs once more to the promenade, and head back to the other side of the Charles River. Though people gave up swimming in the gorge back in the 1970s, the water flowing through is becoming healthier every year. Thanks to environmental cleanup efforts, the air wafting from the turbulent river smells fresh and fortifying.

Once back on the western side, take the path to the left, which leads back down to the river's edge. Here, where the river narrows and bends in an oxbow, you will find a small sandy beach edged with crabapple trees. The trail takes you close to a second dam and a reclaimed mill on the opposite bank. From here, follow the path up a hill behind a brick building and then down again to a field that stretches along the river. Traverse this acre of green to arrive back at the parking lot.

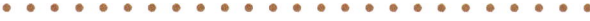

• • • • • • • • • • • • • • • • • • • • • • • • • • • •

**GPS TRAILHEAD COORDINATES** N42° 18.767'  W71° 13.667'

**DIRECTIONS**  From Boston, take MA 9 W. Exit at Boylston Street, before the MA 128 overpass. Take a left onto Chestnut Street and a right onto Eliot Street. Make an immediate right onto Hamilton Place. Park at the small lot near the Hemlock Gorge Reservation bulletin board. There's also a small parking area on Ellis Street closer to MA 9.

The view of the falls makes this walk well worth it.

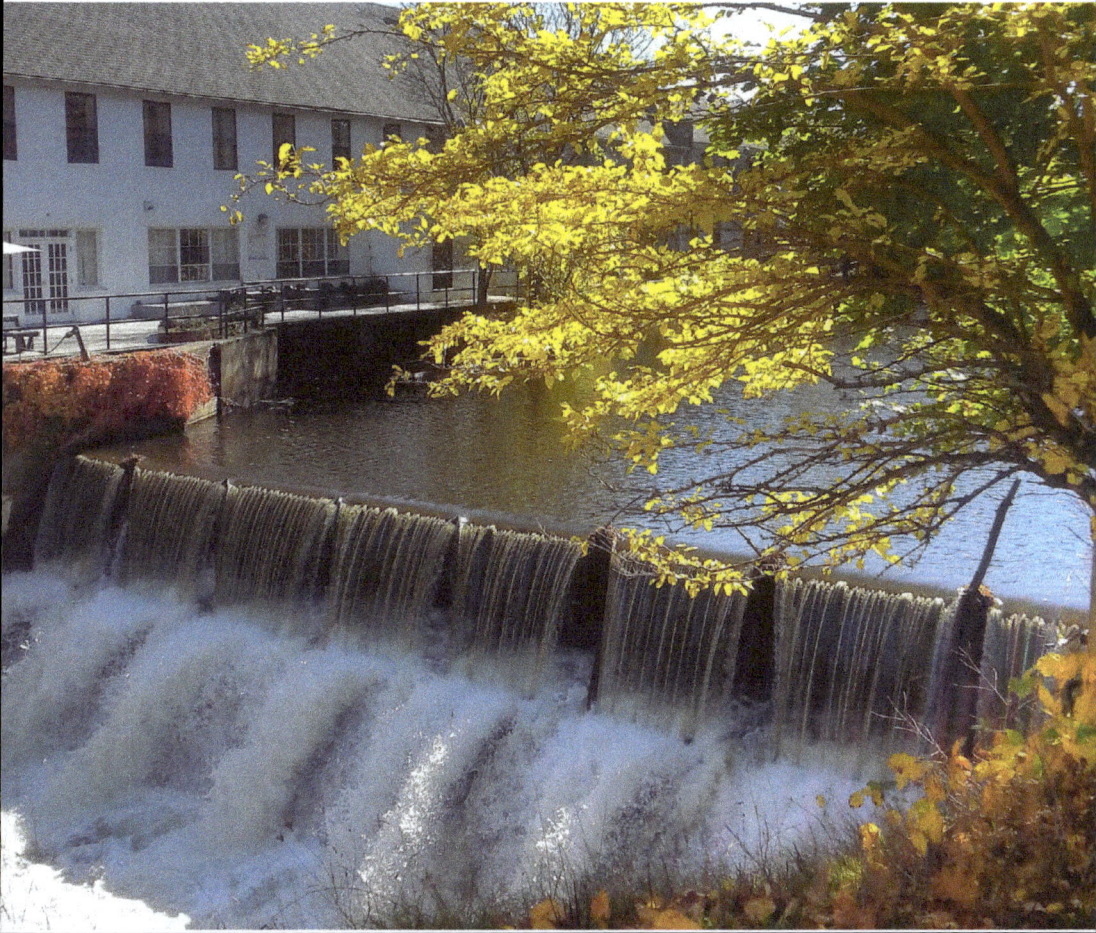

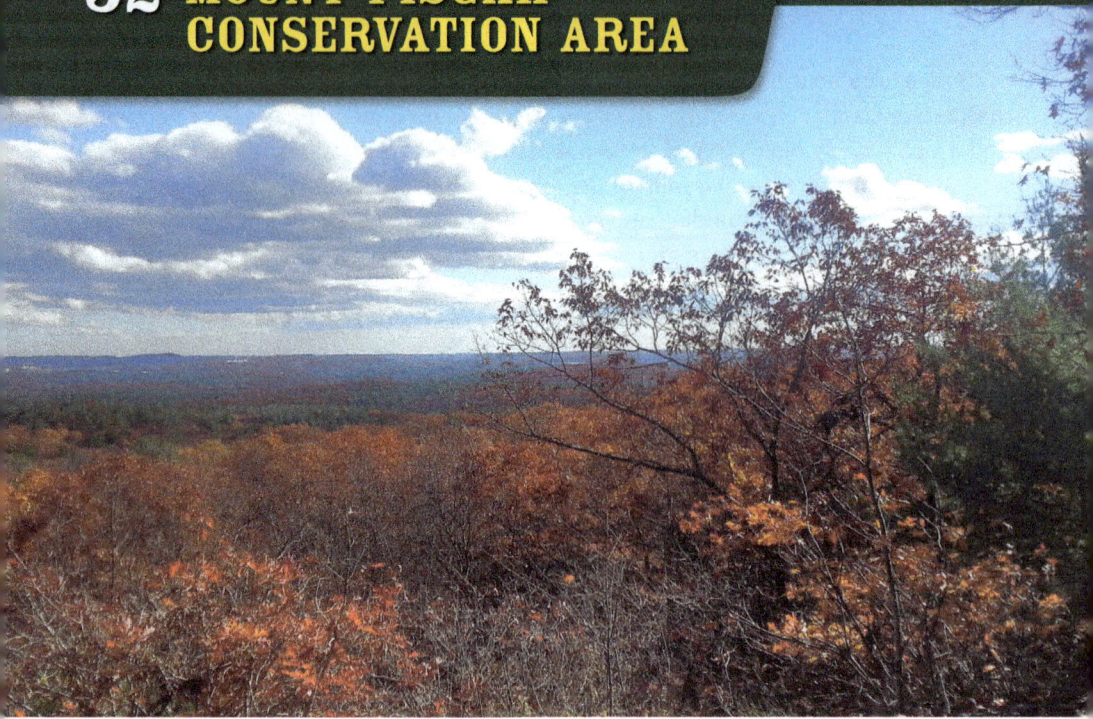

You'll be rewarded with sweeping views from atop Mount Pisgah.

**LOCATED IN ONE** of the more rural areas near Boston, this hike travels through a dense forest and rolling hills that have the feel of unfettered wilderness, despite once being mostly farmland.

## DESCRIPTION

Begin your hike by setting out from the Smith Road parking lot on the Mentzer Trail. Aiming straight toward the summit, this broad trail ascends ever so gently through the dense, tall forest. A stone wall, proof of the hill's former life as pastureland, runs parallel 20 feet or so to the right.

Approaching wetland as it dips and bends northeast, the trail crosses over Howard Brook. Highbush blueberry, swamp azalea, sweet pepperbush, arrowwood, pungent skunk cabbage, and rare swamp oak grow here, supporting game such as fierce fisher cats, coyotes, bobcats, and black bears.

Shortly after crossing the brook, the trail will come to a split. Bear right on the red-blazed Sparrow Trail. Continue south along the base of the hill. The trail becomes a bit narrower as it rises and falls through the forest. This section of trail serves as a warm-up as it winds through a fairly dense forest of pine, oak, birch, beech, and, most notably, thriving sugar maple.

**DISTANCE & CONFIGURATION:** 4.75-mile double loop

**DIFFICULTY:** Moderate

**SCENERY:** Hardwood forest on abandoned farmland, 2 gorges, 2 scenic vistas, Boston's skyline on clear days

**EXPOSURE:** Mostly shade

**TRAFFIC:** Light

**TRAIL SURFACE:** Packed dirt, some rocky areas

**HIKING TIME:** 3 hours

**DRIVING DISTANCE FROM BOSTON COMMON:** 39 miles

**ELEVATION:** 579' at trailhead, 702' at highest point

**SEASON:** Year-round

**ACCESS:** Sunrise–sunset; free

**MAPS:** Available at tinyurl.com/mount pisgahmap

**WHEELCHAIR ACCESS:** No

**FACILITIES:** None

**CONTACT:** Sudbury Valley Trustees, svtweb.org, 978-443-5588

**LOCATION:** Berlin, MA

**COMMENTS:** Fisher cats, a ferocious relative of the weasel, are frequently seen on the trails. These dark-brown, nimble animals can weigh up to 30 pounds. Do not try to catch or corner one of these critters.

Shortly after winding eastward, the Sparrow Trail meets the blue-blazed Berlin Road Trail. Turn right to head south again. Here, in late summer, you might catch the lemony smell of witch hazel (*Hamamelis virginiana*) wafting on the air.

Coasting downhill on an easy grade, the Berlin Road Trail soon enters a wildlife-management area. Here the trail arches east, passing a kiosk and the start of the yellow-blazed Howard Ridge Trail. Turn right at this junction and continue southeast along the rocky spine of an esker, the left side of which falls precipitously into a deep ravine.

A short distance ahead, the trail meets the blue-blazed Howard Brook Trail, which diverges to the right. Follow this trail to descend the esker's western slope. A few feet farther, at another split, continue left and hike downhill on a particularly twisty route. Winding among ash, birch, and hemlock trees and up and over glacial debris, the trail eventually leads to Howard Brook and then reunites with the Howard Ridge Trail. Here you'll pass the Green Street Trail, oddly marked with red blazes, on the right.

From this intersection hike east, following the yellow blazes of the Howard Ridge Trail a few yards to find the red-blazed South Gorge Trail. Turn right to leave the ridge and head for the dramatic gorge beside the esker. Near the start of the trail sits a wooden footbridge looking like a barge on a sandbar. Once past the bridge, the trail bends sharply northeast and climbs out of the gorge along its far banking. Almost sheer rock, this slope has a forbidding feel.

Looping right at a twisted oak high above the gorge, the trail divides at an intersection. Add the South Ridge Loop to your hike by continuing southwest, or stay with the South Gorge Trail, heading south.

After the split, the South Gorge Trail settles on level ground and enters a forest of mostly beech and pine. Winding left and east, the trail reaches another junction.

## Mount Pisgah Conservation Area

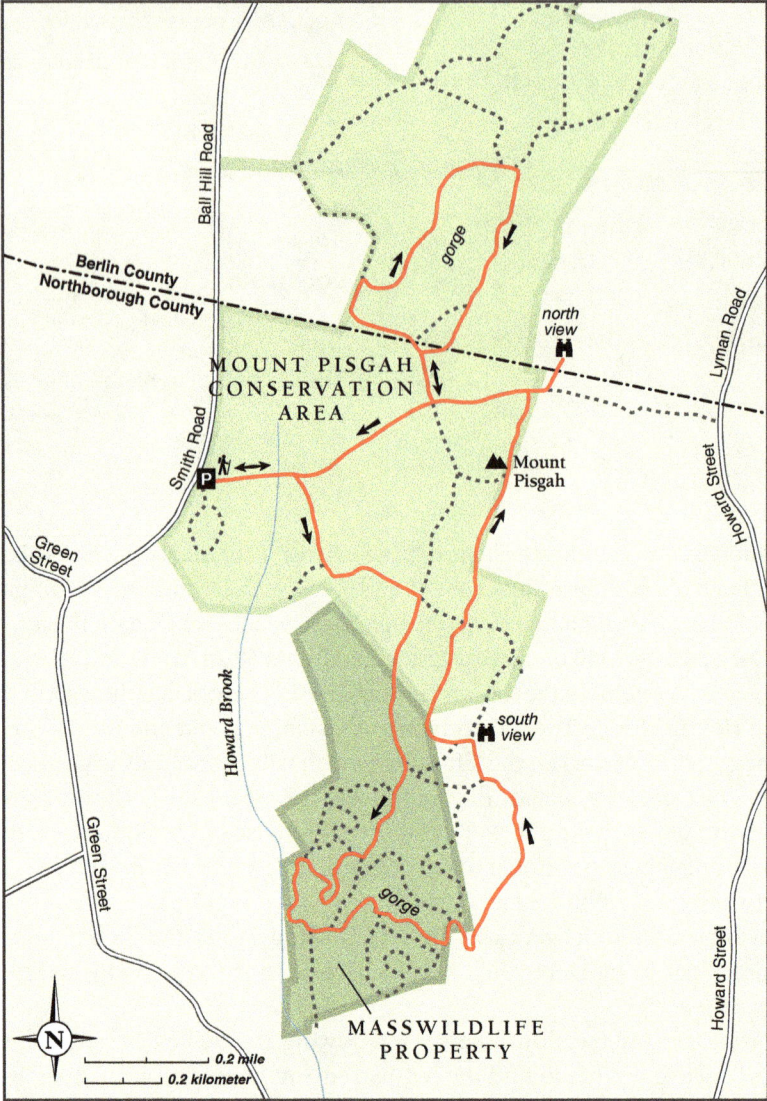

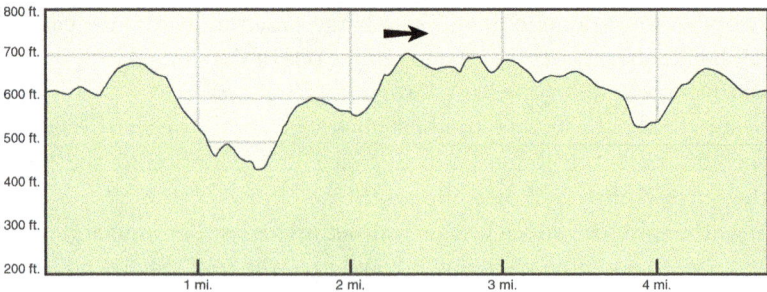

Ball Hill Road

gorge

Berlin County
Northborough County

north
view

MOUNT PISGAH
CONSERVATION
AREA

Smith Road

Lyman Road

P

Mount
Pisgah

Howard Street

Green
Street

Howard Brook

south
view

Green Street

gorge

Howard Street

MASSWILDLIFE
PROPERTY

N

0.2 mile
0.2 kilometer

800 ft.
700 ft.
600 ft.
500 ft.
400 ft.
300 ft.
200 ft.

1 mi.     2 mi.     3 mi.     4 mi.

The Vernal Pool Trail forks off in two directions from this spot, and the South Gorge Trail veers right to feed into the Fisher Trail.

Getting under way, the Fisher Trail jogs left to make a near-straight run north. Except for minor bumps and dips, the trail stays level and dry, crossing through sun-lit groves of young birch, beech, and sometimes hemlock. Someone with a keen eye might even single out American chestnuts sprouting here.

Leaving a decrepit stone wall behind, the trail curves northwest and arrives at a stack of stones with a trail marker. Look for the red triangles of the Fisher Trail and make a quick turn to head up a steep slope. Winding over packed earth, the trail soon reaches a grassy plateau.

From this peak, pick up the Tyler Trail, heading northwest away from the Sparrow Trail (also marked with red blazes). A half mile along, when these two trails intersect, continue on along the Tyler Trail. The hiking is fairly easy as the trail follows along the top of this hill. When the blueberry bushes are full of ripe fruit late in the summer, there's no need to hurry.

Ahead the land slopes gently. Tracing the contour, the Tyler Trail edges higher and soon reaches Mount Pisgah's highest point. The view was probably more impressive back in the farming days, when the 715-foot peak was cleared of trees, but it is still the highest point in Northborough.

Continuing north beyond the summit, the Tyler Trail rubs shoulders with remnant stone walls as it tapers downhill to meet the top end of the Mentzer Trail. Before following the yellow markers of this trail west, take a few more steps east for a view from Mount Pisgah's northernmost point. From the northern lookout, return to the Mentzer Trail, and follow its rocky course to a nearby intersection with the Berlin Road Trail.

The parking lot lies less than 0.5 mile ahead on the Mentzer Trail, so if the sun is low, hike on through. If you have plenty of daylight, plenty of energy, and the weather is fine, veer right onto the rutted cart road running northwest to the Northborough–Berlin border, and continue your exploration.

A short distance ahead, the road reaches a stone wall along the town line. A gap in the wall makes way for the road as it continues northwest, passing a trail to the right and a sign posted by the Berlin Conservation Commission.

Once you are in Berlin, the Berlin Road Trail narrows and looks more like a footpath than a cart road. Although its course remains clear, trail markers are few and far between. Making its way through pinewoods, the path soon swings abruptly right, zigzagging around two mammoth pines. A few yards farther along, the path passes a house on the left that is well concealed by trees.

Beyond the house, the trail reaches a junction. One route, marked with yellow, continues along a stone wall. The other cuts right to head east. Choose the latter, following it downhill to where it meets the North Gorge Trail, splitting to the right at a tree decorated with three markers—two yellow and one white.

Rough, wild, and haunting, the view within the gorge is the most beautiful of the hike. Pale-yellow blazes mark the route as it weaves south along a rocky ridge above a brook and a broad floodplain. Toward the southernmost end of the gorge, the trail descends to the brook and a chaotic convergence of stone walls. From this deep cleft in the land, the trail bends west as it climbs free of the shadowy recesses. Reaching level ground, the trail arrives back at the Northborough–Berlin border.

From here, bear left to return to where the Mentzer Trail bisects the Berlin Road Trail. At the junction, follow yellow markers southwest down an easy grade through forest that transitions from pine to red oak. White pine is known to grab a foothold soon after farmland is abandoned. Once the pines thin out, fast-growing red oak takes over. As time passes and the woods mature, other shade-tolerant species will supplant the red oak, and the forest becomes more diverse.

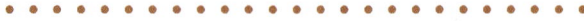

• • • • • • • • • • • • • • • • • • • • • • • • • • • • •

**GPS TRAILHEAD COORDINATES** N42° 21.583'  W71° 40.267'

**DIRECTIONS**  From Boston take I-90 W to Exit 11A and merge onto I-495 N toward Marlborough. Follow I-495 N to Exit 26 and MA 62. Follow MA 62 west into Berlin to Linden Street. Bear left on Linden Street. Follow this to Ball Hill Road and turn left. Ball Hill Road becomes Smith Road. A sign on the right designates a parking area for the trails.

Deeper into the forest at Mount Pisgah

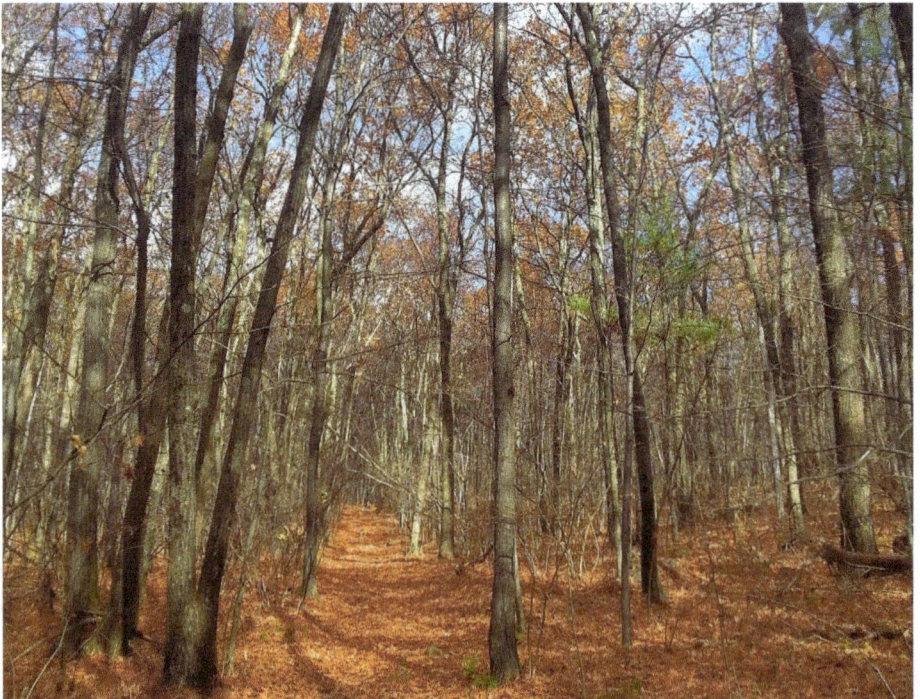

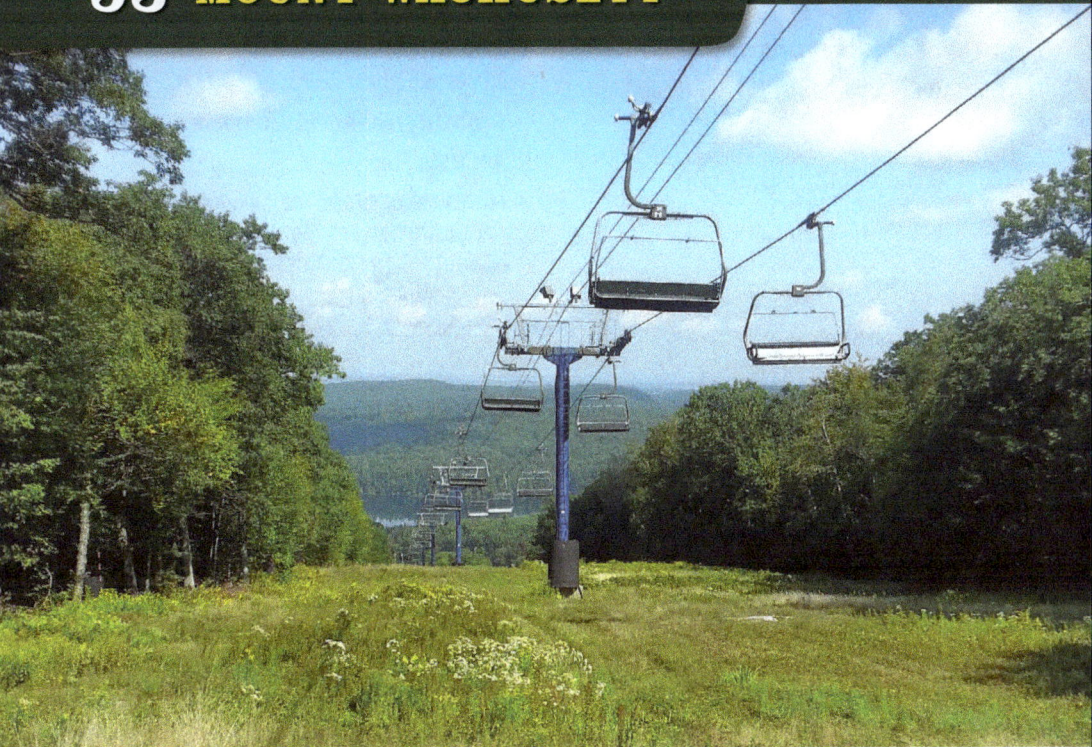

Mount Wachusett is a spectacular place to be in all seasons.

**LOOPING AROUND MOUNT WACHUSETT,** this hike eventually climbs its northeastern face to reach a spectacular view from the peak.

## DESCRIPTION

A popular ski area during the winter months, Mount Wachusett also has an impressive network of hiking trails winding up and around the mountain. From the parking lot beside the Mount Wachusett base lodge, walk right, past the base of the Monadnock Chairlift and the snowmaking garage, to find the start of Balance Rock Trail, located to the right of the magic carpet ski lift that serves the learning area.

As you step into the woods on a quiet morning, you may be lucky enough to hear the sound of loon calls from the lake across the parking lot. A few feet onto the trail, thanks to the quiet of the forest and the shade of hardwoods, the resort atmosphere vanishes. Two diamond-shaped markers—one blue, one yellow—identify the trail as two routes, blue for Balance Rock Trail and yellow for the 92-mile Midstate Trail that passes over Mount Wachusett.

Rising steeply at first, the broad trail of firmly packed dirt and rocks winds as it climbs under hemlock bows. Mountain laurels punctuate the underbrush in wetter areas. About 0.25 mile into the woods, the trail is interrupted by a sandy, unpaved

**DISTANCE & CONFIGURATION:** 5.74-mile loop

**DIFFICULTY:** Moderate, with some easy and some strenuous sections

**SCENERY:** This hike loops around the 2,006-foot Mount Wachusett. The top offers a spectacular view of the Berkshires to the west, Mount Monadnock to the north, and Boston's skyline to the east.

**EXPOSURE:** Mostly shaded

**TRAFFIC:** Moderate

**TRAIL SURFACE:** Packed dirt and some rocky sections

**HIKING TIME:** 3.5 hours

**DRIVING DISTANCE FROM BOSTON COMMON:** 59 miles

**ELEVATION:** 1,026' at trailhead, 2,000' at highest point

**SEASON:** Year-round without restrictions

**ACCESS:** Free

**MAPS:** Available at mass.gov/eea/docs/dcr /parks/trails/wachusett.pdf

**WHEELCHAIR ACCESS:** The trails in this hike are not wheelchair traversable; however, the peak is accessible by a paved service road.

**FACILITIES:** Picnic tables at the summit

**CONTACT:** Massachusetts Dept. of Conservation and Resources, tinyurl.com/wachusettmountain, 617-626-1250

**LOCATION:** Princeton, MA

road. Turn right at this intersection, and follow the road a few yards to a sign on the left for Balance Rock. Leave the road here, and take this short path for a look at this geological spectacle.

Loop back to the road on the Balance Rock Trail, and look south to find the start of Old Indian Trail. The trail is well worn from the passage of many moccasins and boots over the years. It makes a steep climb over roots and rocks 1.3 miles to the summit. For a less direct route on this hike, switch to the Semuhenna Trail when the two trails break. The Old Indian Trail continues straight while the Semuhenna Trail turns to the right, heading southwest. Quite a few turns and different trails make up this hike, so if you can, get your hands on a map before setting out.

At this slightly higher elevation, the wind whistles through the bare treetops. Soon the trail passes between a gap in an old stone wall that runs seemingly without purpose through the trees. There is frequent evidence of the stone walls that once defined the landscape here when it was all farmland.

After making its way south through the shelter of hemlocks, the trail reaches the auto road to the top of Mount Wachusett. Cross over the road to stay with the Semuhenna Trail. From here, the trail levels out and passes through a stand of young beeches. A series of small bridges offers dry passage over a muddy area as the path climbs just short of the peak. Coming into the open, the Semuhenna Trail passes a group of picnic tables and signs for other trails. Having approached the mountain's highest point, the Semuhenna Trail again crosses the paved summit access road and then ducks off to the southeast.

Circling around the mountaintop at a fairly constant elevation just shy of the peak, the Semuhenna Trail turns east. Dark flanks of granite make a wall to the left, and moss-covered fallen trees and displaced boulders lie to the right on the downhill slope.

# Mount Wachusett

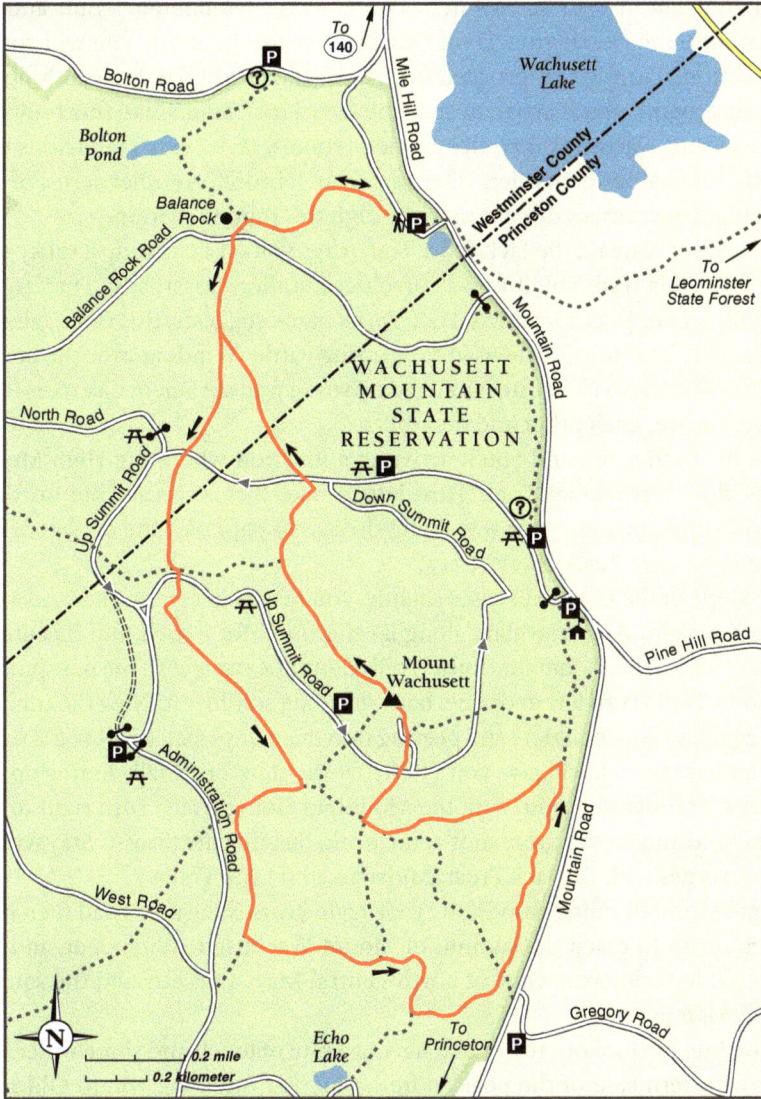

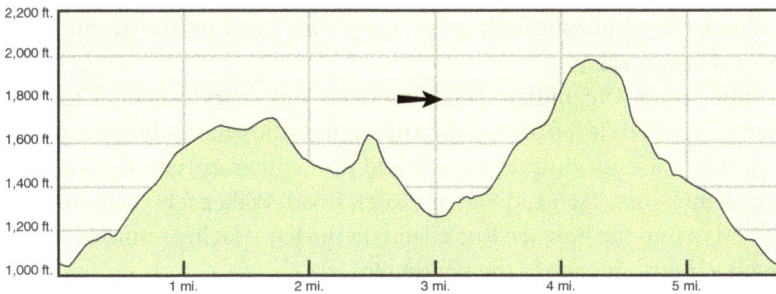

To 140

*Wachusett Lake*

Bolton Road

*Bolton Pond*

Mile Hill Road

Westminster County
Princeton County

*Balance Rock*

Balance Rock Road

To
Leominster
State Forest

Mountain Road

WACHUSETT
MOUNTAIN
STATE
RESERVATION

North Road

Up Summit Road

Down Summit Road

Up Summit Road

Pine Hill Road

*Mount Wachusett*

Administration Road

West Road

Echo Lake

To Princeton

Gregory Road

N

0.2 mile
0.2 kilometer

2,200 ft.
2,000 ft.
1,800 ft.
1,600 ft.
1,400 ft.
1,200 ft.
1,000 ft.

1 mi.    2 mi.    3 mi.    4 mi.    5 mi.

When the trail arrives at an intersection, leave Semuhenna Trail, and turn right (west) onto the Harrington Trail. Shortly after this junction, you will come to another junction. Turn left to proceed on Lower Link Trail. Hiking south now on relatively flat ground, you'll arrive next at the Jack Frost Trail. Take this trail to the left and travel east. Narrower than the previous routes, Jack Frost Trail winds uphill past laurels growing beside rivulets diverting from a brook. Another series of short wooden bridges guarantees dry crossing through this muddy section.

From this wet plateau, the Jack Frost Trail takes you on a climb up a rocky slope. Emerging from this trail, you'll find yourself at another crossroads. Turn right to hike downhill on the High Meadows Trail. As its name suggests, this route takes you southwest across land previously used for grazing cattle. Winding over the curve of the hill, the trail leads to two plateaus edged by stone walls. Ancient oak trees lean in to spread shade over each other and the trail.

Hike a bit farther on, and you'll arrive at a junction where the High Meadow Trail meets the Bicentennial Trail. Turn left to take Bicentennial Trail northeast. Continue downhill, picking your way along the rough path past the occasional wizened oak and younger black cherry trees.

As the slope of the mountain eases slightly, you may hear cars on the road a short distance to the right. After traveling along level ground for a spell, the Bicentennial Trail intersects with the Mountain House Trail. Continue straight to the next junction, with the Loop Trail. Turn left to double back, heading southwest. Now the trail takes you uphill again, scaling boulders and peering into the many small caves you'll pass.

This rigorous stretch will give you a hefty workout before finally letting up upon your arrival at another junction, with the Mountain House Trail. Turn right to leave the rocks behind and take a direct shot at the peak, heading northwest. Stay with this trail as it converges with the Jack Frost, Midstate, and Link Trails.

Emerging from thinning woods, the trail again crosses the auto road then makes one last run north to reach the summit of Mount Wachusett. Wide open and bare, the peak provides a fantastic view of north-central Massachusetts and the southern edge of New Hampshire.

After scaling the lookout tower and having a bite of lunch and some water, cross to the northwestern side of the peak to find a marker directing you to Old Indian Trail. Following this gentle path through the woods, you soon come to a ski lift, which in all seasons—but especially when there's no snow on the ground—resembles some kind of spaceship.

From here, trace Old Indian Trail's crooked trajectory downhill to where it crosses the auto road. Hike left and resume the trail on the other side of the pavement. Continuing, the trail leads through woods and three times crosses ski slopes before meeting the Semuhenna Trail and Balance Rock Road. Walk a few yards downhill on the sandy road to find the Balance Rock Trail on the left. Having returned to the first trail of the hike, follow it back to the parking lot.

*Note:* Mount Wachusett is a superb hawk-watching venue from September to November, with as many as 12,000 hawks sighted per season over the last 24 years. Autumn is a wonderful time to hike Mount Wachusett, but if you are planning to venture into the woods between mid-October and mid-December, play it safe and wear bright colors, preferably orange. Avoid wearing white or brown.

## NEARBY ATTRACTIONS

Those spending a weekend in the area might consider visiting the Wachusett Meadow Wildlife Sanctuary, located at 113 Goodnow Road, Princeton. Managed by the Massachusetts Audubon Society, the sanctuary offers 12 miles of trails and an abundance of wildlife in addition to a wheelchair-accessible nature center. Admission is $4 for nonmember adults and $3 for nonmember children ages 3–12 and senior citizens. For more information, call 978-464-2712.

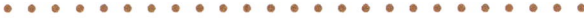

· · · · · · · · · · · · · · · · · · · · · · · · · · ·

**GPS TRAILHEAD COORDINATES** N42° 30.317'  W71° 53.067'

**DIRECTIONS**  From Boston, take MA 2 to Exit 25 (MA 140 S). Follow MA 140 south 2 miles. Turn right onto Park Road at the Mount Wachusett Ski Area sign. Follow Park Road 0.5 mile to the split in the road. Bear left at fork onto Mountain Road. Follow Mountain Road another 0.5 mile or so. The reservation entrance is clearly marked on the right. The Mount Wachusett ski lodge and visitor center are immediately on the left once you enter the reservation.

Don't forget your supplemental oxygen to summit Mount Wachusett.

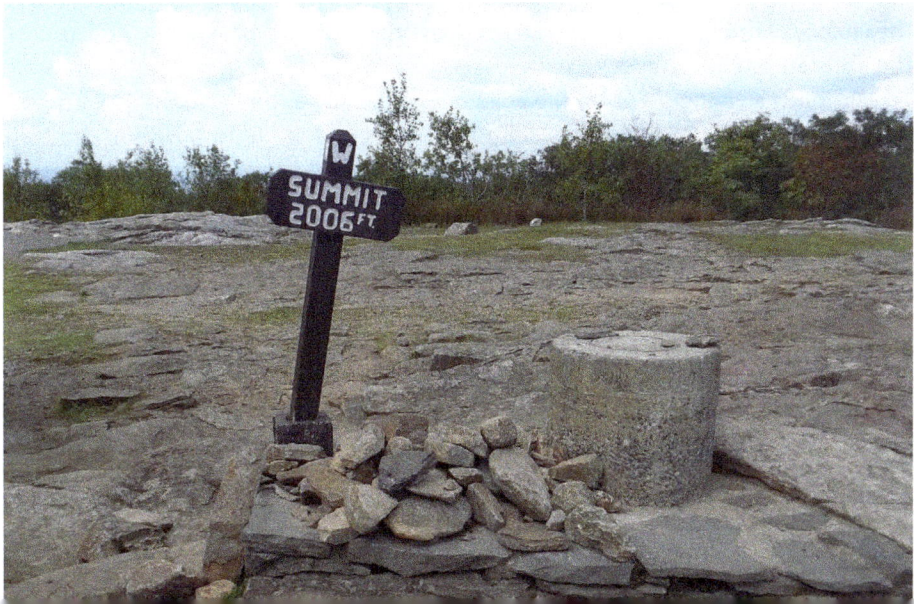

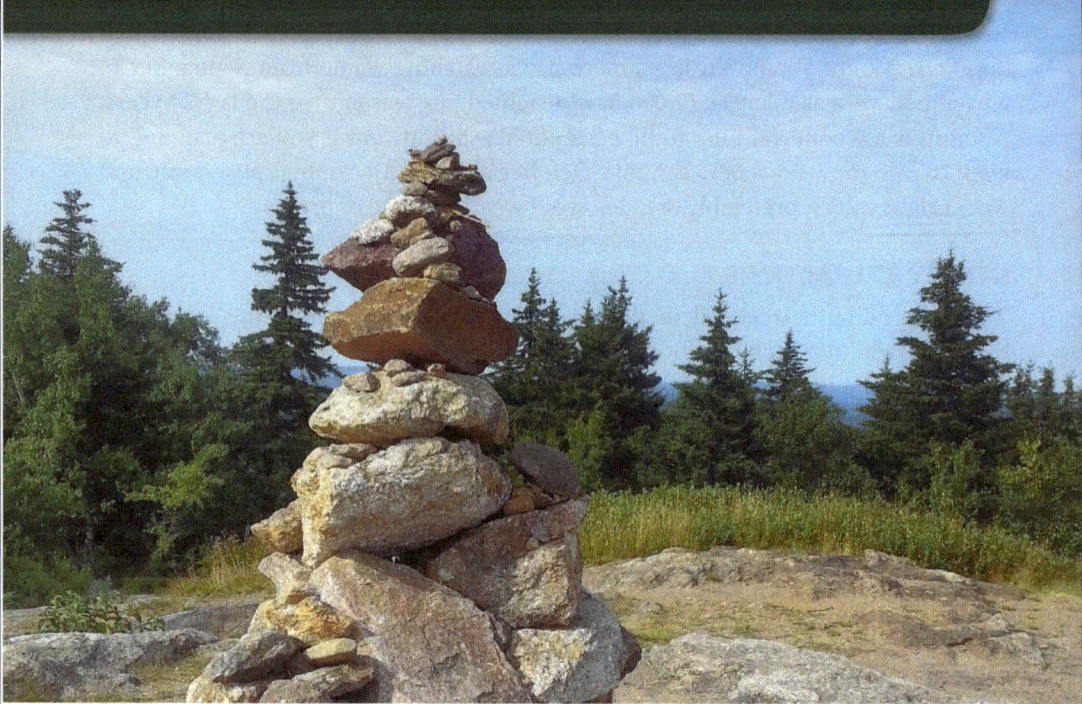

This elaborate cairn marks the summit of Mount Watatic.

**AFTER MAKING A** strenuous ascent to the peak of Mount Watatic, you continue north to scale the lesser peak of Nutting Hill, swing west to the Massachusetts–New Hampshire border, and then ease back to the start.

## DESCRIPTION

Mount Watatic offers not only an exhilarating get-away-from-it-all day hike but also the chance of doing as Henry David Thoreau urged. It is a portal to two epic routes, the Midstate and the Wapack Trails.

From its starting point on the edge of Rhode Island, the Midstate Trail travels north 95 miles, clear across Massachusetts, to its end at Nutting Hill on the New Hampshire border. At 21 miles long, the Wapack Trail is comparatively modest in length but equally inspired and worthy.

This hike starts out on the logging road behind the metal gate at the far side of the parking lot. From this point to the border of New Hampshire, the recently rerouted Midstate Trail and the Wapack Trail follow the same course, identified by yellow triangles. After dipping to wetland dammed by beavers, the logging road reaches a turnoff at 0.23 mile. Bear right and continue uphill over an obstacle course of tree roots to a map kiosk. After this gentle warm-up and adjustments to clothing or backpack straps, follow the trail as it drops to cross a stream then climbs east under hemlocks.

**DISTANCE & CONFIGURATION:** 3.5-mile loop

**DIFFICULTY:** Moderate

**SCENERY:** Woods of hemlock, birch, and beech, with a view from the peak of Mount Watatic

**EXPOSURE:** Mostly shaded

**TRAFFIC:** Light–heavy, depending on the season and day of the week

**TRAIL SURFACE:** Packed dirt and granite in the form of gravel, glacial erratics, or exposed sheets

**HIKING TIME:** 2 hours

**DRIVING DISTANCE FROM BOSTON COMMON:** 54 miles

**ELEVATION:** 1,250' at trailhead, 1,830' at highest point

**SEASON:** Year-round

**ACCESS:** Sunrise–sunset; free

**MAPS:** Available through Friends of Wapack at wapack.org

**WHEELCHAIR ACCESS:** No

**FACILITIES:** None

**CONTACT:** Massachusetts Dept. of Conservation and Resources, tinyurl.com/mountwatatic, 617-626-1250

**LOCATION:** Ashburnham, MA

**COMMENTS:** The peak of Mount Watatic is a fabulous place to watch hawks migrate from September through the first weeks of November. More than 7,000 often fly over Mount Watatic in a given season. Hikers are advised to not leave valuables in their cars.

As it progresses up the side of Mount Watatic, the trail broadens, and the trail surface becomes much rockier, with lengths seemingly paved with loose cobblestones. After becoming markedly steeper and exposed, the trail bends to a gentler pitch and, slinking back under hemlock cover, emerges at an outcropping the size of an opera box, with a view of Mount Monadnock.

Beyond the lookout, the trail rises to meet a stone wall along a ridge, evidence that these lands were all once farmed. In fact, when Thoreau visited the area in 1852, the rolling landscape was virtually treeless.

Once at this stone wall, the trail levels off to offer another terrific view, looking out over what was likely pasture but is now a sparse wood of wind-whipped oaks. A few feet farther on, if the weather obliges, Mount Wachusett is visible to the southwest. Overlapping peaks spread across the horizon.

Turning east again, the trail cuts over the stone wall and heads back into the hemlock wood, passing a swampy grove thick with vivid green ferns. To the left, maple saplings mix with young effervescent pines. Ahead, a boggy glade emerges and provides a surprise respite. Continuing southeast, the trail makes a stumbling ascent over granite chunks to the remains of a shelter crumbled amid hemlocks.

Climb from this plateau up one more thigh-testing slope to reach the top. The almost bald 1,832-foot peak provides a stunning panoramic view. Since a fire tower was removed in 1997, and the lifts from the ski area that once operated on the western side of the mountain were dismantled, the monadnock has been free of man-made obstructions. And as of July 10, 2002—thanks to a Herculean effort by the Massachusetts Division of Fisheries and Wildlife, the Ashby Land Trust, and the Ashburnham Conservation Trust—the mountain is forever protected from development.

## Mount Watatic Reservation

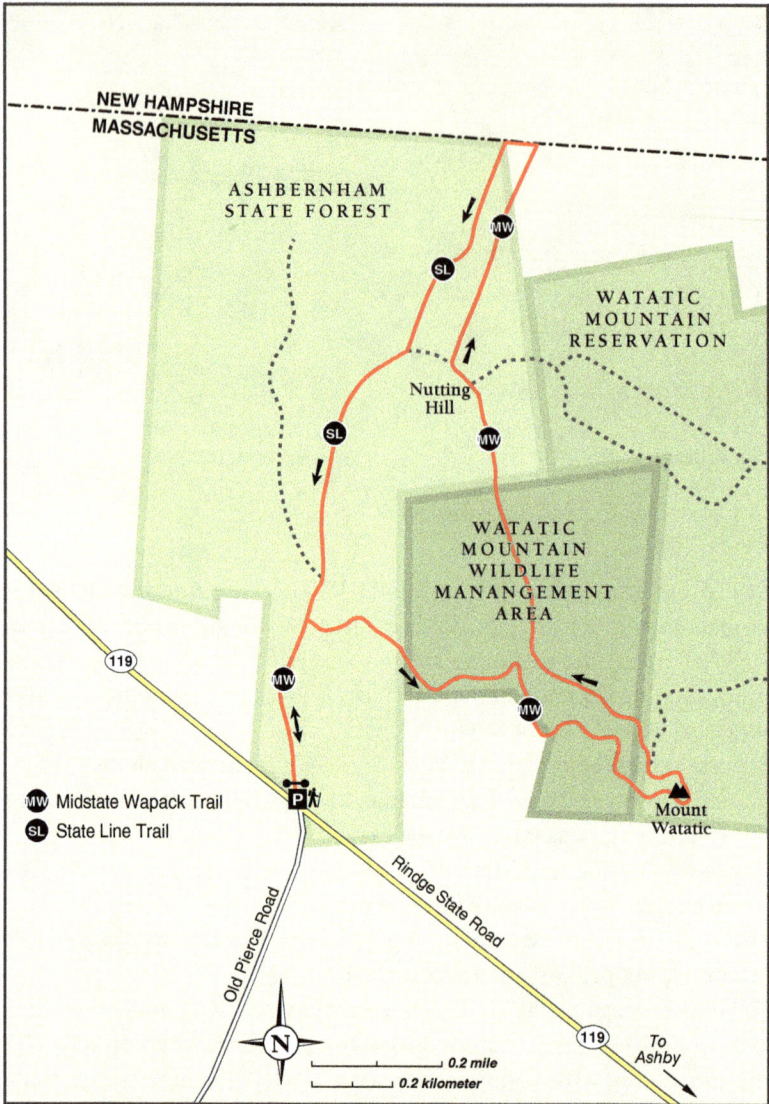

NEW HAMPSHIRE
MASSACHUSETTS

ASHBERNHAM
STATE FOREST

MW

SL

WATATIC
MOUNTAIN
RESERVATION

Nutting
Hill

SL

MW

WATATIC
MOUNTAIN
WILDLIFE
MANANGEMENT
AREA

119

MW

MW

**MW** Midstate Wapack Trail
**SL** State Line Trail

P

Mount
Watatic

Old Pierce Road

Rindge State Road

N

0.2 mile

0.2 kilometer

119

To
Ashby

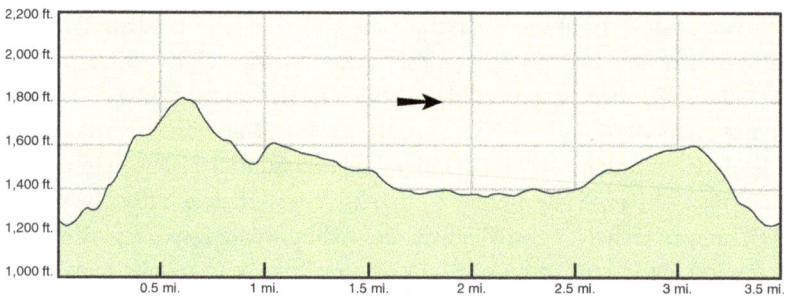

2,200 ft.
2,000 ft.
1,800 ft.
1,600 ft.
1,400 ft.
1,200 ft.
1,000 ft.

0.5 mi.    1 mi.    1.5 mi.    2 mi.    2.5 mi.    3 mi.    3.5 mi.

From the meadowlike peak, take the partially constructed gravel road north several yards to a narrow path to the left. Starting downhill, this trail joins a stone wall as it fixes on a northwest trajectory. Forming a U like the humps of a camel, the trail links the peak of Watatic to the knob of Nutting Hill. If hiking in early summer, plan to picnic here on the hill's granite flanks. Abundant blueberries will be your dessert.

Here and there, minor paths feed in from the edges. Continue over the contours of Nutting Hill, following the yellow triangle blazes. Ahead at the intersection, heed the arrows pointing right, toward New Hampshire. Cut wide to accommodate cross-country skiers. This grassy, relatively rock-free section eases downhill a short way then nearly levels as it projects northeast.

Stone walls on either side pencil in this well-traveled road. Farther on to the left, it passes the foundation of what might have been a shepherd's shelter. Farther still, the trail passes a T junction, where a path marked with white enters to the right through a gap in a stone wall. Continue past these to the junction at the New Hampshire border.

Those interested in a longer hike north to New Ipswich, Pack Monadnock, and beyond would continue north here. Sprightly arrows pointing straight ahead to a road-wide path make such wanderlust hard to resist. However, stick with the plan, and bear left (northwest). A trail marked MIDSTATE EXPRESS barrels in from the left and right, conveying hikers to the start or the finish of their cross-state trek. A hundred yards or so ahead, flush with a stone wall, the trail leads to two granite blocks, one engraved A&A MASS 1894, and the other, THE MIDSTATE TRAIL 1985.

To finish the circuit back to the parking lot, bear away from the stone wall, and hike southwest under hemlocks that practically shut out daylight. Follow the blue blazes as this spindly trail meanders along the gentle slope of Nutting Hill. At the next junction, double blue arrows point right, to MA 119 and the parking lot 0.79 mile away. Pick up this rugged logging trail—on which the hike began—and follow it south to the start.

## NEARBY ATTRACTIONS

The Windblown Ski Touring Center (windblownxc.com) is 10 miles up the road (NH 123A) from the Wapack trailhead off MA 119 in Ashburnham. It has 25 miles of trails and offers rental equipment, a lodge, and hearty food. The telephone number is 603-878-2869, and the owners request you call only between 7 a.m. and 9 p.m.

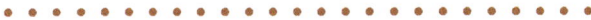

• • • • • • • • • • • • • • • • • • • • • • • •

**GPS TRAILHEAD COORDINATES** N42° 41.817' W71° 54.267'

**DIRECTIONS** From Boston, take MA 2 W 22 miles. Turn right at the Abbott Avenue Exit. Go about 0.8 mile and turn right on Bemis Road/John Fitch Highway. Continue 2.9 miles to a traffic circle. Keep straight on Rindge Road. Go 7.4 miles and turn right onto MA 101. Turn left onto MA 119. The difficult-to-spot parking lot is 1.4 miles ahead on the right.

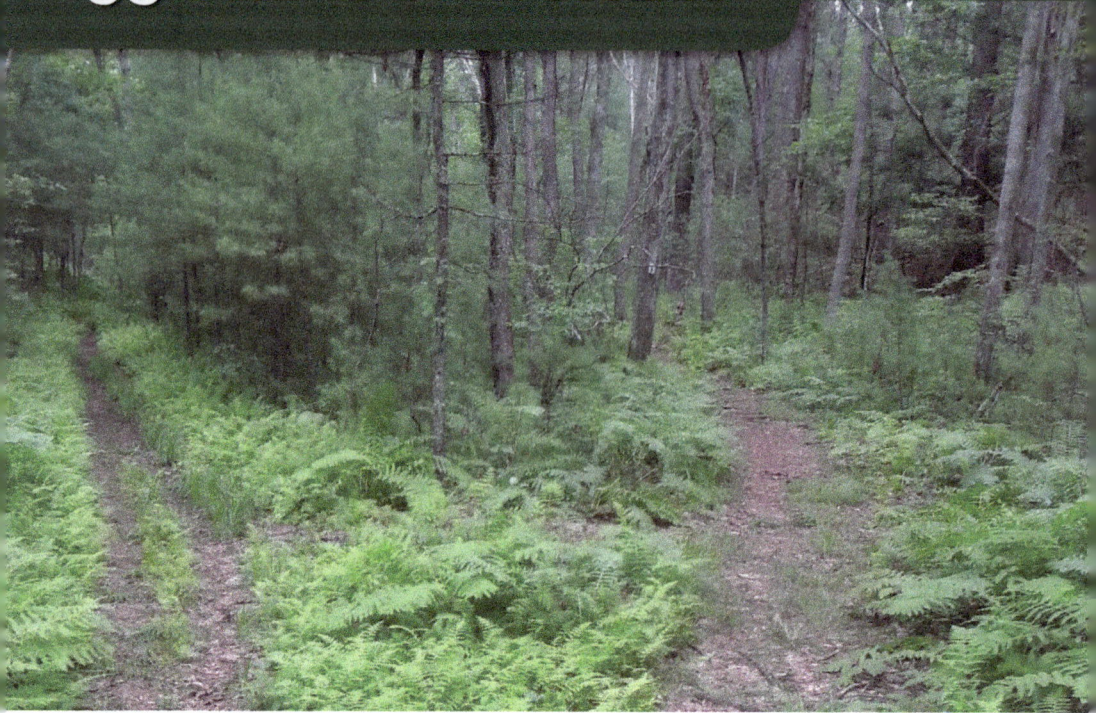

Ogilvie Town Forest takes you through dense swampland and even a quicksand pit.

**STARTING OUT IN** a dense pine grove, this hike becomes more beautiful and intriguing as it ventures along a ridge formed by the collision of continental plates and leads to the swamp-filled corner of a fault line.

## DESCRIPTION

With 2,000 acres of protected open space, an extensive trail network, and active sustainable forestry and community agriculture programs, the former farming town of Weston is a national leader in land conservation and stewardship. In 1955 the town began acquiring large tracts of unbuilt land and established the Weston Forest and Trail Association to maintain trails and educate the townspeople about the forests and forest ecology. The result is neighborhoods woven together by vast tracts of unspoiled land and miles of public trails.

From the small parking spot on the shoulder of Sudbury Road, locate the trailhead near a small green Weston Forest trail marker, and head north into a grove of pine. Traveling in a nearly straight line past a stone wall on the left, the trail arrives at a two-way junction. Bear right, continuing slightly uphill on a wider path edged by pines and a smattering of oaks and other hardwoods.

Rolling northeast, this grassy fire road soon leads to a two-way intersection marked 8. Continue left, hiking north under shade cast by oak, hickory, and white

**DISTANCE & CONFIGURATION:** 3 miles, 2 loops

**DIFFICULTY:** Easy–moderate

**SCENERY:** Reforested farmland, swamp, and a fault zone created when continental plates collided to form the supercontinent Pangaea during the Precambrian–Mesozoic eras

**EXPOSURE:** Mostly shaded

**TRAFFIC:** Light

**TRAIL SURFACE:** Packed dirt, with rugged areas of loose gravel and exposed rock

**HIKING TIME:** 1.5–2 hours

**DRIVING DISTANCE FROM BOSTON COMMON:** 19 miles

**ELEVATION:** 220' at trailhead, no significant gain

**SEASON:** Year-round

**ACCESS:** Sunrise–sunset; free

**MAPS:** Can be purchased at the Weston Town Hall and are available from the Weston Forest and Trail Association at westonforesttrail.org.

**WHEELCHAIR ACCESS:** No

**FACILITIES:** None

**CONTACT:** Town of Weston, weston.org/489 /weston-trail-maps, 781-786-5000

**LOCATION:** Weston, MA

**COMMENTS:** This forest is a veritable cornucopia of mushrooms, both edible and inedible.

pine. You are deep in the woods now, so you'll hear none of the jarring sounds of suburbia. Nuthatches, chickadees, and other woodland birds twitter in the mid-canopy, and occasionally a red-tailed hawk perches high on a dead oak limb long enough to attract a mob of crows. Otherwise, you'll enjoy the peacefulness of the "wise silence" of the natural world. Emerson would approve.

As the trail descends through a void created by two ridges, note the bedrock. As extraordinary as it seems, the bedrock you see extruding from the slopes is consolidated volcanic rock and ash, called tuff. Its source is even more extraordinary. According to geologists, distinct sections of New England, including several in the Boston area, are pieces of faraway lands, including Africa and a chain of volcanic islands that once protruded from the sea above the South Pole. The volcanic rock then is either of foreign origin or a local product created when one plate of Earth's crust rode up over another. All told, Massachusetts has experienced no fewer than three such momentous collisions in the past 500 million years. Although all lies quiet today, a certain amount of instability exists, along with the many fault lines that radiate from these points of impact.

Tumbling in stop-motion, a stone wall crosses down one slope, lets the trail through, then climbs to the right. Ahead, where the trail splits at another junction, hike left (northwest) under hemlock cover. Rolling gradually northwest in easy undulations over gravel footing, the trail soon reaches junction 4. A hemlock stands at the crook of the V next to an umbrella-shaped sassafras tree. Bear right, continuing alongside intriguing ridges.

Departing the fire road at junction 3, climb over the mounded chunks of microcontinents, crystallized volcanic ash, and organic detritus to descend to the swamp below. In crossing this spot, you'll find that flooding dictates the way. Follow the markers pointing right. The trail sidles along the swamp only temporarily; a moment later it edges back up onto the flank of another ridge.

## Ogilvie Town Forest

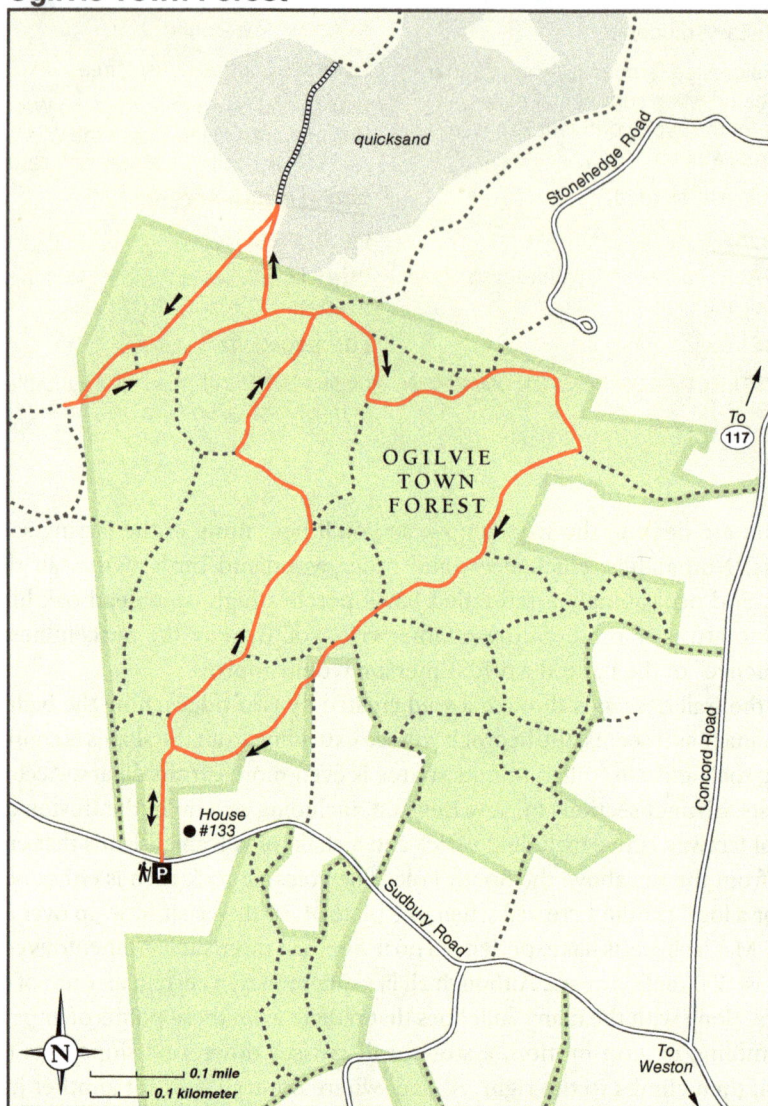

Ahead you'll come to a sign bearing a warning you wouldn't expect to see in New England: quicksand in the lowland area beyond. The treacherous zone is an outlying tract of the Bloody Bluff Fault. For a cautious look, follow the trail down into the swamp, being sure to stop on the near side of logs serving as a makeshift bridge. On returning to the orange warning sign, hike uphill to the right and follow the path as it switches back over the top of the ridge traced earlier. The view looking southeast from this static mass is something like that of the view from the crest of a rogue wave.

Several paths feed in from the edges, but you stay with the main trail as it continues straight along the ridge beneath black oaks. As it begins to taper downhill, the trail bows left and right. Choose the right-hand route to descend along a pit used as a rifle-training range during World War II.

Beyond that pit, the trail levels off as it continues on its southwest run along the border of Weston and Wayland. Across the stone wall demarcating the town line, you can see a meadow through a thin wall of trees. At the T junction ahead, bear right for a brief foray into Wayland, on land owned by the Sudbury Valley Trustees.

Returning to the woods of Weston, continue straight across the top of the T, heading east. The fire road–turned–hiking trail travels alongside a ravine cut by glacial outwash during the formation of Lake Sudbury. Easing into the recess, the trail arrives at junction 2. Continue left, hiking over floodplain to return to junction 3.

At this familiar point, keep left to hike southeast into the southern reaches of Lincoln. The next junction comes quickly. Here, a trail marked with the red sign of the Lincoln Trail System bears left, but bear right to remain in Ogilvie Forest. Midway up a banking, the trail forks; stay right. At the top of the rise, you'll pass another stone wall, and the trail splits yet again. Bear left, hiking east under pines and hemlocks. Encountering the stone wall once more, the trail continues through a gap in the stones, reaches another split, and continues straight.

To round out a tour of the forest, the trail forges northeast toward the Lincoln border, crossing another glacial-outwash plain to access high ground. Houses are visible through trees to the left as the trail arrives at junction 9. Using drumlins and eskers as stepping-stones through wetland, continue on the route as it heads right (southeast).

Just beyond the foundation of a house on the right, the trail forks. Stay right to curve southwest. Grit washed into a mound beneath glacial ice rises to the right, facing a stone wall. Descending from this esker, the trail dips then climbs another, crossing a stream in between. Arriving at a split a moment later, stay on high ground to follow the trail as it arcs southwest.

At the V of junction 6 and the unmarked junction that follows, continue straight, hiking downhill on a gravel-strewn slope. Junction 7 comes quickly; bear left, keeping on a southwest trajectory. The trail now returns to a far tamer landscape. White pine saplings and sassafras fill sunlit spaces, and the ground lies flat.

The trail diverges left, but bear right to continue southwest through the pine groves. On arriving at the next junction, turn left to return to Sudbury Road.

## NEARBY ATTRACTIONS

Land's Sake (781-893-1162, landssake.org) is a private, nonprofit organization devoted to land stewardship, sustainable farming, and forestry. The organization runs a full calendar of events year-round, including maple sugaring in February and

March, and a Strawberry Festival in June. Land's Sake's headquarters is located at the Melone Homestead, 27 Crescent St., Weston.

• • • • • • • • • • • • • • • • • • • • • • • • • •

**GPS TRAILHEAD COORDINATES** N42° 23.167'  W71° 20.050'

**DIRECTIONS**  From Boston Common, take I-90 W and continue 10.3 miles. Take Exit 15A to I-95. At 0.3 mile, exit left to I-95 north. Continue 1.9 miles and take Exit 26 to US 20 and follow signs for US 20 W. Follow US 20 west 1.4 miles. Veer right onto Boston Post Road and at 0.7 mile turn right onto Concord Road. Continue 1.6 miles on Concord Road. Where Concord turns right, stay straight to go onto Sudbury Road. The entrance to Ogilvie Town Forest is ahead 0.4 mile, next to house number 133. There is parking for only one or two cars.

You might want to turn around here.

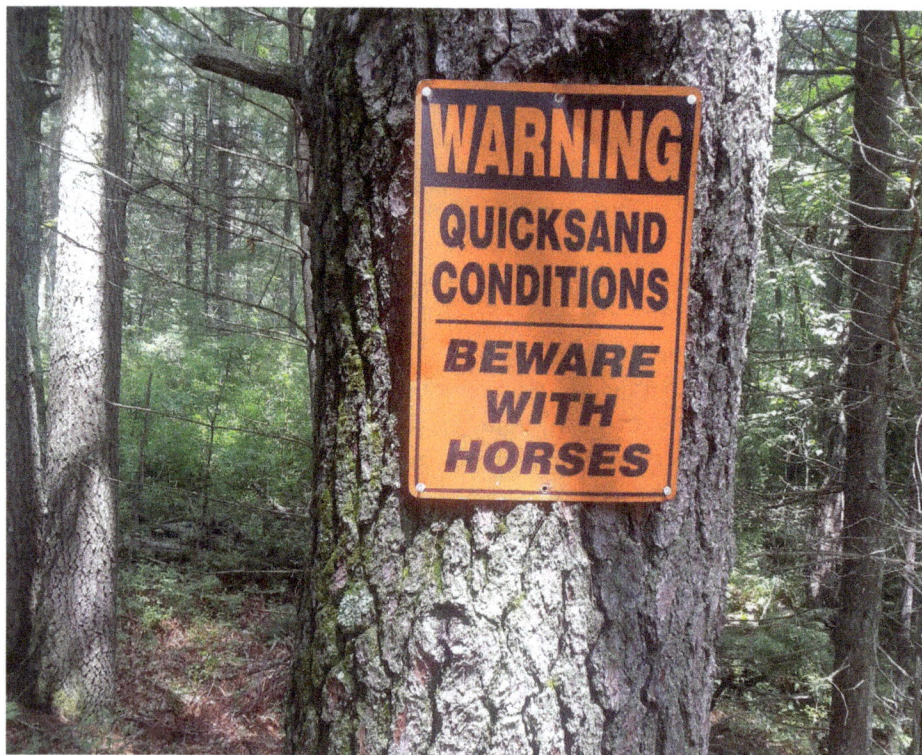

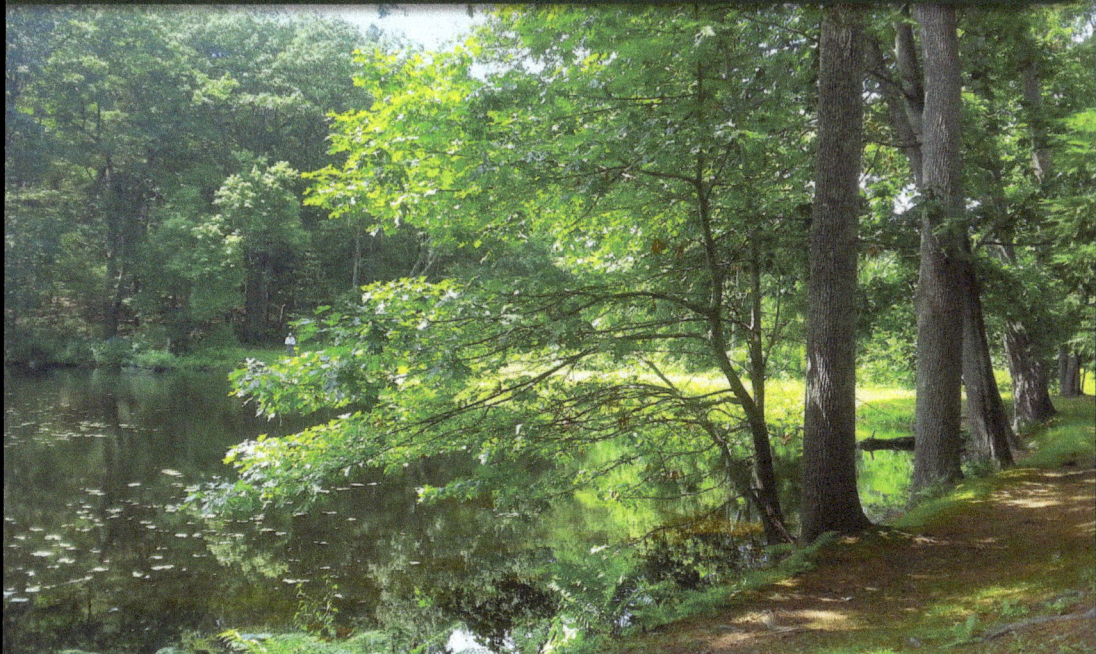

This historic hike retraces some of the steps of Henry David Thoreau.

**THIS HIKE LINKS** three popular hiking destinations: Mount Misery, Adams Woods, and Walden Pond.

## DESCRIPTION

To find the trailhead, cross Oxbow Road and, bearing right, hike to a gap in evergreens framing a field. Look for the insignia of the Lincoln Land Conservation Trust. From this corner, head northeast along the edge of the field to reach a paved drive and woods beyond. Cross the pavement, and resume the trail as it continues north between two massive oaks marked with orange blazes.

Starting where the trail bears left atop an esker nearly in the clouds, the trail swerves, dips, and lurches its way to Farrar Pond below. Having arrived at level ground, proceed left and follow the trail as it traces the pond's perimeter.

Stay with the trail as it continues northwest on its orbit around the pond, passing several trails along the way. Heading directly north, the trail leads to a peninsula then makes a hairpin turn right to continue southwest.

Just before reaching a home the color of redwood, the trail intersects another route jutting in from the left and appears to dead-end at a gushing outlet. Despite the sign reading PRIVATE, the route continues across the abbreviated bridge. A white Bay

**DISTANCE & CONFIGURATION:** 8.67-mile out-and-back with 2 loops

**DIFFICULTY:** Easy–moderate

**SCENERY:** Farrar Pond, Mount Misery, wooded landscape contoured by glacial ice

**EXPOSURE:** Mostly shaded

**TRAFFIC:** Moderate

**TRAIL SURFACE:** Widely varied, including packed dirt, grassland, rocky terrain, and some pavement

**HIKING TIME:** 5 hours

**DRIVING DISTANCE FROM BOSTON COMMON:** 25 miles

**ELEVATION:** 139' at trailhead, 263' at highest point atop Mount Misery

**SEASON:** Year-round

**ACCESS:** Sunrise–sunset; free

**MAPS:** Available through the Lincoln and Concord conservation commissions

**WHEELCHAIR ACCESS:** No

**FACILITIES:** None

**CONTACT:** Lincoln Land Conservation Trust and Rural Land Foundation, lincolnconservation.org

**LOCATION:** Wayland, MA

**COMMENTS:** If you're bringing your dog, be sure to bring a leash. And dogs are not allowed at the Walden Pond State Reservation.

Circuit Trail marker attached to an oak indicates where the trail proceeds between a fenced-in meadow and a wispy wall of evergreens. Be respectful of this passage, and stay on the trail, following the course of the fence toward the road.

The trail follows a driveway to a road at the foot of the hill. Aim for the Bay Circuit Trail marker next to a dirt pulloff across the road, then carefully continue around a blind curve to the right. Noting a white trail marker on a large pine, hike behind the parking area to a boat launch on the Sudbury River.

The trail arcs back to the road where a pair of markers, one white and one yellow, indicates that the trail travels southeast alongside the road, dropping below the traffic as it skirts wetland thick with reeds.

The trail arrives at the base of Mount Misery. The orange trail offers the option of climbing straight north. Take this route several yards to a split, then ease right, following a red arrow to descend back to street level. Across the parking lot in the northeast corner, the Bay Circuit Trail picks up again. Resuming this route momentarily, pass a pond, then bear left on the Kettle Trail.

After shooting straight to the top of an esker, the trail darts through an intersection then rims a kettle pond before plunging down the other side, banking a curve, and then snaking the other way to climb again.

Reaching a plateau, the trail turns southeast and, a moment later, slices across the Bay Circuit Trail and leads to another four-way intersection. Take the yellow trail, which splits left here to spiral to the top of Mount Misery. Though a peaceful spot to enjoy a snack, the peak affords little in the way of a view.

When ready to descend, follow the yellow trail along the edge of a tremendously steep slope. At the base of Mount Misery, bear right, then continue straight to a cultivated field. Trace the field's boundary to the left, and enter the woods where a sign reads PRIVATE TRAIL TO ADAMS WOODS.

# Oxbow Meadows/Farrar Pond/Mount Misery:
# In Thoreau's Footsteps

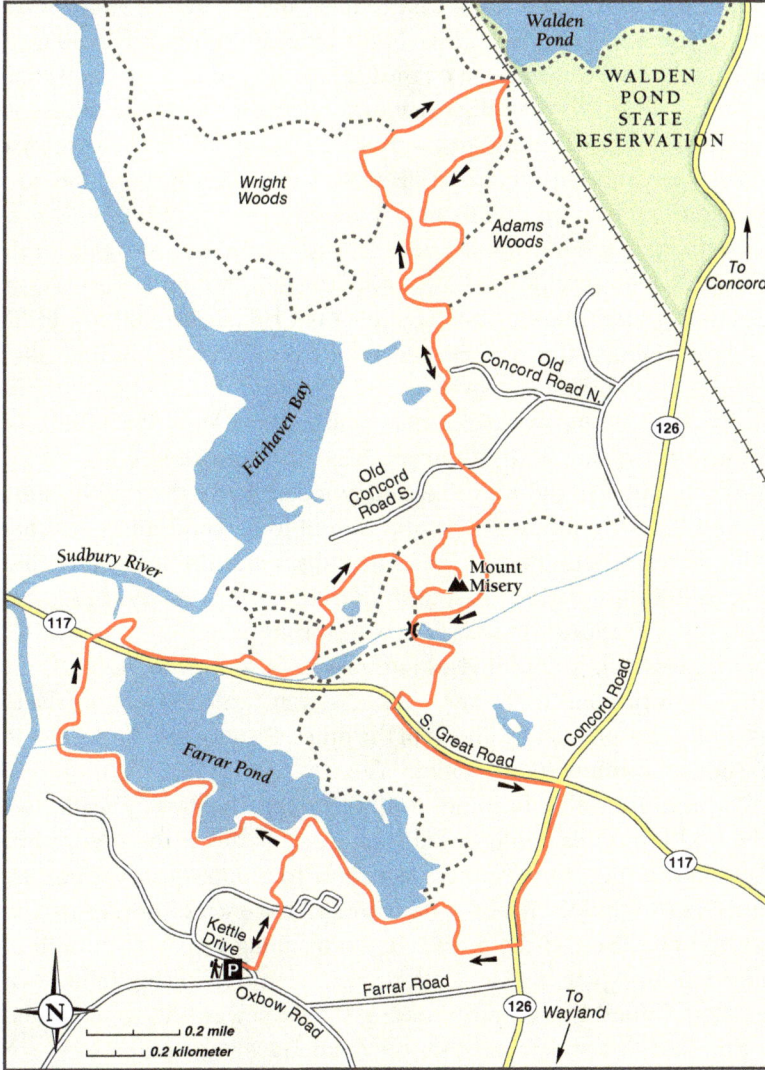

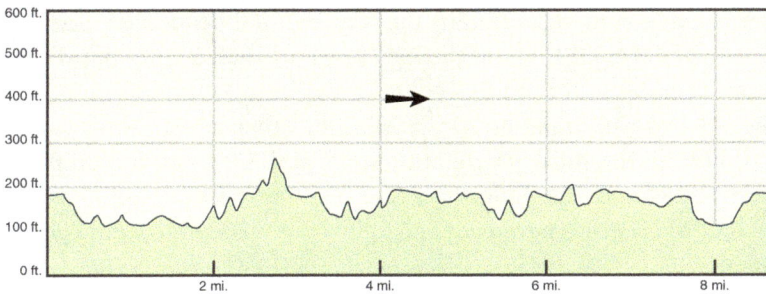

Follow orange dots as they lead past houses across a paved drive. Bear left just short of a horse paddock. This turn is easy to miss, but if you find yourself face-to-face with a horse standing before a brown house on a hill, you've gone too far.

Traveling north between a stream on the left and the paddock, the trail continues across a wooden bridge to meet a driveway a short distance later and Adams Woods beyond. Locate the trail to the right, marked with a hiker symbol and an orange dot.

Departing from the stream, the trail crosses through one junction to reach another distinguished by a gate on the left. When the orange trail forks just ahead, stay on course to continue northwest over sandy ground above wetland. At the top of a slight grade near a kettle pond, a sign points south to Mount Misery. Round the bend to the left to another kettle pond and junction. Hike left uphill to a fork and a sign marking the Lincoln–Concord border. Where the Fairhaven Trail breaks off to the left, veer right to continue northwest.

Having left Lincoln, be aware of a change in trail markers. The steward of the land you're now traversing is the Concord Land Conservation Trust. At each of the next intersections, stay right. The second junction marks the halfway point. To return to Farrar Pond, continue on the orange trail to descend south on a banking far above the outwash field. Follow the orange discs and the white medallions of the Concord Land Conservation Trust to stay on course. At a sprawling intersection where the orange trail appears to split in two, bear right.

Climbing a moraine, the trail rises and proceeds southwest on upland. After running due south through pines and oaks, the trail turns sharply northeast and reaches two junctions, one nearly on top of the other. Bear right at both. The second right sends the trail southwest once more.

On this downhill, fields become visible through the trees ahead, and in a moment the trail intersects another. Turn left here, as this is the orange trail you hiked earlier. Follow the sign to retrace your route to Mount Misery. Upon arriving at the mountain's threshold, where the Bay Circuit Trail enters from across the field, hike left to circle the base of the great hill. Rising along wetland, the trail parts a stone wall then, at an expansive intersection, heads south, following yellow markers.

A small kettle pond lies ahead. Crossing the causeway, the trail arrives at an intersection marked E. Bear left and trace the pond, traveling southeast. Where Wolf Pine Trail appears at the far bank, turn right and continue southwest, paralleling a stone wall. With yellow markers leading the way, the trail bends right just short of South Great Road (MA 117). Brush through ferns to reach a junction, where you turn left to meet the road.

Leaving wooded paths temporarily, cross to the other side. Proceed 0.4 mile to Concord Road (MA 126). Make a right angle south at this intersection. At 0.36 mile, between houses 234 and 239, look for a sign marking a trail traveling east–west across Concord Road. Leave pavement and follow this well-hidden and lightly traveled path west.

For 0.27 mile this delightful orange-marked path slips along the edges of private property to emerge at the southeastern end of bowtie-shaped Farrar Pond. On its final leg before it reaches Farrar's wooded bank, the trail darts diagonally across a driveway.

Once beside the water, the trail picks its way over the root-tangled shore to return to where it first approached the pond hours ago. At this third junction, bear left and make one last push to return to Oxbow Road.

## NEARBY ATTRACTIONS

To see where the "shot heard round the world" was fired (the ground on which the American Revolution began on April 19, 1775), plan a trip to Minute Man National Historical Park (250 N. Great Road, Lincoln; 978-369-6993; nps.gov/mima).

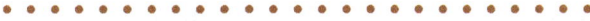

• • • • • • • • • • • • • • • • • • • • • • • • • •

**GPS TRAILHEAD COORDINATES** N42° 24.517'  W71° 21.317'

**DIRECTIONS**  From Boston, take I-90 W 11.4 miles to I-95 via Exit 15A. Bear left to merge onto I-95 N. Continue 1.9 miles to Exit 26/US 20. Bear left onto Stow Street, then turn left onto Main Street/MA 117. Continue 3.8 miles, then turn left onto Old Sudbury Road. Travel 1.4 miles, then turn right onto Concord Road/MA 126. Turn left onto Oxbow Road. There is a parking pulloff on the right.

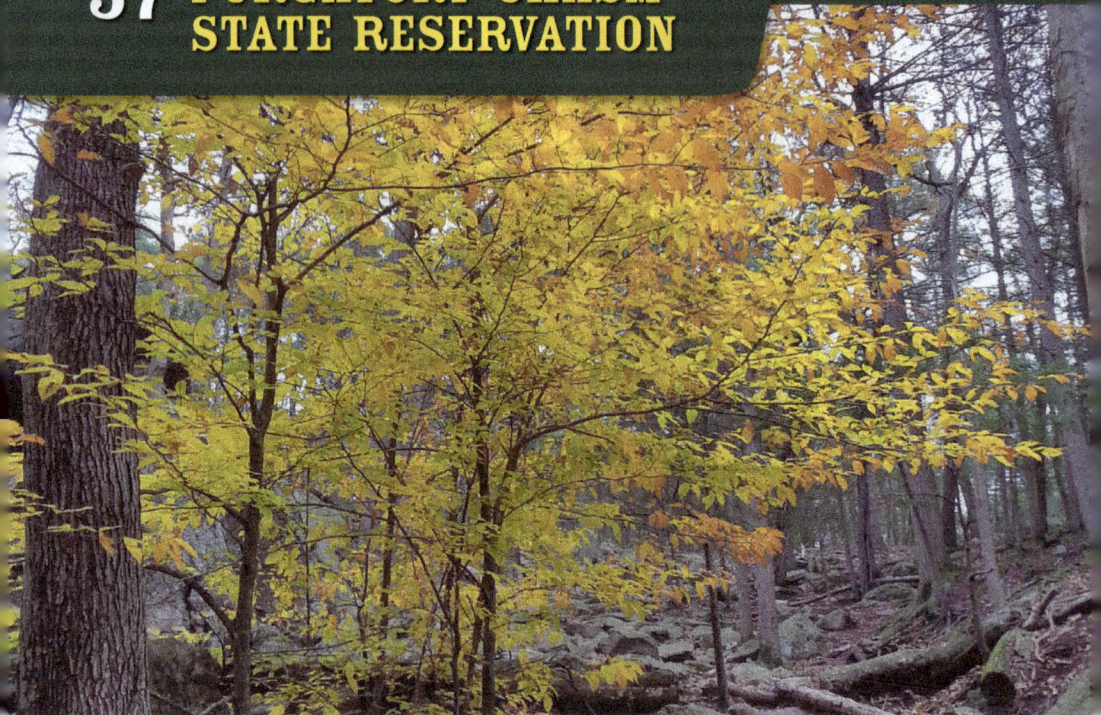

You could spend hours exploring the nooks and crannies of Purgatory Chasm.

**TAKING THE BACK-DOOR ENTRANCE** into the spectacular Purgatory Chasm, this hike explores the geological curiosity from within, surveys the fissure from cliffs above, and explores the surrounding woods. Those interested in lengthier hikes can access the Sutton State Forest from linking trails.

## DESCRIPTION

You will be hard-pressed to find cliff and rock formations as dramatic as those within the Purgatory Chasm State Reservation. This hike explores the chasm and circumnavigates the surrounding forest, but plan to spend as much time as you'd like exploring the cliffs, caves, and fissures as well.

From the map and information board at the head of the parking lot, set out left (southeast). Beyond a large sheltered picnic area and swing, you will find a short stretch of paved road leading to Charlie's Loop trailhead, named for Charles Gravlin, who oversaw the park for many years. Starting off wide and gravel-topped, this route passes under hemlocks as it rises and falls, twists and turns, and then settles to level ground. Stay on the trail here, following the faint yellow markers of Charlie's Loop. Early on, the trail will descend a short, rocky hill with several large granite cliffs off to the left, which are well worth exploring. Farther down, the trail makes a distinct 45-degree right turn. Continue northwest on Charlie's Loop along the nice flat

**DISTANCE & CONFIGURATION:** 2.25-mile loop

**DIFFICULTY:** Easy, with extremely treacherous sections

**SCENERY:** Wooded trails, with views of a rugged chasm with granite cliffs as high as 70'

**EXPOSURE:** Mostly shaded

**TRAFFIC:** Light

**TRAIL SURFACE:** Packed dirt, except inside the chasm, where the trail meanders over and between great slabs of stone

**HIKING TIME:** 1.5 hours

**DRIVING DISTANCE FROM BOSTON COMMON:** 48 miles

**ELEVATION:** 542' at trailhead, 627' at highest point; overall gain is not significant, but the cliffs in the chasm itself are dramatic

**SEASON:** Year-round

**ACCESS:** Sunrise–sunset. Parking is $5 for MA residents, $6 for nonresidents

**MAPS:** Posted near the parking lot and available at visitor center and mass.gov/eea/docs/dcr/parks/trails/purgatory.pdf

**WHEELCHAIR ACCESS:** No

**FACILITIES:** Restrooms at park offices, picnic tables with grills, often an ice-cream truck in summer

**CONTACT:** Massachusetts Dept. of Conservation and Resources, tinyurl.com/purgchasmreservation, 617-626-1250

**LOCATION:** Sutton, MA

**COMMENTS:** Hikers are advised to wear rubber-soled shoes or hiking boots because the rocky path through the chasm can be slippery.

terrain. The trail here is well defined and hard-packed dirt. Charlie's Loop continues straight until it reaches a wide, open junction. Here a trail marked with blue continues straight while two other trails diverge right. Take the more extreme right, and proceed on the gravel path that narrows quickly as it bends around a clutch of two-story-high boulders. This is the far end of Purgatory Chasm.

Some say the chasm was formed by glacial action 14,000 years ago when geological movement let loose meltwater locked within bedrock. American Indian legend attributes the enormous fissure to an incident involving the evil spirit Hobomoko. Another intriguing notion is that the powerful earthquake that ripped across the land on November 18, 1755, forged the chasm. Whichever tale you choose to believe, you'll just be glad this incredible dramatic geological feature is here to explore.

A few yards ahead, the trail delivers you to the Devil's Coffin, a deep, dark void surrounded by slabs of dour quartz-freckled, feldspar-veined granite. Poke your head inside or pass quietly by, following the blue dashes of paint that indicate the recommended path to take over and between the chaos of stone.

Heading north, the crack in the earth deepens, its walls rising higher and higher until they reach upwards of 70 feet. On any given day, you may also see rock-climbers ascending and descending the cliffs as you enter the chasm.

Halfway through the chasm, you come to the Devil's Pulpit, a rock formation favored by the many rock-climbers who come to Purgatory Chasm in all seasons. Beyond the pulpit, a sign on the left alerts you to the heart-quickening cliff known since the very day of Custer's Last Stand as Lover's Leap.

Just before reaching the northern end of the chasm, the trail passes His Majesty's Cave. His Majesty may be an ogre, a bear, or a bat—it's up to anyone gutsy enough

# Purgatory Chasm State Reservation

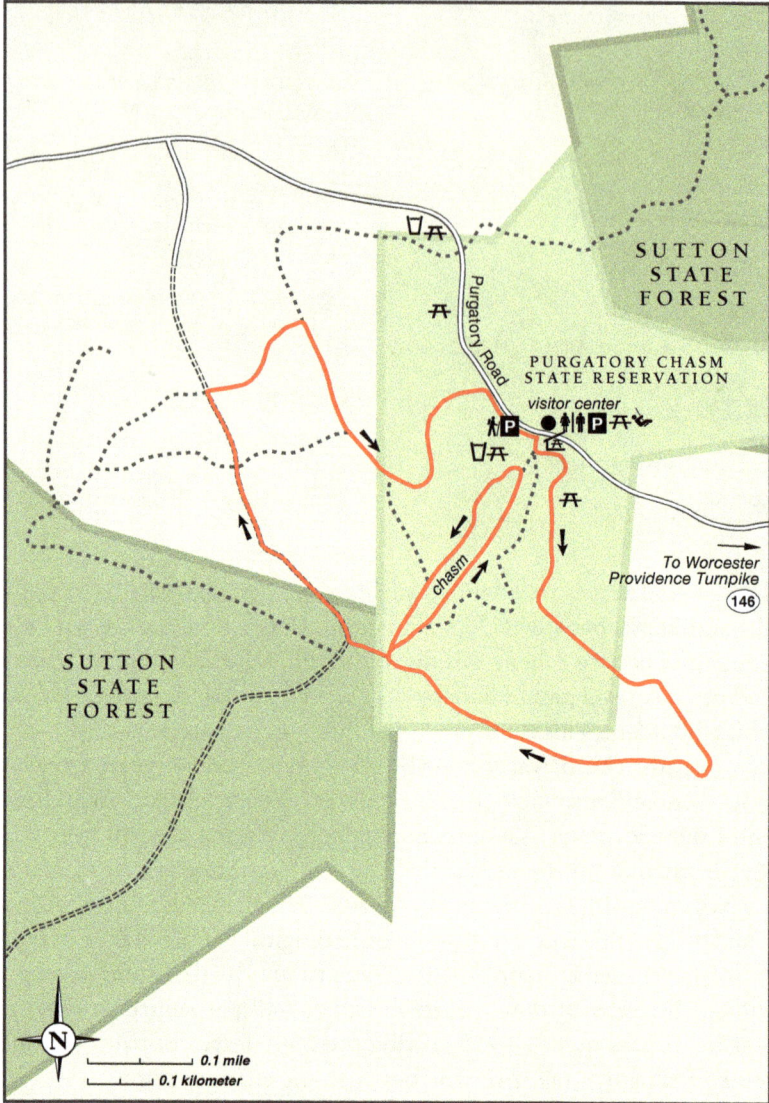

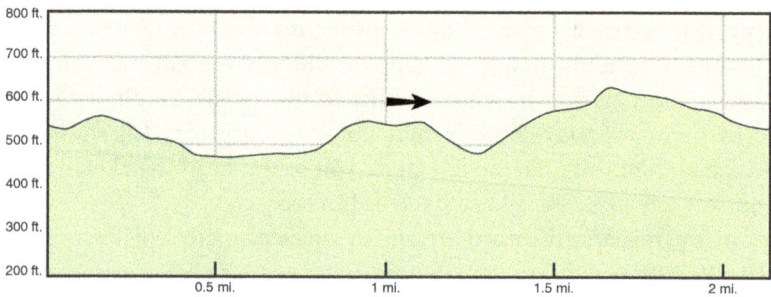

SUTTON
STATE
FOREST

Purgatory Road

PURGATORY CHASM
STATE RESERVATION

visitor center

chasm

To Worcester
Providence Turnpike
146

SUTTON
STATE
FOREST

N

0.1 mile

0.1 kilometer

800 ft.

700 ft.

600 ft.

500 ft.

400 ft.

300 ft.

200 ft.

0.5 mi.          1 mi.          1.5 mi.          2 mi.

and equipped with a headlamp to say. In 1865, word of a "huge beast" at the chasm compelled Henry David Thoreau to investigate. He traveled by horse cart for miles but found no hint of the fierce animal.

Emerging from the chasm, you find yourself back at the park entrance. To continue your hike, turn left and look for a sign for Charlie's Loop. The trail travels west through sparse woods growing on the edge of the cliff far above the chasm. The path veers far enough away from the tear in the earth that nothing within view alerts you.

To get a look down into the chasm, you must leave the trail and tread carefully over uneven sheets of granite. Do so with exceptional caution. There is nothing between the woods and the chasm's void—no wall, handrail, or rope, just an understated warning sign or two. You can get as close to the edge as your nerves and reasonable precautions allow, but it's certainly an impressive view.

Follow Charlie's Loop as it heads south to deliver you back to the far end of the quarter-mile-long chasm. At this broad intersection, which you will recognize from earlier, turn right to pick up the Forest Road Trail, which is marked with blue. This wide fire road makes for easy walking after the rock-scrambling deep within the chasm. Continue uphill, and stay on this trail when it bears right upon meeting another trail that heads left to Purgatory Brook.

Travel north (right). The trail persists up a steep slope for a third of a mile or so. Upon reaching a steel gate, continue to the second of two intersections. Here you will head back into the woods, still on the Forest Trail heading toward the Old Purgatory Trail to the right. The trail here is more like a typical hiking trail—narrow, winding, and punctuated with roots and rocks.

A short distance farther, at another junction, go right again onto the orange-blazed Old Purgatory Trail. This is a narrow trail that weaves through woods over grizzled roots and loosened stones.

The trail soon curves south and emerges at an open pine grove nearly devoid of underbrush. As the trail winds north, the woods thicken again and the trail scales a ridge as it approaches a paved road to the left. Just after a park building on the left, you arrive at a parking lot slightly north of the chasm entrance. Walk along the wide shoulder of Purgatory Road to return to your starting point.

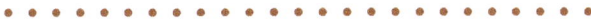

• • • • • • • • • • • • • • • • • • • • • • • • • • • •

**GPS TRAILHEAD COORDINATES** N42° 07.750'  W71° 42.900'

**DIRECTIONS** Take I-90 W 39.8 miles to Exit 10A toward US 20 to Worcester. After 0.9 mile turn right and merge onto MA 146 S. After 7.1 miles take the Purgatory Road ramp toward Northbridge/Whitinsville. Just ahead take the Purgatory Road ramp toward Purgatory Chasm and bear right onto Purgatory Road. Parking is 0.8 mile ahead.

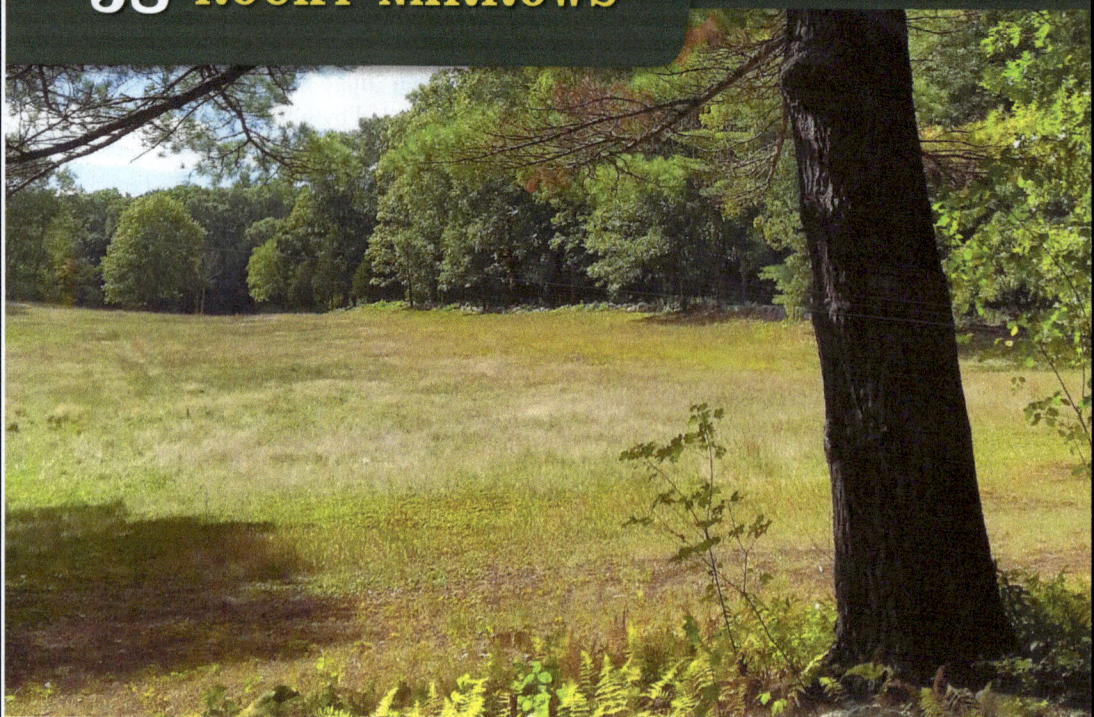

Rocky Narrows is a sublime and peaceful hike.

**YOU'LL SEE THE** Charles River at its finest on this hike. Starting off from a field kept cleared since farming days, the trail leads through reforested agricultural land to a canoe landing before tracking the river.

## DESCRIPTION

In 1897, five years after landscape architect Charles Eliot founded The Trustees of Reservations, Frederick Law Olmsted Jr. oversaw the initial transaction that led to the protection of 227 acres on the Charles River, now called Rocky Narrows. In the years since, others have made similar donations, with the most recent acreage added in 1995 for a current total of 249 acres.

Begin your hike on the slender path called the Red Trail that starts to the left of the Forest Street parking area at the head of a meadow. Crossing the grassy expanse to join a gravel road, bear left at the first intersection, marked 23. From here red dots mark the way. As you hike along this open stretch, you'll see and hear lots of songbirds.

Guided by stone walls on either side, the path quickly heads into woods composed of white pine, oak, cherry, and nut trees that have grown in since Eliot and Olmsted took charge of the land. This part of the hike is gentle and easy as the broad path winds down around soft bends, making a causeway as it passes through wetland.

**DISTANCE & CONFIGURATION:** 3.8-mile loop

**DIFFICULTY:** Easy–moderate

**SCENERY:** Views of the Charles River, forested wetlands

**EXPOSURE:** Mostly shaded

**TRAFFIC:** Light

**TRAIL SURFACE:** Packed dirt, with significant rock outcroppings

**HIKING TIME:** 2 hours

**DRIVING DISTANCE FROM BOSTON COMMON:** 19 miles

**ELEVATION:** 193' at trailhead, 242' at highest point

**SEASON:** Year-round

**ACCESS:** Sunrise–sunset; free

**MAPS:** Kiosk at the trailhead or tinyurl.com /rockynarrowsmap

**WHEELCHAIR ACCESS:** No

**FACILITIES:** None

**CONTACT:** The Trustees of Reservations, thetrustees.org/places-to-visit, 617-542-7696

**LOCATION:** Sherborn, MA

**COMMENTS:** Rocky Narrows is a gateway to the Charles River and the Bay Circuit Trail— a 200-mile continuous greenway around Boston from Kingston and Duxbury on the south shore to Plum Island.

When the path arrives at a split with the number 21 posted on the right, continue left (east). The dominant species of tree shifts to pine as the trail leads to a clearing at a T. From here, turn right (south) at marker 20. Follow as the trail tacks southwest, passing beneath tall conifers through a distinctly wetter zone. Soon you arrive at another fork. At this juncture, bear left to continue on the Red Trail.

The massive pines and hemlocks along this part spread a beautiful canopy overhead. Though old-growth trees were mostly cleared for pasture in New England, a few stands still exist in some areas, such as in this riparian zone. In a moment you arrive at a clearing where the woods end at the sandy bank of the Charles River. The number 19 on a tree identifies this spot as the canoe landing at Rocky Narrows. Concerted efforts to clean up the Charles River have seen impressive results. Fish are jumping again, muskrats are back in force, and there have been claims of otter sightings.

Leave the canoe landing, heading southwest along the river's edge. Eventually the trail turns away from the river and joins a path going right. Keep left and travel west up a hill. The trail is a bit narrower here, but the ground is still firm. You will see the number 18 and a red dot on a tree to the left. Follow these as they direct you up a steep embankment and lead you along a hemlock-sheltered ridge high above the river. Continuing along the ridge, you will pass a trail coming from the right. A little farther on, you meet another trail. Keep right to stay on the Red Trail, leaving the ridge to head west, following the red markers.

The path widens, levels, and soon arrives at a triangular intersection marked 16. Walk straight through, staying with the Red Trail. Elevated above the river basin, the path is surrounded by young woods. Glimpsing the horizon, you see nothing but seemingly untouched land for miles. Follow the path downhill until you come to trail 14. Take this sharp left back uphill to reach King Philip's Overlook, which is worth the detour.

## Rocky Narrows Park

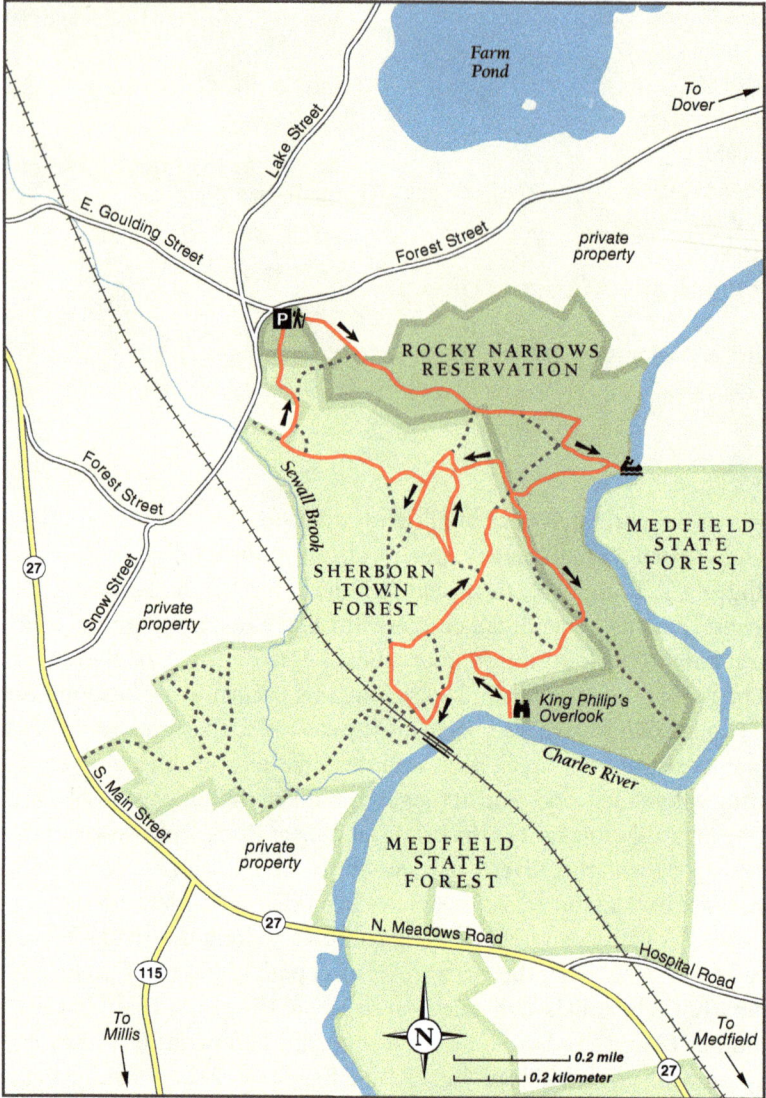

Map showing: Farm Pond, To Dover, Lake Street, E. Goulding Street, Forest Street, private property, ROCKY NARROWS RESERVATION, Sewall Brook, Forest Street, 27, Snow Street, private property, SHERBORN TOWN FOREST, MEDFIELD STATE FOREST, King Philip's Overlook, Charles River, S. Main Street, private property, MEDFIELD STATE FOREST, N. Meadows Road, Hospital Road, 27, 115, To Millis, To Medfield, 27, 0.2 mile, 0.2 kilometer, N

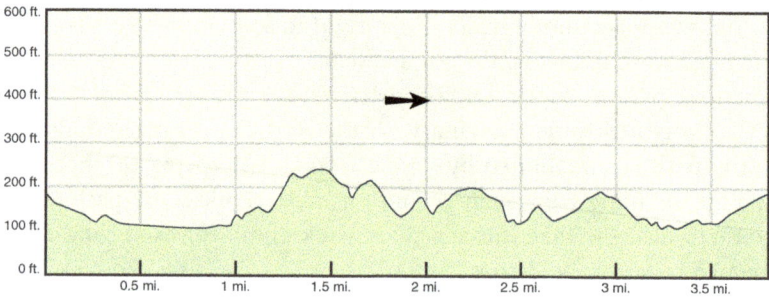

Elevation profile: 600 ft., 500 ft., 400 ft., 300 ft., 200 ft., 100 ft., 0 ft.; 0.5 mi., 1 mi., 1.5 mi., 2 mi., 2.5 mi., 3 mi., 3.5 mi.

After enjoying the view, double back to return to the Red Trail; take it downhill toward railroad tracks. The trail curves right as it nears the tracks then descends another long slope. Farther on, when the trail splits at marker 12, break off to the right and climb back east before arriving at another intersection and continuing north. Shortly you'll arrive at junction 26. Cross here, hiking northeast.

Partway down a rocky slope edged with pine saplings, you will come to a trail running uphill to the right. Climb this link to where you will again reconnect with the Red Trail. Hike left, back to marker 18, then follow the Red Trail to where it cleaves through a stone wall. Here turn left onto a narrower trail.

When you reach a four-way intersection, turn right (northwest) and follow the path straight to marker 24. Bear left to head southwest. You will pass one or two trails leading left, but stay on course to reach marker 25. At this intersection, follow the trail left as it climbs a hill through a dense growth of young white pines. Reaching another junction, continue left and slightly downhill, heading northeast. Passing the Green Trail, continue straight ahead to reach another fork. Stay left here and head left again at the next split. At the next intersection, turn right onto a path running along a stone wall.

This path, marked with orange, treads between wetlands and upland to reach marker 10. From this junction, head northwest on the Red Trail, continuing left at the next fork. After hiking a bit farther, turn right to return to the Red Trail. Having zigzagged your way to marker 8, the last crossroads of the hike, bear left to link back to the parking lot.

As with many hiking areas described in this book, the trail network here at Rocky Narrows is a series of interconnecting loops. Enjoy the hike described here, or equip yourself with a map and just explore. The entire network of trails is diverse, scenic, and captivating.

## NEARBY ATTRACTIONS

After a hike at Rocky Narrows, stop at The Peace Abbey Multi-Faith Retreat Center (2 N. Main St., 508-655-2143). A chapel, pacifist living-history museum, vegan-peace sanctuary, and guesthouse are just a sampling of what you will find. Hours are Monday–Friday, 9 a.m.–5 p.m., and Saturday and Sunday, 10 a.m.–6 p.m.

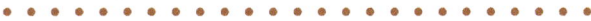

• • • • • • • • • • • • • • • • • • • • • • • •

**GPS TRAILHEAD COORDINATES** N42° 13.550'  W71° 21.233'

**DIRECTIONS**  From Boston take I-90 W 16.9 miles. Take Exit 13 (MA 30 E). Turn right onto Speen Street, then continue 2.8 miles and turn left onto Coolidge Street. After 1.2 miles turn right onto South Main Street. Continue 2 miles and turn left onto Goulding Street. At 0.6 mile turn left onto Forest Street; parking is on the right.

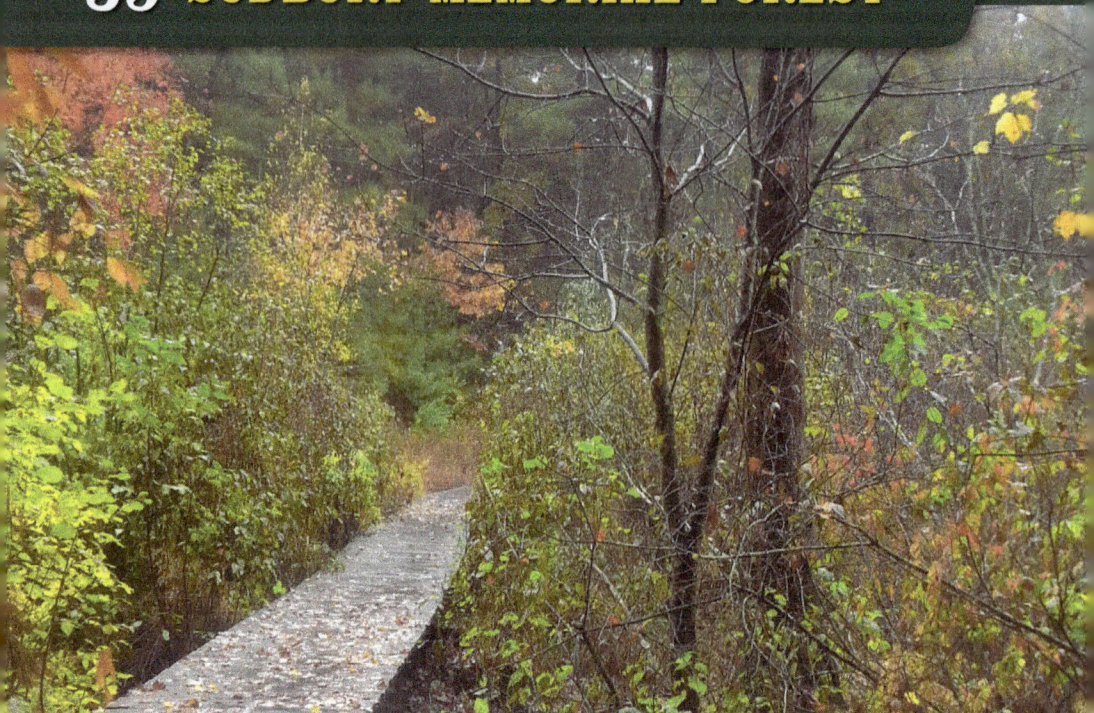

Sudbury Memorial Forest is a fairly gentle and surprisingly diverse hike.

**BECAUSE OF DEEP SAND DEPOSITS** left by glaciers, would-be farmers once deemed the land in the Sudbury Memorial Forest worthless, leaving it comparatively free of the effects of human intervention. Interestingly, much of this land was once owned by one of America's greatest industrialists—Henry Ford, who bought much of the land abutting the western Sudbury border in the 1930s.

## DESCRIPTION

The wildly varied landscape of the Sudbury Memorial Forest is bound to take you by surprise. Predictably, the forest's unusual landscape is the handiwork of the glaciers. After the last glacier retreated north, leaving meltwater in its wake, crushed bedrock washed into low-lying pockets and was buried as the water collected and deepened. Some of the glacial waters remain as swampland on the lake's poorly drained edges, and the Desert Loop and sand pit are further evidence of the glaciers' crushing influence.

The hike begins at the trailhead beside the kiosk just west of the parking lot. Taking the long way around a complex of buildings belonging to the Federation of Women's Clubs, the trail leads through a pine stand flush with the wetland to reach a footbridge spanning Hop Brook. This is a superb gateway to the forest. The bridge offers views north and south of a magnificent wetland landscape animated by brook fish, flycatchers, kingfishers, and countless other wild birds and insects.

**DISTANCE & CONFIGURATION:** 5.75-mile double loop

**DIFFICULTY:** Easy–moderate

**SCENERY:** Wetlands, wildlife pond, pitch-pine forest, sandy "beaches" composed of glacial sediment that settled at the bottom of a lake created by glacial meltwater

**EXPOSURE:** Mostly shaded

**TRAFFIC:** Moderate

**TRAIL SURFACE:** Packed dirt, sand, a few boardwalks

**HIKING TIME:** 3–3.5 hours

**DRIVING DISTANCE FROM BOSTON COMMON:** 24 miles

**ELEVATION:** 163' at trailhead, no significant gain

**SEASON:** Year-round

**ACCESS:** Sunrise–sunset; free

**MAPS:** Available at tinyurl.com/sudbury memorialforestmap

**WHEELCHAIR ACCESS:** No

**FACILITIES:** None

**CONTACT:** Sudbury Valley Trustees, svtweb.org

**LOCATION:** Sudbury, MA

**COMMENTS:** Camping is allowed at Hop Brook Marsh in Sudbury, with the proper permit, available from the Sudbury town clerk or the Sudbury Conservation Commission. Contact Town Hall at 322 Concord Road, Sudbury, MA 01776; 978-639-3351.

From the bridge, the trail continues west across the mud zone emanating from Hop Brook to reach the dry footing of a moraine—a mound of debris shed from the glacier as it retreated north. At the two-way intersection marked J at the base of the slope, stay left to hike over the rise via the Plympton Trail.

Continuing west, the trail leads to junction K, where Ocean Bypass Trail offers an opportunity to hike clear across what were once the lowest depths of Lake Sudbury. Stay on the Plympton Trail for a full tour of the reservation. Before long, you'll come to an esker cut by a gas line, which is also the Marlborough–Sudbury town line. Follow the trail as it jogs left, runs along the ridge of gravel (left from a stream running beneath glacial ice), and then hikes right to junction L. If you went straight here and stayed on the Plympton Trail, it would take you to the northern border of the forest.

Proceed straight at junctions M and N on the Hanson Trail. Then bear right, away from the red maple swamp of Trout Brook. Although still distinctly sandy underfoot, Marlborough State Forest is a good deal less austere than the central portion of the forest.

As the Hanson Trail continues west, the earth becomes more fertile. On what was once the outskirts of Lake Sudbury, glacial till (a mix of clay, sand, and gravel collected over drumlins and ledge) supports a vigorous oak forest and an understory of lowbush blueberry and huckleberry. The abundance of acorns, pinecones, succulent berries, and peaceful acres also supports a wide variety of wild birds. Keep an eye out for scarlet tanagers, hermit thrushes, ovenbirds, and ruffed grouse, all favoring distinct niches. While habitats near brooks appeal to warblers, bluebirds and whippoorwills prefer the more open meadows.

A lively assortment of fur-bearing animals lives here as well. Think twice about dog footprints you may find in the sand; they are just as likely those of a coyote.

## Sudbury Memorial Forest

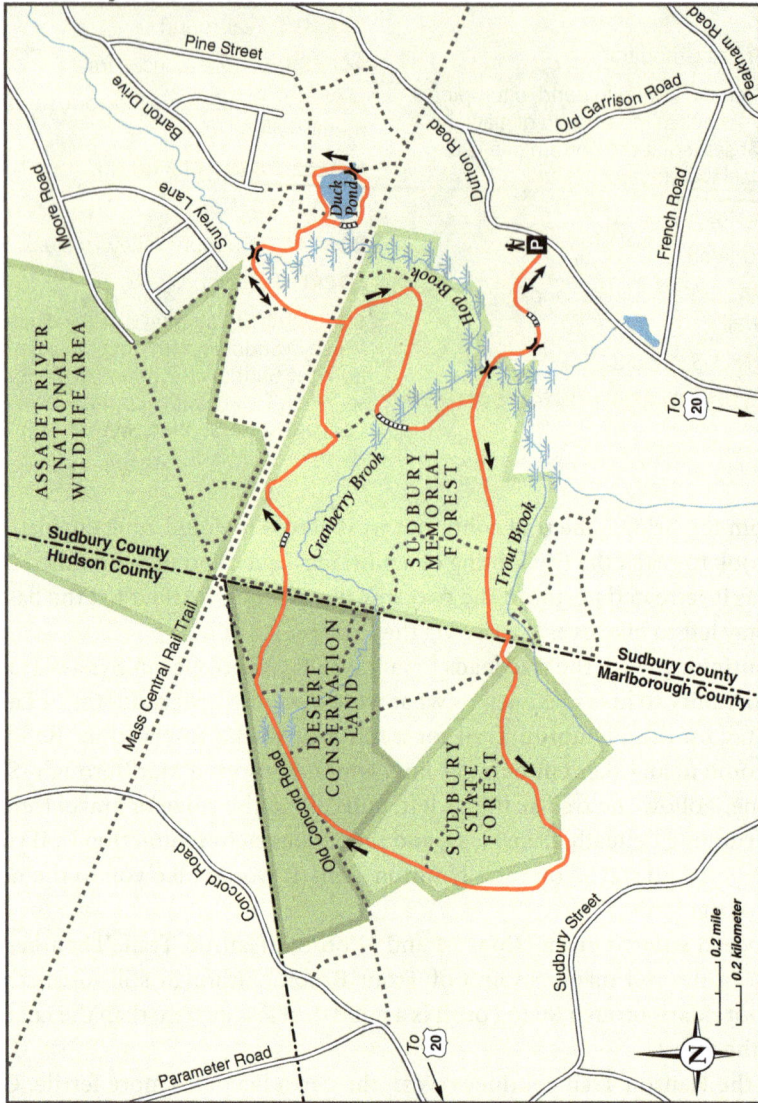

Skunks, raccoons, opossums, and fisher cats are no strangers to these woods, and, of course, deer are never far away.

At junction N, a route with the intriguing name Witches' Cove Trail departs to the right. The Hanson Trail broadens the tour by dipping south then climbing north along the reservation's border to junction O, where once again it converges with the Witches' Cove Trail.

Farther along the trail, junction A marks where the Hanson Trail joins Old Concord Road, an old horse and oxcart throughway. Taking up this new route, bear right and hike northeast on a beeline to cross Cranberry Brook not once but twice. The first crossing is by way of a massive stone bridge just off Hanson Trail, the next via a causeway just a hair beyond where the Plympton Trail emerges, at junction B. Here enterprising beavers have transformed the trickling brook into a swollen marshland, so you are likely to get your feet wet traversing this section.

The two trails that split off from Old Concord Road up ahead offer markedly different hiking experiences. The first, the Cranberry Brook Trail at junction C, travels through a dense forest traversing swampland. The Desert Trail bears east at junction D and brings you to a dry landscape of sand and dunes.

Don't miss the chance to check out one of eastern Massachusetts's most unusual places. Continue to the Desert Trail. Once you are across the northern end of the gas line, the ground grows increasingly sandy. The trail swings north then south again as it opens to a great circular beach with an island of pitch pine in the center.

Hike farther east, and you'll find reassuring Sudbury Valley Trustees (SVT) trail markers. Continue through woods of pitch pine and scrub oak. The Desert Trail splits at junction G to become the Desert Loop. Bear left to reach the impressive glacial sand pit.

Arcing east over flat ground carpeted by fallen pine needles, the trail reaches junction H, which presents a link to Hop Brook Marsh. Take a little side tour here, if you'd like, between an increasingly dense pine forest and the rusted tracks of an abandoned railroad piercing the sand.

Beyond the railroad, conditions change dramatically from parched to lush in remarkably few steps. Soon after bearing left at a fork, the trail finds itself on a bridge straddling spongy land punctuated by Hop Brook. Bear right at the junction on the sandy slope ahead, and cross to the east side of Hop Brook. Following the Ridge Trail south above the wetland, bear right at the second junction. In a moment the trail arrives at a V, where the trail splits to embrace Duck Pond.

To circle the pond counterclockwise, choose the path to the right. The trail never wanders more than a few feet from the water's edge. On the pond's north side, the trail veers wide to meet other trails, but stay left to complete a full circle. Leaving this picturesque spot, retrace your steps to the Desert Loop at junction H.

Bear left to hike into the old sandpit. Staying on track with the help of SVT markers, continue over undulating terrain, following the trail east until it approaches the marshes of Hop Brook and winds south. The trail makes a bold turn west and shoots up a gentle incline to junction I. Turn left and ease downhill to an abbreviated boardwalk to cross the vibrant floodplain of Cranberry Brook. Climbing the swell of the upland opposite, the trail soon jogs east to once again meet the Plympton Trail at junction J. Back at this familiar location, turn left and follow the trail to its end beside the parking lot.

## NEARBY ATTRACTIONS

No visit to the area is complete without a meal or stayover at the historic Wayside Inn (72 Wayside Inn Road, Sudbury, MA; 978-443-1776; wayside.org). The inn was renamed to capitalize on the success of Henry Longfellow's book of poems titled *Tales of a Wayside Inn,* published in 1863. Longfellow visited Howe's Inn in 1862 and based many of his characters on the inn's colorful proprietor and patrons.

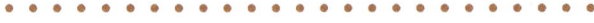

• • • • • • • • • • • • • • • • • • • • • • • • • •

**GPS TRAILHEAD COORDINATES** N42° 22.283'  W71° 27.733'

**DIRECTIONS**  From Boston, take I-90 W 11.4 miles to Exit 15B; bear left toward MA 30. Turn right onto Park Road then left onto South Avenue. South Avenue becomes Highland Street. Continue 1.3 miles and turn left onto Love Lane then left onto US 20 toward Waltham/Weston. Turn right onto Peakham Road. After 0.4 mile turn left onto Old Garrison Road. At 0.1 mile turn left onto French Road, then after 0.5 mile turn right onto Dutton Road; continue to the parking lot on the right.

The canals and marshlands of Sudbury Memorial Forest

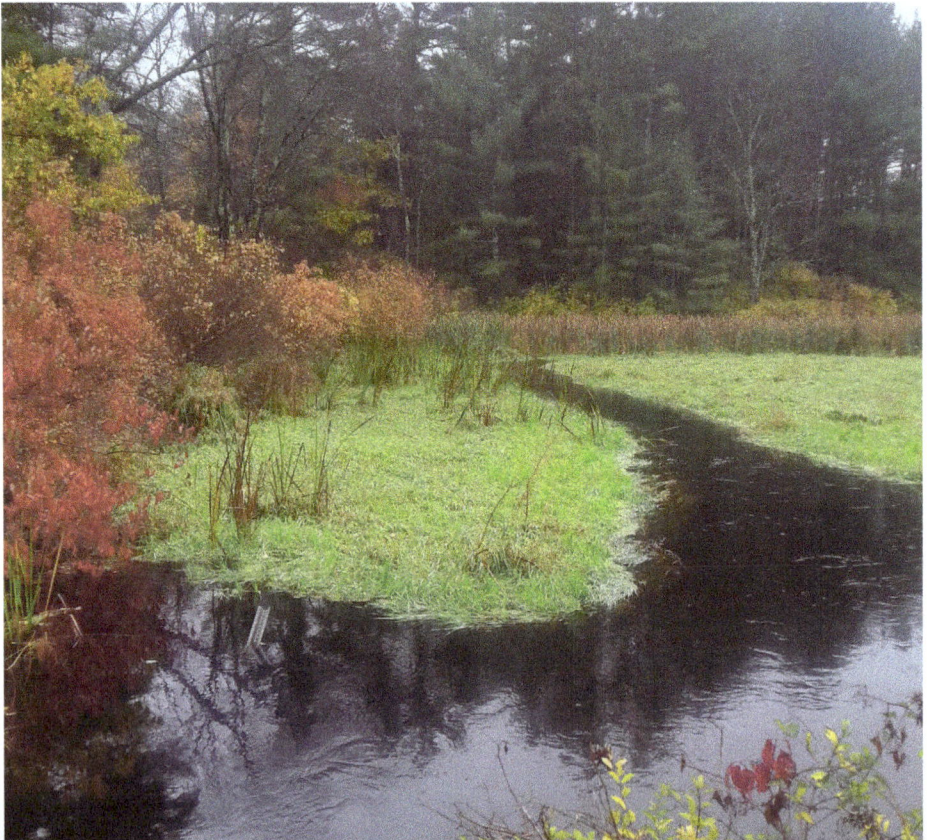

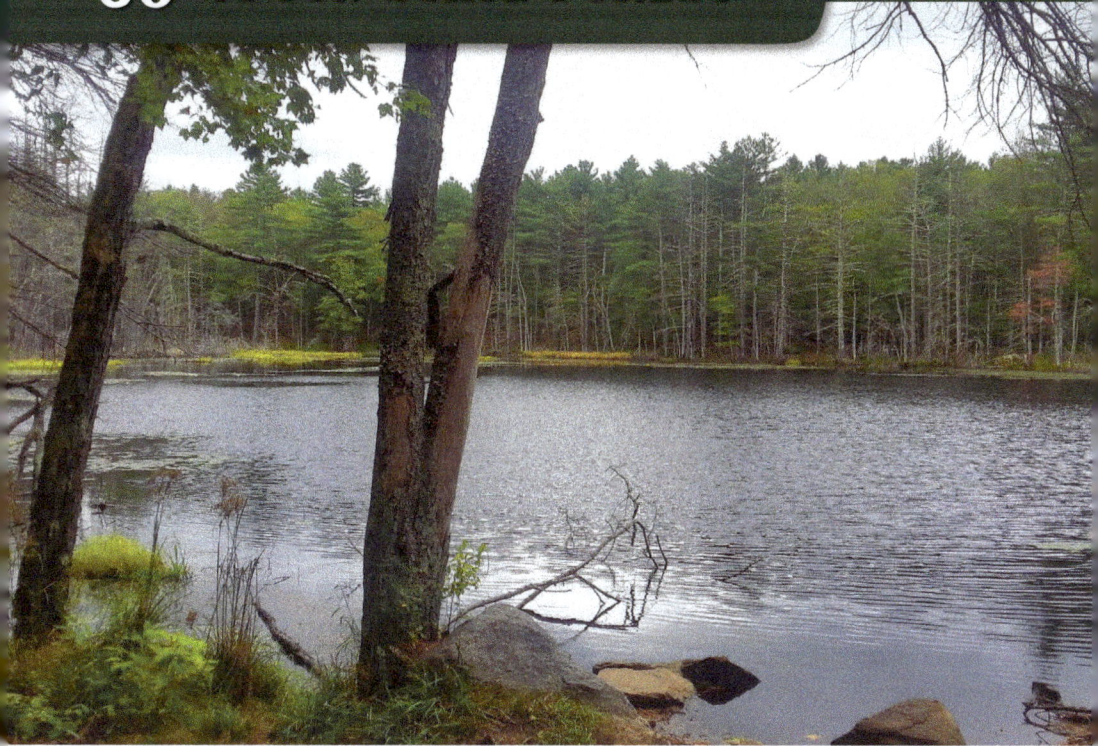

Dean Pond is set deep within Upton State Forest.

**THE 2,660-ACRE** Upton State Forest takes you deep into the woods and to the shores of the swampy but scenic Dean Pond.

## DESCRIPTION

Like many Massachusetts Department of Conservation and Resources properties, Upton State Forest is a varied mix of wider, firm, flat trails resembling an old fire road and narrow, winding true hiking trails. You can mix it up as you see fit. And as with any hike in this book, you can either follow the prescribed hike or explore on your own.

Start off from the parking area, which has room for 15–20 cars. You will hike through a closed metal gate (intended to keep out ATVs and other motorized vehicles). You start off on the wide, firmly packed Civilian Conservation Corps (CCC) road. This is a wide, flat dirt road passing through a moderately dense young forest of mostly deciduous trees with several tall stately pines standing guard over them.

Just a few minutes in on this wide relaxing trail, bear right onto Park Road. The character of the trail is similar to the CCC road; it's still a wide fire road. This takes you on a mostly flat traverse through the forest. After the trail begins a slight ascent, watch for the Nuthatch Trail on the right, which is clearly marked with a sign posted on a tree. While you will eventually take this trail, wait until you are a bit farther

**DISTANCE & CONFIGURATION:** 3.2-mile loop

**DIFFICULTY:** Moderate

**SCENERY:** Deep woods and Dean Pond

**EXPOSURE:** Shaded forest

**TRAFFIC:** Light–moderate

**TRAIL SURFACE:** Mostly packed dirt, with a few rough areas

**HIKING TIME:** 2 hours, 15 minutes

**ELEVATION:** 432' at trailhead, 557' at highest point

**SEASON:** Year-round

**DRIVING DISTANCE FROM BOSTON COMMON:** 37.9 miles

**ACCESS:** Sunrise–sunset; free

**MAPS:** Available at kiosk in parking lot or at mass.gov/eea/docs/dcr/parks/trails/upton.pdf

**CONTACT:** Massachusetts Dept. of Conservation and Resources, mass.gov/locations/upton-state -forest, 617-626-1250

**WHEELCHAIR ACCESS:** Parts of Park Road are somewhat accessible.

**FACILITIES:** None

**LOCATION:** Upton, MA

down. Continue straight on Park Road. You will also pass Middle Road on the left. The trail is still gently rising here but flattens out after about 10 minutes. The next trailhead you will pass is the Whistling Cave Trail, on the left. The trailheads are well marked with signs posted on trees.

After 25 minutes or so, Park Road bends slightly left and gently descends. Start looking for the Nuthatch Trail again on the right, and enter the forest here. Initially the Nuthatch Trail is moderately wide, with a rugged surface of roots and rocks. There are no trail blazes to speak of, but the trail is quite well defined and easy to follow. It takes a gentle rise and fall as it winds through the woods. The dense under-growth helps define the trail.

After 35 minutes, you pass through a grove of lush white pine. The trail con-tinues winding gently through the woods, with a slight rise and fall. There is a deep sense of solitude in this corner of the woods. After this reverie, the trail ensures you're paying attention with a short, steeper descent. The trail then winds left, and you'll pass a huge, moss-covered boulder on your right.

You may start to hear a little road noise but not too much. When you come to an unmarked intersection, turn left to stay on the Nuthatch Trail. Turning right will take you out to Westboro Road. After bearing left here, the trail climbs slightly. Shortly after this rise, the trail will take you on a long, gentle descent. At the next intersec-tion, turning left will bring you to Park Road, and right will stay on Nuthatch. Turn right to stay on Nuthatch and continue this loop. After the next intersection, the trail smooths out and flattens considerably. You'll cross over a natural-gas line clearing and head right back into the woods. The trail continues its gentle nature here and eventu-ally brings you back to Park Road. Turn left and follow Park Road to Dean Pond Road.

Turn left on Dean Pond Road. You'll pass the Chickadee Trail on the right and another entrance to the Nuthatch Trail on the left. Keep going straight until you come to a triangular intersection (where Park Road bears left); turn right to head toward Dean Pond.

# Upton State Forest

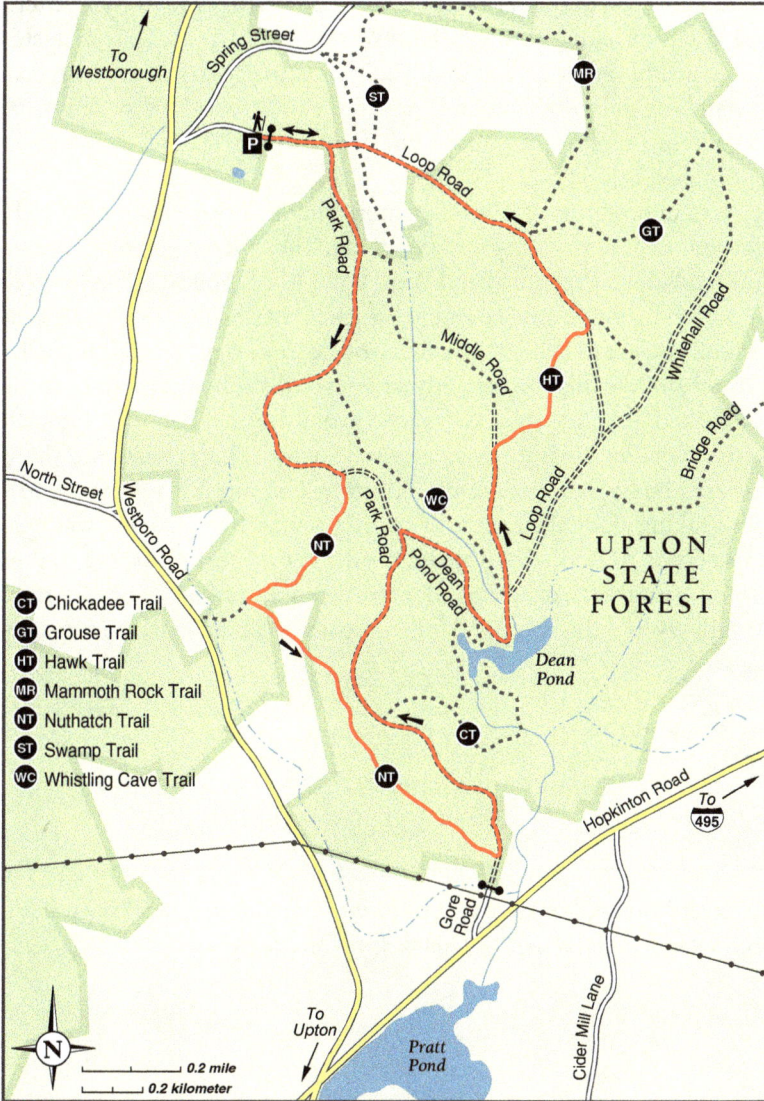

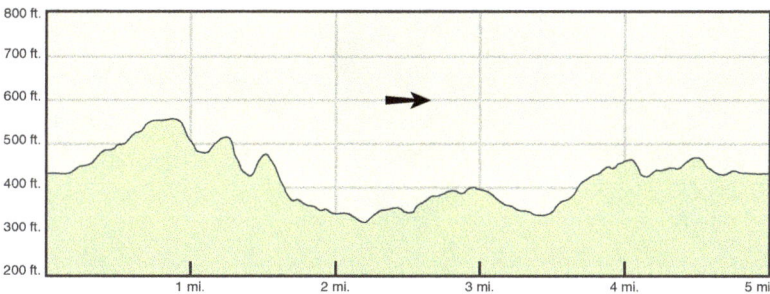

**To Westborough**

Spring Street

ST

MR

P

Loop Road

GT

Park Road

Whitehall Road

Middle Road

HT

Bridge Road

North Street

Westboro Road

WC

Loop Road

**UPTON STATE FOREST**

Park Road

NT

Dean Pond Road

Dean Pond

CT Chickadee Trail
GT Grouse Trail
HT Hawk Trail
MR Mammoth Rock Trail
NT Nuthatch Trail
ST Swamp Trail
WC Whistling Cave Trail

CT

NT

Hopkinton Road

To 495

Gore Road

Cider Mill Lane

N

0.2 mile
0.2 kilometer

To Upton

Pratt Pond

800 ft.
700 ft.
600 ft.
500 ft.
400 ft.
300 ft.
200 ft.

1 mi.   2 mi.   3 mi.   4 mi.   5 mi.

Like Park Road, Dean Pond Road is a wider fire road–type of trail. After about an hour and a half of hiking through the lush woods of Upton State Forest, you'll come to the small and serene Dean Pond. You'll want to spend some time relaxing on the shores, watching the woodland birds darting in and around the swampy marsh of Dean Pond. When you're ready to move on, circle around, leaving the pond on your right to continue on Loop Road.

At the next intersection you'll encounter, Middle Road heads left, and Loop Road heads right. Bear right to stay on Loop Road. The trail here is still fairly wide but definitely not as wide as Park Road and Dean Pond Road. Follow Loop Road toward Whitehall Road on the right. You'll pass the Bridge Road trailhead on the right. Stay on Loop Road until you get to Whitehall. When you do, turn right onto Whitehall.

The Whitehall Road narrows slightly and descends. The trail surface is still firm and densely packed dirt and rocks, so it's pretty easy footing. Follow Whitehall Road to the Sparrow Trail on the left. Turn left on Sparrow. This is back into the woods and a narrower hiking trail. Follow the Sparrow Trail until it rejoins Loop Road. Here you'll be hiking along the course of an old stone wall most of the way.

Once you come to Loop Road again, head right to start returning to the parking area. You'll pass the Grouse and Mammoth Rock trailheads on the right, but stay on the yellow-blazed Loop Road for a relaxing walk through the forest back to the parking area.

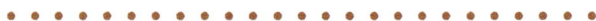

• • • • • • • • • • • • • • • • • • • • • • • • • • •

**GPS TRAILHEAD COORDINATES** N42° 12.557'  W71° 36.364'

**DIRECTIONS** From Boston, take I-90 W to I-495 S. From I-495, take Exit 21B for West Main Street toward Upton. Continue as it turns into Hopkinton Road. Take a sharp right onto Westboro Road, and the park is 2 miles down on the right.

# APPENDIX A: Outdoors Shops

**EASTERN MOUNTAIN SPORTS**
ems.com

**Boston**
855 Boylston St.
Boston, MA 02116; 617-236-1518

**Boston**
1041 and 1045 Commonwealth Ave.
Boston, MA 02215; 617-254-4250

**Cambridge**
Harvard Square
1 Brattle Square, Second Floor
Cambridge, MA 02138; 617-864-2061

**Hingham**
Anchor Plaza
211 Lincoln St.
Hingham, MA 02043; 781-741-8808

**Newton**
300 Needham St., Unit 1
Newton, MA 02464; 617-559-1575

**Peabody**
Northshore Mall
MA 128 and MA 114
Peabody, MA 01960; 978-977-0601

**FJÄLLRÄVEN**
304 Newbury St., Upper Level
Boston, MA 02115; 857-702-3075
fjallraven.us

**HILTON'S TENT CITY**
565 Mass Ave.
Cambridge, MA 02139; 617-227-9242
hiltonstentcity.com

**MAYNARD OUTDOOR STORE**
24 Nason St.
Maynard, MA 01754; 978-897-2133
maynardoutdoor.net

**NATICK OUTDOOR STORE**
38 North Ave.
Natick, MA 01760; 508-653-9400
natickoutdoor.com

**NEW ENGLAND BACKPACKER**
6 E. Mountain St.
Worchester, MA 01606; 508-853-9407
newenglandbackpacker.com

**NORTH RIVER OUTFITTER (NRO)**
39 Charles St.
Boston, MA 02114; 617-742-3900
northriveroutfitter.com/sport

**REI**
rei.com

**Boston**
401 Park Drive
Boston, MA 02215; 617-236-0746

**Framingham**
375 Cochituate Road
Framingham, MA 01701; 508-270-6325

**Hingham**
98 Old Derby St., Ste. 470
Hingham, MA 02043; 781-740-9430

**Reading**
279 Salem St. (Exit 40 off MA 128)
Reading, MA 01867; 781-944-5103
847-720-4105

## APPALACHIAN MOUNTAIN CLUB

Main Office
10 City Square
Boston, MA 02129; 617-523-0636
**outdoors.org**

## MASSACHUSETTS AUDUBON SOCIETY

208 S. Great Road
Lincoln, MA 01773
781-259-9500 or 800-AUDUBON (283-8266)
**massaudubon.org**

## THE ANDOVER VILLAGE IMPROVEMENT SOCIETY (AVIS)

**avisandover.org**

## BAY CIRCUIT TRAIL AND GREENWAY

**baycircuit.org**

## ESSEX COUNTY GREENBELT

82 Eastern Ave.
Essex, MA 01929; 978-768-7241
**ecga.org**

## MASSACHUSETTS DEPARTMENT OF CONSERVATION AND RESOURCES

251 Causeway St., Ste. 900
Boston, MA 02114; 617-626-1250
**mass.gov/orgs/department-of -conservation-recreation**

# APPENDIX C: Hiking Clubs

**APPALACHIAN MOUNTAIN CLUB**
AMC Main Office
10 City Square
Boston, MA 02129; 617-523-0636
outdoors.org

**BOSTON HIKING MEETUP GROUP**
meetup.com/boston-hiking

**CHARLES RIVER CONSERVANCY**
43 Thorndike St., S3-3
Cambridge, MA 02141; 617-608-1410
thecharles.org

**DARTMOUTH NATURAL RESOURCES TRUST**
318 Chase Road
Dartmouth, MA 02747; 508-991-2289
dnrt.org

**FRIENDS OF THE BLUE HILLS**
781-828-1805
friendsofthebluehills.org

**FRIENDS OF HEMLOCK GORGE**
1094 Chestnut St.
Newton Upper Falls, MA 02464
hemlockgorge.org

**FRIENDS OF LYNN WOODS**
lynnwoods.org

**FRIENDS OF THE MIDDLESEX FELLS RESERVATION**
235 W. Foster St.
Melrose, MA 02176; 781-662-2340
friendsofthefells.org

**FRIENDS OF THE WAPACK**
wapack.org

**MANCHESTER ESSEX CONSERVATION TRUST**
978-890-7153
mect.org

**MIDSTATE TRAIL**
midstatetrail.org

**MASSACHUSETTS SIERRA CLUB**
50 Federal St., Third Floor
Boston, MA 02110; 617-423-5775
sierraclub.org/massachusetts

**SUDBURY VALLEY TRUSTEES**
18 Wolbach Road
Sudbury, MA 01776; 978-443-5588
svt@svtweb.org
svtweb.org

**THE TRUSTEES OF RESERVATIONS**
Main Office
200 High St.
Boston, MA 02110; 617-542-7696
thetrustees.org

# ABOUT THE AUTHORS

## ABOUT THE ORIGINAL AUTHOR

**Helen Weatherall** is a writer, sculptor, and environmentalist who prefers to spend her time outdoors. Having explored wildlands from Mount Washington to Montana, the Amazon to Sri Lanka, and much in between, Weatherall now lives in Ipswich, Massachusetts, with her husband, cat, and terrier.

## ABOUT THE REVISING AUTHOR

**Lafe Low** is a lifelong New Englander. He spends nearly all his free time outside skiing, hiking, skiing, camping, skiing, kayaking, skiing . . . you get the picture. He has nearly reached his goal of having his garage look like an REI or EMS basement sale. He has worked as a writer and editor for decades, launching his own magazine, *Explore New England,* in 1995. After that, he went on to be the editor of *Outdoor Adventure.* Most of his career has been with various technology and business publications. The tech stuff pays the bills; the outdoor stuff feeds the soul. He is also the author of *Best Tent Camping: New England* (fourth edition) and *Best Hikes of the Appalachian Trail: New England.*

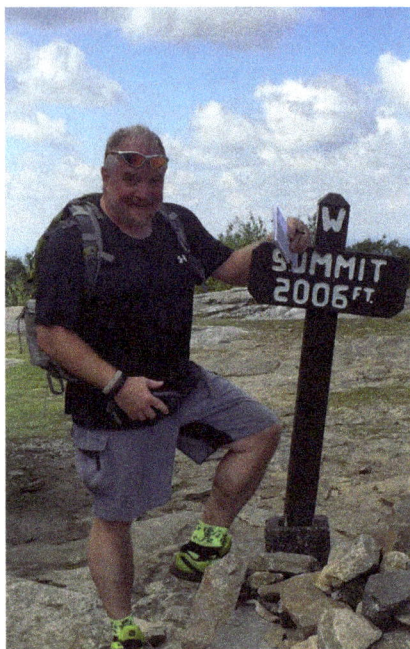